AF710098

Combining Targeted Biological Agents with Radiotherapy

Current Status and Future Directions

Combining Targeted Biological Agents with Radiotherapy

Current Status and Future Directions

EDITED BY
William Small, Jr., MD

Demos
MEDICAL PUBLISHING
New York

Acquisitions Editor: R. Craig Percy
Cover Design: The Book Designers
Copyeditor: Joann Woy
Compositor: Patricia Wallenburg
Printer: Malloy Litho

Visit our website at www.demosmedpub.com

© 2008 Demos Medical Publishing, LLC. All rights reserved. This book is protected by copyright. No part of it may be reproduced, stored in a retrieval system, or transmitted in any form or by any means, electronic, mechanical, photocopying, recording, or otherwise, without the prior written permission of the publisher.

Medicine is an ever-changing science. Research and clinical experience are continually expanding our knowledge, in particular our understanding of proper treatment and drug therapy. The authors, editors, and publisher have made every effort to ensure that all information in this book is in accordance with the state of knowledge at the time of production of the book. Nevertheless, the authors, editors, and publisher are not responsible for errors or omissions or for any consequences from application of the information in this book and make no warranty, express or implied, with respect to the contents of the publication. Every reader should examine carefully the package inserts accompanying each drug and should carefully check whether the dosage schedules mentioned therein or the contraindications stated by the manufacturer differ from the statements made in this book. Such examination is particularly important with drugs that are either rarely used or have been newly released on the market.

Library of Congress Cataloging-in-Publication Data

Combining targeted biological agents with radiotherapy : current status and future directions / edited by William Small Jr.
p. ; cm.
Includes bibliographical references and index.
ISBN-13: 978-1-933864-34-1 (pbk. : alk. paper)
ISBN-10: 1-933864-34-6 (pbk. : alk. paper)
1. Cancer—Radiotherapy. 2. Combined modality therapy. 3. Growth factors—Receptors. I. Small, William.
[DNLM: 1. Neoplasms—therapy. 2. Antineoplastic Agents—therapeutic use. 3. Combined Modality Therapy. 4. Radiotherapy—methods. QZ 266 C7315 2008]
RC271.R3C66 2008
616.99'40642—dc22

2008001694

Special discounts on bulk quantities of Demos Medical Publishing books are available to corporations, professional associations, pharmaceutical companies, health care organizations, and other qualifying groups. For details, please contact:

Special Sales Department
Demos Medical Publishing
386 Park Avenue South, Suite 301
New York, NY 10016
Phone: 800–532–8663 or 212–683–0072
Fax: 212–683–0118
Email: orderdept@demosmedpub.com

Made in the United States of America

08 09 10 11 5 4 3 2 1

To all the scientists, both basic and clinical, who strive every day to advance our knowledge and treatment of cancer. Your dedication does not go unnoticed and is truly appreciated.

To the past and present members of the armed services who have dedicated their lives to another battle. Without your efforts, we would not have the freedom that makes our work possible.

Contents

Preface

Cancer remains a significant cause of morbidity and mortality in the United States. Current standard cancer therapy utilizes surgery, chemotherapy, and radiotherapy, either alone or in combination. Radiotherapy plays a prominent role in the palliative and curative therapy for many malignancies, with a large proportion of cancer patients receiving radiotherapy during the course of their treatment. Attempts to improve tumor response and control with radiotherapy have increasingly included the addition of cytotoxic chemotherapy. Although this strategy is often successful, the combination of chemotherapy and radiotherapy invariably leads to an increase in toxicity. The ideal radiosensitizer would enhance the antitumor effects of radiotherapy without increasing injury to normal tissue. In recent years, a number of agents have been developed that are directed at specific molecular targets of malignant transformation. These agents most commonly are antibodies to specific tumor-associated antigens or small-molecule inhibitors of the tyrosine kinase pathway. There is growing excitement that combining these agents with cytotoxic therapies will lead to increased tumor control without significantly increased treatment-related toxicity.

This book is designed to review both the basic science and current clinical status of combining targeted biologic agents with radiotherapy. The authors of the chapters included in *Combining Targeted Biological Agents with Radiotherapy* are some of the premier investigators in the field and will provide a strong background for what promises to be the next significant breakthrough in cancer therapy. Chapter 1 is a comprehensive introduction to the subject that provides a solid background for the rest of the book. Chapters 2 and 3, with lead authors Michael Hagan and Andrew Fontanella, provide the basic science rationale behind the two most important current targeted agents: epidermal growth factor receptors and vascular epithelial growth factor receptors. This is followed by a chapter discussing the dermatologic manifestations of targeted agents—especially as they apply to the combination of these therapies with radiotherapy. Mario Lacouture is an international expert in this field, and Chapter 4 is essential to the day-to-day management of patients. The final general chapter, expertly handled by Lanea Keller, introduces the reader to radioimmunotherapy—a treatment that has the ability to combine targeted agents directly with radiotherapy. The remaining six chapters focus on specific disease sites, including malignant gliomas, head and neck, lung, pancreatic, cervical, and endometrial cancers. Each of these chapters includes authors who are at the forefront of the oncologic field in general and in biologically targeted agents in particular.

In summary, I believe *Combining Targeted Biological Agents with Radiotherapy* will help to introduce and define the role of combining targeted agents and radiotherapy. It is hoped that this fourth weapon in cancer therapy—in addition to surgery, chemotherapy, and radiotherapy—will lead to improved outcomes for our patients. I want to thank all the contributors for helping to assemble a truly state-of-the-science textbook for a rapidly evolving subject.

William Small, Jr.

Contributors

Mark Agulnik, MD, CM
Associate Professor
Department of Medicine, Division of Hematology/Oncology
Northwestern University Feinberg School of Medicine
Chicago, Illinois
Chapter 4: Dermatologic Manifestations of Targeted Therapies

Christopher J. Anker, MD
Resident
Department of Radiation Oncology
Huntsman Cancer Hospital
University of Utah
Salt Lake City, Utah
Chapter 10: Targeted Therapies in Cervical Cancer

Yiting Cao, MD, PhD
Research Associate
Departments of Radiation Oncology and Surgery
Duke University Medical Center
Durham, North Carolina
Chapter 3: Vascular Epithelial Growth Factor (VEGF) Receptors

Jergin Chen, MD
Chief Resident
Department of Radiation Oncology
Huntsman Cancer Hospital
University of Utah
Salt Lake City, Utah
Chapter 11: Targeted Therapies in Endometrial Cancer

Roger B. Cohen, MD
Senior Member
Department of Medical Oncology
Director, Phase I Clinical Trials Program
Fox Chase Cancer Center
Philadelphia, Pennsylvania
Chapter 7: Targeted Therapies in Head and Neck Cancer

Christopher H. Crane, MD
Associate Professor, Program Director and Section Chief GI Service
Department of Radiation Oncology
MD Anderson Cancer Center
Houston, Texas
Chapter 9: Targeted Therapies in Pancreatic Cancer

David T. Curiel, MD, PhD
Professor and Director
Division of Human Gene Therapy
Gene Therapy Center
University of Alabama at Birmingham
Birmingham, Alabama
Chapter 2: Epidermal Growth Factor Receptors (EGFR)

Paul Dent, PhD
Professor
Departments of Biochemistry and Molecular Biology
Virginia Commonwealth University School of Medicine
Richmond, Virginia
Chapter 2: Epidermal Growth Factor Receptors (EGFR)

Mark W. Dewhirst, DVM, PhD
Gustavo S. Montana Professor of Radiation Oncology
Professor of Pathology
Professor Biomedical Engineering
Department of Radiation Oncology
Duke University Medical Center
Durham, North Carolina
Chapter 3: Vascular Epithelial Growth Factor (VEGF) Receptors

Paul B. Fisher, MPH, PhD
Professor and Chairman
Department of Human Genetics
Virginia Commonwealth University School of Medicine
Richmond, Virginia
Chapter 2: Epidermal Growth Factor Receptors (EGFR)

Andrew N. Fontanella, BS
Graduate Research Assistant
Department of Biomedical Engineering
Duke University Medical Center
Durham, North Carolina
Chapter 3: Vascular Epithelial Growth Factor (VEGF) Receptors

David K. Gaffney, MD, PhD
Professor and Medical Director
Department of Radiation Oncology
Huntsman Cancer Hospital
University of Utah
Salt Lake City, Utah
Chapter 10: Targeted Therapies in Cervical Cancer
Chapter 11: Targeted Therapies in Endometrial Cancer

Leo I. Gordon, MD
Abby and John Friend Professor of Cancer Research
Professor of Medicine
Director, Lymphoma Program
Division of Hematology/Oncology
Department of Medicine
Northwestern University Feinberg School of Medicine
Chicago, Illinois
Chapter 5: Radiolabeled Monoclonal Antibody Therapies

Steven Grant, MD
Professor of Medicine, Biochemistry, and Pharmacology
Department of Internal Medicine
Virginia Commonwealth University School of Medicine
Richmond, Virginia
Chapter 2: Epidermal Growth Factor Receptors (EGFR)

Sean Grimm, MD
Assistant Professor
Department of Neurology
Northwestern University Feinberg School of Medicine
Chicago, Illinois
Chapter 6: Targeted Therapies in Malignant Gliomas

Michael P. Hagan, MD, PhD
Professor
Department of Radiation Oncology
Virginia Commonwealth University School of Medicine
Massey Cancer Center
Richmond, Virginia
Chapter 2: Epidermal Growth Factor Receptors (EGFR)

Paul M. Harari, MD
Jack Fowler Professor and Chairman
Department of Human Oncology
University of Wisconsin School of Medicine
Madison, Wisconsin
Chapter 7: Targeted Therapies in Head and Neck Cancer

Philip B. Hylemon, PhD
Professor of Microbiology and Medicine
Department of Microbiology and Immunology
Virginia Commonwealth University School of Medicine
Richmond, Virginia
Chapter 2: Epidermal Growth Factor Receptors (EGFR)

Antonio Martin Jimenez, MD
Resident
Department of Internal Medicine
Rush University Medical Center
Chicago, Illinois
Chapter 5: Radiolabeled Monoclonal Antibody Therapies

Lanea M. M. Keller, MS
Medical Student
Rush Medical College
Rush University Medical Center
Chicago, Illinois
Chapter 5: Radiolabeled Monoclonal Antibody Therapies

Sunil Krishnan, MD
Assistant Professor, Director GI Translational Research
Department of Radiation Oncology
MD Anderson Cancer Center
Houston, Texas
Chapter 9: Targeted Therapies in Pancreatic Cancer

Mario E. Lacouture, MD
Assistant Professor
Director, Cancer Skin Care Program
Department of Dermatology
Robert H. Lurie Comprehensive Cancer Center
Northwestern University Feinberg School of Medicine
Chicago, Illinois
Chapter 4: Dermatologic Manifestations of Targeted Therapies

Ranee Mehra, MD
Associate Member
Department of Medical Oncology
Fox Chase Cancer Center
Philadelphia, Pennsylvania
Chapter 7: Targeted Therapies in Head and Neck Cancer

Bharat B. Mittal, MD
Professor and Chairman
Department of Radiation Oncology
Northwestern University Feinberg School of Medicine
Chicago, Illinois
Chapter 4: Dermatologic Manifestations of Targeted Therapies

Vishal Rana, MD
Research Assistant
Department of Radiation Oncology
MD Anderson Cancer Center
Houston, Texas
Chapter 9: Targeted Therapies in Pancreatic Cancer

William Small, Jr., MD
Professor and Vice Chairman
Department of Radiation Oncology
Associate Medical Director
Robert H. Lurie Comprehensive Cancer Center
Northwestern University Feinberg School of Medicine
Chicago, Illinois
Chapter 1: Targeted Therapies: Definitions, Limitations, and Future Directions
Chapter 5: Radiolabeled Monoclonal Antibody Therapies

Tamara Z. Vern, BA, DO
Doctor of Osteopathic Medicine
Department of Pediatrics
Advocate Christ Medical Center
Hope Children's Hospital
Oak Lawn, Illinois
Chapter 1: Targeted Therapies: Definitions, Limitations, and Future Directions

Gregory M.M. Videtic, MD, CM, FRCPC
Staff Physician
Residency Program Director
Department of Radiation Oncology
The Cleveland Clinic
Cleveland, Ohio
Chapter 8: Targeted Therapies in Lung Cancer

Adly Yacoub, PhD
Assistant Professor
Department of Radiation Oncology and Biochemistry
Virginia Commonwealth University School of Medicine
Massey Cancer Center
Richmond, Virginia
Chapter 2: Epidermal Growth Factor Receptors (EGFR)

I Targeted Therapies: Definitions, Limitations, and Future Directions

TAMARA Z. VERN
WILLIAM SMALL, JR.

Start by doing what is necessary, then do what's possible, and suddenly you are doing the impossible.

—St. Francis of Assisi

Through the centuries, Hippocrates, Galen, Celsius, Halsted, Paget, and others considered cancer an incurable disease, even when the original tumor was removed, because it inevitably recurred. (1,2). The first documented cases of cancer were eight cases of breast cancer, recorded on papyrus in 1500 B.C., in Egypt (3). Hormonal therapy was discovered in the nineteenth century by Thomas Beatson, when he decreased breast tumor size by removing ovaries, and by Charles Huggins, who found the same results for prostate cancer by removing testes (1). At the end of the nineteenth century, Wilhelm Conrad Roentgen ignited worldwide anticipation with the discovery that the "X-ray" could be used for medical diagnosis and in the treatment of cancer (2,3). The start of the twentieth century brought new therapeutic modalities to the aid of cancer patients with the discovery of radioactivity by Henri Becquerel in 1903, the isolation of polonium and radium by Pierre and Marie Curie, and Marie Curie's work in the identification of the therapeutic properties of radium (2,3). Chemotherapy emerged as a cancer treatment with the discovery of nitrogen mustard as a treatment for lymphoma by the U.S. Army after World War II, and Sidney Farber's use, in 1956, of aminopterin (a precursor of methotrexate) to treat choriocarcinoma (1,2). Although many cancer patients were cured in the twentieth century using surgery, chemotherapy, and radiotherapy, many also suffered the consequences of subsequent morbidity, since these modalities all had side effects. The twenty-first century presents new challenges, with the characterization of the human genome and the potential of treatment to target the cancer cell itself.

In 2007, an estimated 1,444,920 new cases of cancer will be diagnosed, and more than 559,650 individuals will die from the disease in the United States alone (4). Cancers of the lung, prostate, breast, and colon continue to be the most common fatal cancers, accounting for approximately half of the cancer deaths among men and women (4). Radiation therapy has become a valuable player in the treatment of many solid tumors because of its ability to assist in tumor control and improve survival. The response of solid tumors to radiation depends on multiple factors including tumor cell oxygenation, radiosensitivity, and proliferation between radiation treatments. Changes in any of these features can enhance or diminish tumor response to radiation (5). The combination of cytotoxic chemotherapy and radiotherapy has been one approach to increase radiosensitivity and the therapeutic index, although the toxicity associated with chemoradiotherapy often limits treatment benefit and increases morbidity.

Targeted biologic agents that optimize the benefits and limit the risks of conventional cancer treatments are emerging as an exciting and hopeful new "fourth weapon" against cancer (after surgery, radiation therapy, and chemotherapy).

Clinical trials of cancer treatment continue to focus on examining strategies to determine the safety and effectiveness of new and current therapies, identify potential radiation modifiers, and improve survival and the human condition (6).

DEFINITION OF BIOLOGICALLY TARGETED AGENTS

Cancer cells are not subject to the normal maintenance of vital cellular pathways. With their unpredictable and infinite ability to replicate, malignant cells acquire insensitivity to growth inhibitory signals, the ability to avoid apoptosis, the capacity to trigger angiogenesis, and invade healthy tissue. Biologically targeted therapies are designed to address those specific molecular pathways of cancer cell growth and metastases. These therapies focus on different pathways, including genetic mutations, apoptosis, gene expression, DNA repair, angiogenesis, transformation of hypoxic states, structural changes in proteins that are products of mutated genes, and alterations in signaling pathways (6). The goal of combining biologic modifiers with radiotherapy is to increase antitumor efficacy while limiting toxicity. Targeted agents can also be conjugated with cytotoxic agents, such as radiolabeled antibodies, thus making them directly toxic to tumor cells.

A number of biologically targeted therapies have undergone preclinical and clinical trials with some success: monoclonal antibodies and small-molecule inhibitors of the tyrosine kinase (TK) pathways are two critical approaches that have been studied and developed through extensive preclinical and clinical trials. Epidermal growth factor receptor (EGFR) signaling has been the most investigated pathway to date (7). Angiogenesis inhibitors prevent tumor cells from signaling the surrounding normal tissue for new sprouting blood vessels that would deliver nutrients and oxygen to the enlarging tumor cell mass through proangiogenic factors such as vascular endothelial growth factor (VEGF). Inhibition of these signaling pathways may prevent the target tumor cell from multiplying, migrating, maturing, or surviving. This chapter briefly reviews the current major biologic targets, agents, and future directions. Many of these topics are discussed in detail elsewhere in the book.

■ EPIDERMAL GROWTH FACTOR RECEPTOR

The EGFR has received extensive recognition for its proliferative and cytoprotective traits. The EGFR is a transmembrane glycoprotein that consists of an extracellular ligand-binding domain, a transmembrane region, and a cytoplasmic domain that contains a TK region (7). It is expressed in cells from all embryonic layers, but predominately in cells of epithelial origin such as skin, respiratory tract, gastrointestinal tract, urinary tract, and liver (8). The EGFR is part of four closely related TK receptors that make up the ERBB family: EGFR (or ERBB1/HER-1), HER-2/*neu* (ERBB2), HER-3 (ERBB3), and HER-4 (ERBB4) (9). Ligand binding to the EGFR, either by epidermal growth factor (EGF) or transforming growth factor (TGF)-α, activates TK activity, causing receptor autophosphorylation and initiating signal transduction pathways that lead to cell proliferation, inhibition of apoptosis, and angiogenesis. Dysregulation can result in oncogenesis and cancer extension (7,10).

Several studies have revealed that the EGFR-mediated signals are involved in a number of processes contributing to cancer development and progression (11,12). Normal EGFR-containing cells have approximately 20,000–200,000 copies per cell. However, in various neoplasms, EGFR can be overexpressed or mutated, and this has been linked with more aggressive tumors, poorer prognosis, increased rate of recurrence, and diminished survival (13–17). These tumors include non-small cell lung (NSCL) carcinoma, head and neck, pancreatic, colorectal, breast, kidney, ovarian, prostate, and bladder cancers, and gliomas of the brain (12,18,19). Mechanisms of cancer cell resistance to radiotherapy are important. Overexpression of EGFR has been associated with resistance to hormonal treatments, chemotherapeutic agents, and radiotherapy (18,20,21). Radiation can increase the expression of EGFR in cancer cells (22,23). Schmidt-Ullrich and colleagues (24) demonstrated that ionized radiation increased EGFR TK phosphorylation and was linked to several essential branches of the mitogenic and proliferative response. They also showed that radiation exposures in 0.5- to 5-Gy dose ranges can counteract growth inhibition by either activating EGFR, which leads to growth stimulation, or by triggering EGFR upregulation, within 24 hours of ionized radiation exposure. By blocking the EGFR signaling pathway, further growth is inhibited and radiosensitivity is increased. Another reason to inhibit EGFR in fractionated radiotherapy is to prevent accelerated repopulation, which occurs during radiotherapy (17,25). Tumor cell proliferation during radiotherapy is estimated to reduce the efficiency of 2 Gy/day fractions of head and neck cancer by approximately 0.6 Gy/day (17, 25). In vitro studies have demonstrated that radiation causes the release of TGF-α, which further stimulates tumor cell proliferation (26).

MONOCLONAL ANTIBODIES TO EGFR

Cetuximab (IMC-C225, Erbitux)

Cetuximab (IMC-C225, Erbitux) is a chimeric human–mouse monoclonal IgG_1 antibody against the ligand-binding domain of EGFR. It is the first anti-EGFR targeted therapy to participate in phase II/III studies of oncology patients as a single therapy or as adjuvant therapy to traditional therapies such as chemotherapy and radiotherapy. It targets specifically the EGFR with high affinity and competitively inhibits endogenous ligand binding. In vitro studies have shown that cetuximab induces dimerization and internalization of the EGFR, contributing to the inhibitory effects of the antibody (20,27). In mice, it also inhibits the growth of epidermoid, prostate, colon, and renal cell carcinoma in xenografts in vivo, with significantly increased mouse survival (20,27). Tumor growth inhibitory effects have also been demonstrated with several other human tumor xenografts in vivo, such as tumors derived from the vulva, stomach, head and neck, and breast (28). Harari and colleagues (29) studied the in vivo response of squamous cell carcinoma (SCC) xenografts in athymic mice to combined therapy using radiation and cetuximab. Their results suggest that radiation therapy in conjunction with cetuximab elicits marked inhibition of tumor extension as well as complete tumor regression for up to 100 days of study, interference with post-radiation damage repair, and inhibition of tumor angiogenesis (29). Decreased EGFR activity by antibody-mediated receptor blockade or genetic alteration can lead to increased tumor radiosensitivity (30–32). Blockade of EGFR with the cetuximab monoclonal antibody enhances in vitro radiosensitivity of cultured tumor cells (33).With cetuximab in the treatment regimen, the inhibition of radiation-induced DNA repair mechanisms and a decrease in VEGF production by cancer cells, are two possible mechanisms by which increased radiation sensitivity is achieved in the tumors treated (20,29,33,34).

Bonner and colleagues (35) performed a study evaluating cetuximab in combination with radiotherapy, which demonstrated that 13 of 15 patients with locally advanced head and neck cancer had complete response, and one patient had a partial response after receiving combination therapy; this was a significantly higher response rate than with radiotherapy alone. One of the most important phase III randomized studies in targeted therapies included 424 patients with loco-regionally advanced SCC of the head and neck (SCCHN), who received either radiotherapy with weekly cetuximab or radiotherapy alone. A statistically significant median progression-free survival improvement was noted in the group treated with cetuximab and radiotherapy, as compared with the group treated with radiotherapy alone (17.1 months versus 12.4 months). The overall median survival was 49 months with combination therapy versus 29.3 months with radiotherapy alone. This study provided a foundation for further studies and a critical proof of principle (36).

Nimotuzumab (THERACIM, hR3, CIMAher)

Nimotuzumab (THERACIM, hR3, CIMAher) is a humanized IgG_1 monoclonal antibody derived from human placenta. It is directed against the extracellular domain of EGFR. With its high affinity to EGFR, it interrupts binding of EGF and TGF-α to the receptor, thus preventing TK activity, which in turn reduces cell proliferation. Nimotuzumab exhibits antitumor activity in nude mice xenografted with A461 human carcinoma cells (37). It has been tested in phase II head and neck cancer clinical trials, in conjunction with radiotherapy. Complete responses were obtained in 60% of cases. No cases of skin rash have been reported in more than 70 patients treated with nimotuzumab. If proven to be consistent in future studies, this may give it an advantage over other monoclonal antibodies (38).

Toxicity

The most common adverse effect associated with monoclonal antibodies is a skin rash. Saltz and colleagues (39) reviewed four phase II studies evaluating multiple different tumor types. Patients who had a rash after receiving cetuximab had longer survival rates than did those without a rash. Furthermore, those patients with higher-grade skin rash had greater survival rates than those with a less-severe rash. Reports also exist of hypersensitivity reaction with the administration of the chimeric monoclonal antibody cetuximab, which is made of 65% human and 35% murine components. Some of the newer, fully humanized monoclonal antibodies (panitumumab, nimotuzumab) have a decreased risk of allergic reaction.

TYROSINE KINASE INHIBITORS TO ENDOTHELIAL GROWTH FACTOR RECEPTOR

Tyrosine kinase inhibitors present as either receptor TKs (gefitinib, erlotinib) or nonreceptor TKs (ZD6474/vandetanib). As transmembrane proteins, receptor TKs have a ligand-binding extracellular domain and a catalytic intracellular kinase domain. Nonreceptor TKs are located in the plasma membrane, cytosol, and nucleus (40). Dysregulation of TKs in cancer occur by overexpression and mutations, which disrupt autoregulation of the kinase, and by depletion of factors that limit TK activity, such as decreased expression of TK inhibitor proteins. The goal of TK inhibitor treatment is to introduce ways to block the catalytic activity of the kinase by interrupting the binding of adenosine triphosphate (ATP) and other substrates. Interference can be achieved by either neutralization of ligand, prevention of ligand binding, receptor internalization, or antibody-mediated cytotoxicity (41). Kormantsky and colleagues (42) performed a phase I trial using erlotinib (Tarceva) with gemcitabine and radiotherapy in patients with pancreatic cancer. Of the eight patients treated, seven had stable disease and one required resection. Aside from gefitinib and erlotinib, other EGFR-TK inhibitors are being investigated in phase I/II clinical trials. CI-1033 is an innovative TK inhibitor that is active against all four members of the ERBB receptor TK family (7,43).

Gefitinib (ZD1839, Iressa)

Gefitinib (ZD1839, Iressa) is a low-molecular-weight synthetic anilinoquinazoline and acts as a reversible inhibitor of EGFR TK. Preclinical studies have demonstrated cytostatic growth-inhibiting activity in many human cancer cell lines that present functional EGFRs, including breast, ovarian, colon, epidermoid, prostate, small-cell lung, and NSCL (20). In vitro studies have shown that gefitinib in combination with radiotherapy has a synergistic effect in several NSCL cancer cell lines (44). It enhanced effectiveness of radiotherapy in LoVo human colon carcinoma xenograft models, and blocked tumor-induced angiogenesis (41,45). She and colleagues (46) treated human xenograft models with gefitinib and demonstrated a significant increase in radiation-induced tumor growth delay. However, data also suggested that no correlation existed between the extent of radiosensitization and the amount of EGFR or ERBB2 expression.

Toxicity

Tyrosine kinase inhibitors are generally not associated with severe toxicities. The two most common ones include an acneiform skin rash and severe diarrhea. Skin toxicity is an acne-like rash in the upper chest, face, and forearms, which is reversible after discontinuation of drug; it has the potential to cause grave discomfort, and many patients refuse continuation of treatment (19,47–50). A primary concern involving another TK inhibitor, trastuzumab, is an increased risk of cardiac dysfunction (51). Some studies have noted increased cardiotoxicity with frequent dosing or when combined with chemotherapeutic agents, whereas others have found no statistical significance (51–56).

■ ANGIOGENESIS INHIBITORS

Under normal circumstances such as wound healing and embryogenesis, angiogenesis is highly ordered, tightly controlled, and arrests when construction is complete (57). The formation of new blood vessels occurs in abnormal pathologic conditions. In these situations, angiogenesis is uninhibited and willing to take on its own regulation. Judah Folkman was the first to suggest that tumor advancement is dependent on new blood vessel formation (58). Angiogenesis is an intricate and essential process for tumor growth, expansion, and metastasis. Vessels provide oxygen and metabolites, and allow tumors to continue on with malignant progression to distant sites. Because tumors rely on blood supply to subsist, they can express various proangiogenic factors that support their own evolution, such as VEGF, interleukin (IL)-8, endothelial growth factor (EGF), platelet-derived growth factor (PDGF), and basic fibroblast growth factor. In animal models, radiotherapy had increased antitumor effect when used in combination with angiostatin (59). Because of its strong angiogenic qualities, the VEGF pathway has become a major target for new developing angiogenesis inhibitors. Vascular endothelial growth factor has two receptor TKs (VEGFR-1 or VEGFR-2), both of which are overexpressed in many NSCL, prostate, renal cell, breast, and colorectal cancers (40,60). Different isoforms of VEGF can interact with VEGFR-3, which can stimulate lymphogenesis (61).

■ ANTIBODIES TO VASCULAR ENDOTHELIAL GROWTH FACTOR

In the 1990s, the first clinical trials were initiated to test the efficacy of anti-angiogenic agents for cancer. Bevacizumab (Avastin) was the first U.S. Food and Drug Administration (FDA)-approved biologic therapy created to inhibit blood vessel formation in tumors. It is a monoclonal antibody developed to inhibit VEGF and thus cause the destruction of blood vessel networks. It was approved in February 2004, based on a phase III clinical trial that showed benefit in the first-line treatment with chemotherapy for metastatic colon cancer (*www.cancer.gov*). Preliminary results using bevacizumab with concurrent radiotherapy and capecitabine in patients with locally advanced pancreatic cancer showed 21% partial response, median survival time (MST) of 11.6

months, and a 1-year survival of 45% of the patients (62,63). These results inspired a RTOG PA 04-11 phase II randomized study testing capecitabine and radiotherapy (50.4 Gy) followed by gemcitabine and either bevacizumab or erlotinib until progression of disease. In addition, Small and colleagues and investigators at Northwestern University have nearly completed a study utilizing gemcitabine and bevacizumab with concurrent radiotherapy in locally advanced pancreatic cancer (64).

■ TYROSINE KINASE INHIBITORS TO VASCULAR ENDOTHELIAL GROWTH FACTOR

Vatalanib (PTK787/ZK222584)

Vatalanib (PTK787/ZK222584) is an oral TK inhibitor that specifically targets VEGFR TK signaling. Preclinical in vitro studies showed that vatalanib selectively inhibited VEGF-mediated endothelial cell proliferation, survival, and migration. In rodent models, vatalanib selectively inhibited angiogenesis and development of lung and lymph node metastases (65). Vatalanib was also able to slow glioma development in rats (66). Currently, the European Organization for the Research and Treatment of Cancer (EORTC) is conducting a clinical trial evaluating vatalanib with concurrent temozolomide and radiotherapy in newly diagnosed glioblastoma patients (67).

■ LIMITS OF BIOLOGICALLY TARGETED THERAPIES

Many tumors have a molecular phenotype that may be the cause of therapy resistance and, ultimately, treatment failure. Receptor downregulation and loss of TK-inhibitory pathways are two suggested mechanisms of resistance to monoclonal antibody therapies targeting receptor TKs; however, these still remain poorly understood (68).

In research evaluating the use of gefitinib and erlotinib in patients with NSCL cancer, it became apparent that a subset of patients had a higher response rate. Patients with bronchoalveolar carcinoma, patients who never smoked, females, and Japanese patients had a greater clinical response. Pao and Miller (69) pursued these findings and revealed somatic mutations in exons encoding the TK domain of the EGFR and a close correlation with clinical response.

Among patients with glioblastoma, a small group seems to benefit from EGFR kinase inhibitors such as erlotinib and gefitinib (70). However, discordance is noted between the overexpression of the EGFR gene and the responsiveness to EGFR kinase inhibitors (70,71). Many glioblastomas express a deletion variant of EGFR, EGFRvIII, which strongly activates the phosphatidylinositol 3' kinase (PI3K) signaling pathway, which provides access for cell survival, proliferation, and extension (70,72–74). The PTEN (phosphatase and tensin homologue deleted in chromosome 10) tumor-suppressor protein inhibits the PI3K signaling pathway. Its absence in glioblastoma may encourage resistance to EGFR kinase inhibitor therapy by disrupting EGFR inhibition from the downstream PI3K pathway inhibition (70,75,76). Mellinghoff and colleagues (70) evaluated EGFRvIII and PTEN in glioblastomas from patients before treatment with EGFR kinase inhibitors. They found a strong correlation between responsiveness to EGFR kinase inhibitors and coexpression of EGFRvIII and PTEN by the tumor. Lack of PTEN in gliomas was associated with resistance to EGFR kinase inhibitors (70). These data suggested that further studies of molecular determinants of tumor sensitivity to molecular targeted therapies are necessary to ensure proper patient selection and tumor screening to prevent therapy resistance.

Endothelial cell proliferation seems to be stimulated by tumor cells, which in turn has an indirect effect over tumor growth. Brem and colleagues (77) revealed a possible hierarchy that exists between various tumors and their dependence on endothelial cell proliferation. Brain tumors appeared to be the most dependent, followed by carcinomas and sarcomas, with chondrosarcomas having the least dependence on endothelial cell proliferation. This may be an explanation for angiogenesis inhibitor resistance and may promote individually tailored cancer treatment research.

■ CONCLUSIONS

Although new therapies continue to show promise, much is still to be discovered about cancer cells and their microenvironment, especially in advanced metastatic disease. Biologically targeted therapies have the potential to be less toxic than traditional cytotoxic agents and improve the therapeutic ratio. The EGFR seems to be an ideal target, but we still struggle to discover how to inhibit the pathway to make it respond successfully to monotherapy and to optimize its power with concurrent radiotherapy. Ongoing research now attempts to uncover how to best incorporate anti-EGFR therapies with concurrent radiotherapy. The promising outcome seen with anti-EGFR antibodies combined with radiotherapy in SCCHN provides the foundation for future studies in other epithelial EGFR-dependent and radiotherapy-sensitive cancers such as rectal and esophageal tumors (8). Further research needs to be done to discover predictors of response and identify patient subsets for whom the treatment should be most effective.

Multiple signaling pathways exist; inhibiting one pathway is unlikely to be as effective as targeting a tumor from multiple approaches. An area of ongoing research is the incorporation of either anti-EGFR or anti-HER-2 growth factor inhibitors with other molecular-targeted therapies. It is unlikely that tumor growth and continued existence is dependent on one signaling pathway or receptor. Also, the synergistic capabilities are endless (8). Because the therapeutic results occur through nonoverlapping signal pathways, radiotherapeutic and biologically targeted agents have the potential to limit toxicity for patients and allow for more efficient treatment regimens. A link exists between angiogenesis and ERBB receptor signaling in the progression of solid tumors. Preclinical data has supported the hypothesis of increased therapeutic benefit when ERBB inhibitors are used in conjunction with VEGFR inhibition. In vivo studies revealed prolonged tumor growth inhibition and vascularization with combination blockade of the two signaling pathways (78–81). Sini and colleagues (81) investigated the effects of Erb1 inhibitors given alone or in combination with PTK787/ZK222584 (VEGF inhibitor) in several tumor models in vitro and showed that the ERBB inhibitors significantly enhanced the antitumor activity of PTK787 by blocking tumor cell release, release of proangiogenic factors, and proliferation of tumor and endothelial cells.

Many evolving roles are developing for the synergistic use of radiotherapy and targeted agents to optimize the efficacy and decrease toxicity of current therapies (82). Targeting tumor glycans, heparinase inhibitors, conjugated vaccines, cyclo-oxygenase (COX)-2 inhibitors, endostatin, and matrix-metalloproteinase inhibitors (MMP) are a few of the many current drug delivery systems being studied that identify cell surface molecules as therapeutic targets of metastasis. Studies are being performed to analyze new gene products for potential use in cancer vaccines and to develop ways to increase immunogenicity. There are ongoing clinical trials on the efficacy of vaccines, assessing patient immune response and testing their efficacy when used in combination with chemotherapy, humoral, or local radiotherapy (6).

Radiotherapy, although proven to be very beneficial, has recognized limitations in treatment dosage and toxicities. The combination of radiotherapy with biologically targeted agents has the potential to suppress tumor growth and overcome the obstacles that lead to treatment resistance and failure. It may be essential to combine therapies targeting several diverse pathways for optimal success. The new targeted therapies show striking promise.

■ REFERENCES

1. American Cancer Society. Available at: http://www.cancer.org?docroot?CRI/content/CRI_2_6x_the_history_of_cancer_72.asp?site. Accessed Dec. 29, 2007.
2. Diamandopoulus GT. Cancer: An historical perspective. *Anticancer Res* 1996;16:1595–1602.
3. Gallucci BB. Selected concepts of cancer as a disease: From the Greeks to 1900. *Oncol Nurs Forum* 1985;12:67–71.
4. Jemal A, Siegel R, Ward E, et al. Cancer Statistics, 2007. *CA Cancer J Clin* 2007;57: 43–66.
5. Colevas AD, Brown JM, Hahn S, et al. Development of investigational radiation modifiers. *J Natl Cancer Instit* 2003;95(9):646–651.

6. National Cancer Institute. Molecular targets of prevention and treatment. National Cancer Institute: Plans & Priorities for Cancer Research. Available at: http://plan2004.cancer.gov/discovery/targets.htm. Accessed Dec. 29, 2007.
7. Silvesteri GA, Rivera MP. Targeted therapy for the treatment of advanced non-small cell lung cancer: A review of the epidermal growth factor receptor antagonists. *Chest* 2005;128:3975–3984.
8. Baselga J, Arteaga CL. Critical update and emerging trends in epidermal growth factor receptor targeting cancer. *J Clin Oncol* 2005;23:2445–2459.
9. Macias A, Azavedo E, Perez R, et al. Receptors for epidermal growth factor in human carcinomas and their metastases. *Anticancer Res* 1986;6:849–852.
10. Raymond I, Faivre S, Armand JP. Epidermal growth factor receptor tyrosine kinase as a target for anticancer therapy. *Drugs* 2000; 60(Suppl 1):15–23.
11. Noonberg SB, Benz CC. Tyrosine kinase inhibitors targeted to the epidermal growth factor receptor subfamily. *Drugs* 2000;59:753–767.
12. Woodburn JR. The epidermal growth factor receptor and its inhibition in cancer therapy. *Pharmacol Ther* 1999;82:241–250.
13. Bonner JA, Harari PM, Giralt J, et al. Radiotherapy plus Cetuximab for squamous-cell carcinoma of the head and neck. *N Engl J Med* 2006;354:567–578.
14. Dancey JE, Freidlin B. Targeting epidermal growth factor receptor: Are we missing the mark? *Lancet* 2003;362:62–64.
15. Hale RJ, Buckley CH, Gullick W J, et al. Prognostic value of epidermal growth factor receptor expression in cervical carcinoma. *J Clin Pathol* 1993;46:149–153.
16. Eriksen JG, Steiniche T, Askaa J, et al. The prognostic value of epidermal growth factor receptor is related to tumor differentiation and the overall treatment time of radiotherapy in squamous cell carcinomas of the head and neck. *Int J Radiat Oncol Biol Phys* 2004;58:561–566.
17. Brown JM. Therapeutic targets in radiotherapy. *Int J Radiat Oncol Biol Phys* 2001;49:319–326.
18. Salomon DS, Brandt R, Ciardiello F, Normanno N. Epidermal growth factor-related peptides and their receptors in human malignancies. *Crit Rev Oncol Haematol* 1995;19:183–232.
19. Lage A, Crombert T, Gonzalez G. Targeting epidermal growth factor receptor signaling: early results and future trends in oncology. *Ann Med* 2003;35:327–336.
20. Ciardiello F, Tortora G. A novel approach in the treatment of cancer: Targeting the epidermal growth factor. *Clin Cancer Res* 2001;7:2958–2970.
21. Nicholson RI, Gee JM, Barrow D, et al. Endocrine resistance in breast cancer can involve a switch towards EGFR signaling pathways and a gain of sensitivity to an EGFR-selective tyrosine kinase inhibitor, ZD1839. Proceedings of AACR-NCI-EORTC Meeting. Washington, DC, 1999;7.
22. Liang K, And KK, Milas L, et al. The epidermal growth factor receptor mediates radioresistance. *Int J Radiat Oncol Biol Phys* 2003;57:246–254.
23. Bonner JA, Maihle NJ, Folven BR, et al. The interaction of epidermal growth factor and radiation in human head and neck squamous cell carcinoma cell lines with vastly different radiosensitivities. *Int J Radiat Oncol Biol Phys* 1994;29:243–247.
24. Schmidt-Ullrich RK, Mikkelsen RB, Dent P, et al. Radiation-induced proliferation of the human A431 squamous carcinoma cells is dependent of EGFR tyrosine phosphorylation. *Oncogene* 1997;15(10):1191–1197.
25. Maciejewski B, Withers HR, Taylor JM, et al. Dose fractionation and regeneration in radiotherapy for cancer of the oral cavity and oropharynx: Tumor dose-response and repopulation. *Int J Radiat Oncol Biol Phys* 1989;16:831–843.

26. Dent P, Reardon DB, Park JS, et al. Radiation-induced release of transforming growth factor alpha activates the epidermal growth factor receptor and mitogens-activated protein kinase pathway in carcinoma cells, leading to increased proliferation and protection from radiation-induced cell death. *Mol Biol Cell* 1999;10:2493–2506.
27. Goldstein NI, Prewett M, Zuklys K, et al. Biological efficacy of a chimeric antibody to the epidermal growth factor receptor in a human tumor xenograft model. *Clin Cancer Res* 1995;1:1311–1318.
28. Huang SM, Harari PM. Epidermal growth factor receptor inhibition in cancer therapy: Biology, rationale and preliminary clinical results. *Invest New Drugs* 1999;17:259–269.
29. Harari PM, Huang SM. Epidermal growth factor receptor modulation of radiation response: preclinical and clinical development. *Semin Radiat Oncol* 2002;(Suppl 2)12:21–26.
30. Huang SM, Harari P. Modulation of radiation response after epidermal growth factor receptor blockade in squamous cell carcinomas: Inhibition of damage repair, cell cycle kinetics, and tumor angiogenesis. *Clin Cancer Res* 2000;6:2166–2174.
31. Huang S-M, Li J, Armstrong EA, Harari PM. Modulation of radiation response and tumor-induced Angiogenesis after epidermal growth factor receptor inhibition by ZD1839 (Iressa). *Cancer Res* 2002;62:4300–4306.
32. Solomon B, Hagekyriakou J, Trivett MK, et al. EGFR blockade with ZD 1839 ("Iressa") potentiates the antitumor effects of single and multiple fractions of ionizing radiation in human A431 squamous cell carcinoma. Epidermal growth factor receptor. *Int J Radiat Oncol Biol Phys* 2003;55:713–723.
33. Huang SM, Bock JM., Harari PM. Epidermal growth factor receptor blockade with C225 modulates proliferation, apoptosis, and radiosensitivity in squamous cell carcinomas of the head and neck. *Cancer Res* 1999;15:1935–1940.
34. Milas L, Mason K, Hunter M, et al. In vivo enhancement of tumor radioresponse by C225 antiepidermal growth factor receptor antibody. *Clin Cancer Res* 2000;6:701–708.
35. Bonner JA, Ezekiel MP, Robert F, et al. Continued response following treatment with IMC-225, and EGFR MoAb, combined with RT in advanced head and neck malignancies. *Proc Am Soc Clin Oncol* 2000;19:4.
36. Bonner JA, Giralt PM, Harari R. Phase III study of high dose radiation with or without cetuximab in the treatment of locoregionally advanced squamous cell cancer of the head and neck (SCCHN) [abstract]. *Am Soc Clin Oncol* 2004. Available at: http://www.asco.org/ac/1,1003,_12-002636-00_18-0026-00_19-00213,00.asp. Accessed July 1, 2004.
37. Mateo C, Moreno E, Amour K, et al. Humanization of a mouse monoclonal antibody that blocks the EGF-R: Recovery of antagonistic activity. *Immunotechnology* 1997;3:71–81.
38. Crombet T, Osorio M, Cruz T, et al. Use of the anti-EGFR antibody h-R3 in combination with radiotherapy in the treatment of advanced head and neck cancer. *J Clin Oncol* 2004;21:22(9):1646–1654.
39. Saltz LB, Kies M, Abbruzzese L, et al. The presence and intensity of the cetuximab-induced acne-like rash predicts increased survival in studies across multiple malignancies [abstract]. *Proc Am Soc Clin Oncol* 2003;22:204.
40. Krause DS, Van Etten RA. Tyrosine kinases as targets for cancer therapy. *N Engl J Med* 2005;353:172–187.
41. William K, Telfer BA, Stratford IJ, Wedge SR. An evaluation of the EGFR tyrosine kinase inhibitor ZD1839 (Iressa) in combination with ionizing radiation. 11th NCI-EORTC-AACR Symposium on New Drugs in Cancer Therapy, Abs. LB3. Amsterdam, November 7–10, 2000.
42. Kortmansky JS, O'Reilly EM, Minsky BD, et al. A phase I trial of erlotinib, gemcitabine and radiation for patients with locally advanced, unremarkable pancreatic cancer. *Proc Am Soc Clin Oncol* 2005;23:4107a.

43. Slichenmyer WJ, Elliot WL, Fry DW. CI-1033, a pan-erbB tyrosine kinase inhibitor. *Semin Oncol* 2001;5(Suppl 16):80–85.
44. Raben D, Helfrich B, Phistry M, Bunn P. ZD1839 (Iressa), and EGFR-TKI, potentiates radiation/chemotherapy cytotoxicity in human non-small cell lung cancer (NSCLC) cell lines. 11th NCI-EORTC-AACR Symposium on New Drugs in Cancer Therapy, Abs. LB4. Amsterdam, November 7–10, 2000.
45. Ciardiello F, Caputo R, Damiano V, et al. Inhibition of growth factor production and Angiogenesis in human cancer cells by ZD1839 (Iressa), a selective epidermal growth factor receptor tyrosine kinase inhibitor. *Clin Cancer Res* 2001;7:1459–1465.
46. She Y, Lee F, Chen J, et al. The epidermal growth factor receptor tyrosine kinase inhibitor ZD1839 selectively potentiates radiation response of human tumors in nude mice, with a marked improvement in therapeutic index. *Clin Cancer Res* 2003;9:3773–3778.
47. Fukuoka M, Yano S, Giaccone G, et al. Multi-institutional randomized phase II trial of gefitinib for previously treated patients with advanced non-small-cell lung cancer. *J Clin Oncol* 2003;21:2237–2246.
48. Kris MG, Natale RB, Herbert RS, et al. Efficacy of gefitinib, an inhibitor of the epidermal growth factor receptor tyrosine kinase, in symptomatic patients with non-small cell lung cancer: A randomized trial. *JAMA* 2003;290:2149–2158.
49. Herbert RS, LoRusso PM, Perdom M, et al. Dermatologic side effects associated with gefitinib therapy: clinical experience and management. *Clin Lung Cancer* 2003;4:366–369.
50. Giaccone G, Johnson G, Manengold C, et al. A phase III clinical trial of ZD1839 (Iressa) in combination with gemcitabine and cisplatin in chemo-naive patients with advanced non-small cell lung cancer (INTACT 1). *Ann Oncol* 2002;13:2.
51. Romond EH, Perez A, Bryant J, et al. Trastuzumab plus adjuvant chemotherapy for operable HER2-positive breast cancer. *N Engl J Med* 2005;353:1673–1684.
52. Cobleigh MA, Vogel CL, Tripathy D, et al Multinational study of the efficacy and safety of humanized anti-Her2 monoclonal antibody in women who have HER2-overexpressing metastatic breast cancer that has progressed after chemotherapy for metastatic disease. *J Clin Oncol* 1999;17:2639–2648.
53. Seidman A, Hudis C, Pierri MK, et al. Cardiac dysfunction in the trastuzumab clinical trials experience. *J Clin Oncol* 2002;20:1215–1221.
54. Joensuu H, Hellokumpu-Lehtinen P, Bono P, et al. Adjuvant docetaxel or vinorelbine with or without trastuzumab for breast cancer. *N Engl J Med* 2006;354:809–820.
55. Vogel CL, Cobleigh MA, Tripathy D, et al. Efficacy and safety of trastuzumab as a single agent in first–line treatment of HER2-overexpressing metastatic breast cancer. *J Clin Oncol* 2002;20 (3):719–726.
56. Belkacemi Y, Gligorov J, Laharie-Mineur H, et al. Concurrent administration of weekly trastuzumab and adjuvant breast radiotherapy increases skin, esophageal, and cardiac acute toxicities. ASCO Annual Meeting Proceedings. *J Clin Oncol* 2006.;24(18S):630.
57. Nam N, Parang K. Current targets for anticancer drug discovery. *Curr Drug Targets* 2003;4:159–179.
58. Folkman J. Tumor angiogenesis: Therapeutic implications. *N Engl J Med* 1971;285(21):1182–1186.
59. Mauceri HJ, Hanna NN, Beckett MA, et al. Combined effects of angiostatin and ionizing radiation in antitumour therapy. *Nature* 1998;394:287–291.
60. Ferrara N, Gerver HP, LeCouter J. The biology of VEGF and its receptors. *Nat Med* 2003;9:669–676.
61. Hicklin DJ, Ellis LM. Role of the vascular endothelial growth factor pathway in tumor growth and angiogenesis. *J Clin Oncol* 2005;23:1011–1027.

62. Cardenes HR, Chiorean EG, DeWitt J, et al. Locally advanced pancreatic cancer: Current therapeutic approach. Oncologist 2006;11:612–623.
63. Crane CH, Ellis LM, Abbruzzese JL. Phase I trial of bevacizumab with concurrent radiotherapy and capecitabine in locally advanced pancreatic adenocarcinoma. *Proc Am Soc Clin Oncol* 2005;23:4033a.
64. Small W Jr., Mulcahy M, Benson A, et al. A phase II trial of weekly gemcitabine and bevacizumab in combination with abdominal radiation therapy in patients with localized pancreatic cancer. *J Clin Oncol* 2007;24 (18 Suppl):637.
65. Wood JM, Bold G, Buchdunger E, et al. PTK787/ZK222584, a novel and potent inhibitor of vascular endothelial growth factor receptor tyrosine kinases, impairs vascular endothelial growth factor-induced responses and tumor growth after oral administration. *Cancer Res* 2000;60:2178–2189.
66. Goldbrunner RH, Bendszus M, Wood J, et al. PTK787/ZK222584, an inhibitor of vascular endothelial growth factor receptor tyrosine kinases, decrease glioma growth and vascularization. *Neurosurgery* 2004;55:426–432.
67. Brandes AA, Franceschi E. New molecular targets and novel anticancer treatments: Emerging trends in neuro-oncology. *Expert Rev Anticancer Ther* 2006;6(8):1129–1131.
68. Nagata Y, Lan KH, Zhou X, et al. PTEN activation contributes to tumor inhibition by trastuzumab, and loss of PTEN predicts trastuzumab resistance in patients. *Cancer Cell* 2004;6:117–127.
69. Pao W, Miller VA. EGFR mutations, small molecule kinase inhibitors, and non-small cell lung cancer: Current knowledge and future directions. *J Clin Oncol* 2005;23:2556–2568.
70. Mellinghoff IK, Wand MY, Vivanco I, et al. Molecular determinants of the response of Glioblastomas to EGFR kinase inhibitors. *N Engl J Med* 2006;354(8):884.
71. Rich JN, Reardon DA, Peery T, et al. Phase II trial of gefitinib in recurrent glioblastoma. *J Clin Oncol* 2004;22:133–142.
72. Sordella R, Bell DW, Haber DA, et al. Gefitinib-sensitizing EGFR mutations in lung cancer activate anti-apoptotic pathways. *Science* 2004;305:1163–1167.
73. Choe G, Horvath S, Cloughesy TF, et al. Analysis of the phosphatidylinositol 3'-kinase signaling pathway in glioblastoma patients in vivo. *Cancer Res* 2003;63:2742–2746.
74. Batra SK, Castelino-Prabhu S, Wikstrand CJ, et al. Epidermal growth factor ligand-independent, unregulated, cell-transforming potential of a naturally occurring human mutant EGFRvIII gene. *Cell Growth Differ* 1995;6:1251–1259.
75. Smith JS, Tachibana I, Passe SM, et al. PTEN mutation, EGFR amplification, and outcome in patients with anaplastic astrocytoma and glioblastoma multiforme. *J Natl Cancer Inst* 2001;93:1246–1256.
76. Bianco R, Shin I, Ritter CA, et al. Loss of PTEN/MMAC1/TEP in EGF receptor-expressing tumor cells counteracts the antitumor action of EGFR tyrosine kinase inhibitors. *Oncogene* 2003;22:2812–2822.
77. Brem S, Cotran R, Folkman J. Tumor angiogenesis: A quantitative method for histologic grading. *J Natl Cancer Inst* 1972;48(2):347–356.
78. Giaccone G, Debruyne C, Felip E, et al. Phase III study of adjuvant vaccination with Bec2/Bacille Calmette-Guérin in responding patients with limited-disease small-cell lung cancer (European Organization for Research and Treatment of Cancer 08971-08971B; Silva Study). *J Clin Oncol* 2005;23:6854–6864.
79. Ciardiello F, Bianco R, Damiano V, et al. Antiangiogenic and antitumor activity of anti-epidermal growth factor receptor C225 monoclonal antibody in combination with vascular endothelial growth factor anti-sense oligonucleotide in human GEO colon cancer cells. *Clin Cancer Res* 2000;6:3739–3747.

80. Jung YD, Mansfield PF, Akagi M, et al. Effects of combination anti-vascular endothelial growth factor receptor and anti-epidermal growth factor receptor therapies on the growth of gastric cancer in a nude mouse model. *Eur J Cancer* 2002;38:1133–1140.
81. Sini P, Wyder L, Schnell C, et al. The antitumor and antiangiogenic activity of vascular endothelial growth factor receptor inhibition is potentiated by ErbB1 blockade. *Clin Can Res* 2005;11(12): 4521–4532.
82. Germanov E, Berman JN, Guernsey DL. Current and future approaches for the therapeutic targeting of metastasis (Review). *Int J Molec Med* 2006;18:1025–1036.

2 Epidermal Growth Factor Receptors (EGFR)

MICHAEL P. HAGAN
ADLY YACOUB
PHILIP B. HYLEMON
DAVID T. CURIEL
PAUL B. FISHER
STEVEN GRANT
PAUL DENT

The exposure of tumor cells to clinically relevant doses of ionizing radiation promotes rapid tyrosine phosphorylation of ErbB family and other tyrosine kinases (TKs). Activation of ErbB receptors causes the activation of RAS proteins and multiple protective downstream intracellular signaling pathways that alter transcription factor function and the apoptotic threshold of cells. The initial radiation-induced activation of extracellular-signal-regulated kinase (ERK1/2) promotes the cleavage and release of paracrine ligands that cause a temporally delayed reactivation of receptors and intracellular signaling pathways in irradiated and unirradiated bystander cells. The consequence of these signaling events after multiple exposures may be to reprogram the irradiated and effected bystander cells in terms of their expression levels of growth-regulatory and cell survival proteins, resulting in altered mitogenic rates and thresholds at which genotoxic stresses cause cell death. We and others have noted that blocking ErbB receptor phosphorylation or ERK1/2 pathway activity for a short period of time following exposure (~3 h) *protects* tumor cells from the toxic effects of ionizing radiation. Prolonged exposure (~48–72 h) of tumor cells to inhibition of ErbB receptor/ERK1/2 function *enhances* radiosensitivity. In animal and clinical studies, prolonged inhibition of ErbB receptors enhances the toxicity of radiation in a wide variety of tumor cell types, thus arguing that inhibition of ErbB receptor function represents a useful therapeutic approach in the treatment of many malignancies.

Ionizing radiation is used as a primary treatment for many types of cancer. Although the irradiation of cells causes death, it also can enhance proliferation in the surviving fraction of cells and promote long-term resistance to multiple cytotoxic stresses (1,2). Exposure of carcinoma cells to clinically relevant low doses of ionizing radiation promotes the generation of reactive oxygen and reactive nitrogen species (ROS and RNS), with subsequent inactivation of protein tyrosine phosphatases, followed by the activation of the substrates of the tyrosine phosphatases, the growth factor receptor TKs in the plasma membrane (e.g., the ErbB family of receptors) (3–6). Receptor activation within several minutes of exposure enhances the activities of RAS family transducer molecules that mediate signaling from the membrane environment, causing the activation of multiple cytosolic signal transduction pathways. Intracellular pathways such as the RAF-1/ERK1/2 and phosphatidylinositol 3' kinase (PI3K)/AKT pathways play a role in the long-term effects of cell survival from toxic stresses and the regulation of cell growth (7–10). This chapter attempts to connect some of the complex interplay between the primary effects of radiation exposure (ROS and RNA generation) to the rapid initial responses of cells, in particular activation of ErbB receptors and signal transduction pathways and regulation of survival. The chapter discusses the delayed secondary responses of irradiated tumor cells as the impact of the initial wave of signaling pathway activation and transcriptional changes ripple outward to further modify cell biology, including the processing and/or synthesis of ErbB regulatory paracrine growth factors, reactivation of ErbB receptors and pathways, and transcription, and the possible long-term outcomes of these processes upon cell signaling, cell survival, and proliferation.

PATHWAYS FOR IONIZING RADIATION–INDUCED SIGNAL TRANSDUCTION PROCESSES

Growth Factor Receptors and Intracellular Signaling Pathways

Radiation generates ionizing events in the water within the cytosol. These events are amplified, possibly through the mediation of mitochondria, which generate large amounts of ROS and RNS that inhibit protein tyrosine phosphatase (PTPase) activities. In addition, radiation activates acidic sphingomyelinase and increases the production of ceramide. Inhibition of PTPases leads to a general de-repression (activation) of receptor and nonreceptor TKs and the activation of downstream signal transduction pathways. Radiation-induced ceramide has been shown to promote membrane-associated receptor activation by facilitating the clustering of receptors within lipid rafts (11).

Activation of Growth Factor Receptors by Radiation

Multiple laboratories have shown that the epidermal growth factor receptor (EGFR, also called ErbB1 and HER-1) is rapidly activated in response to the irradiation of multiple tumor cell types in vitro (12–16). Low-dose, clinically relevant radiation exposure (1–2 Gy) activates ErbB1 and by heterodimerization, other members of the ErbB receptor family (ErbB2, ErbB3, ErbB4). Activation of ErbB1 to -3 has been linked to downstream activation of intracellular signaling pathways, including the RAF-1/mitogen-activated extracellular-regulated kinase (MEK)1/2/ERK1/2 and the PI3K/protein-dependent kinase (PDK)-1/AKT pathways. Studies in the late 1990s argued that a 2-Gy radiation exposure caused levels of ErbB1 and ERK1/2 pathway activation similar to those observed by growth stimulatory, epidermal growth factor (EGF) concentrations (~0.1 nM) 0–30 minutes after exposure (17–19).

An obvious scientific question was then asked: Namely, how did ionizing radiation promote such a rapid activation of ErbB1? It was known that the activity of TKs and proteins regulated by tyrosine phosphorylation (e.g., ErbB1 and RAF-1) are held in check by the actions of PTPases (20). The relative activity of a PTPase is approximately one order of magnitude higher than that of the substrate (i.e., kinase) it dephosphorylates (21). PTPase activity is sensitive to oxidation and/or nitrosylation of a key Cys residue in the active site, and thus any agent that generates ROS or RNS has potential to promote decreased PTPase activity and, hence, the increased tyrosine phosphorylation of multiple proteins (22). Ionizing radiation induces small amounts of ROS by direct interaction with water; these ROS are magnified in a calcium (Ca^{2+})-dependent manner by mitochondria, generating more ROS and RNS, which can act to inhibit multiple PTPase activities. Inhibition of radiation-induced ROS and RNS generation by use of ROS quenching agents such as N-acetyl cysteine or in cells lacking functional mitochondria (Rho zero cells) abrogates the suppression of PTPase activity by radiation (23,24). In general agreement with a role for PTPase inhibition in radiation-induced ErbB1 activation, the expression of dominant negative SHP2 abolishes the radiation-induced phosphorylation of ErbB1; phosphorylation of ErbB1 Y992 in MDA-MB-231 mammary carcinoma cells was noted to be the most radio-responsive site in terms of its amount of (-fold) induction following irradiation (25,26). ErbB1 Y992 phosphorylation has been linked to activation of phospholipase C (PLC)-γ and the ERK1/2 pathway (27). In further support of an important role for the modulation of PTPase activity and changes in tyrosine phosphorylation in radiation responses downstream of growth factor receptors is that RAF-1, a protein whose activity is enhanced by tyrosine phosphorylation, becomes tyrosine phosphorylated and activated following radiation exposure. Of note, B-RAF, which lacks the sites of tyrosine phosphorylation in RAF-1 due to their substitution by acidic amino acid residues in B-RAF, is not potently activated following irradiation (15,28).

Thus, ionizing radiation has the potential to promote the tyrosine phosphorylation and activation of intracellular pathways via PTPase inhibition at the level of the receptor (ErbB family), a membrane proximal kinase (RAF-1), and possibly, though not proven as yet, also at the level of the tyrosine phosphorylated mitogen-activate protein kinase (MAPK) proteins. It has been argued that ROS can inhibit MAPK phosphatase (MKP) enzymes that normally act to dephosphorylate the activating phospho-tyrosine and threonine residues in MAPK proteins, and thus loss of MKP function will also tend to enhance the phosphorylation and activity of MAPK family enzymes (29).

A recent manuscript has argued that MKP enzymes transiently inactivate ERK1/2 after irradiation of carcinoma cells and that this plays a radioprotective role (30). These studies were performed in the presence of serum, in contrast to other studies that generally use serum-starved cells; of note, we have found that radiation activates ERK1/2 in DU145 cells in the presence of serum, whereas it inactivates ERK1/2 in LNCaP cells. As will be noted in subsequent sections, we have observed that transient inhibition of ERK1/2 signaling also protects cells from the toxic effects of radiation exposure (31).

Other agents of physiologic relevance can also generate ROS and RNS, thereby promoting activation of growth factor receptors via PTPase inhibition. For example, bile acids, through ROS-dependent mechanisms, can activate both ErbB1 and the insulin receptor in primary hepatocytes (32–34). Both mitochondria and nicotinamide adenine dinucleotide phosphate (NADPH) oxidase enzymes have been linked to bile acid–induced ROS production (33–35). Activation of ErbB1 and the insulin receptor in hepatocytes can promote ERK1/2 and AKT activation and regulate cell survival as well as other processes, such as glycogen metabolism (36). Arsenic trioxide and hydrogen peroxide can generate ROS in cells and have also been noted to cause activation of growth factor receptors (37,38). Collectively, these observations demonstrate that a wide variety of external stimuli can promote ROS generation in cells and lead to the initiation/activation of intracellular signaling pathways.

After observations demonstrating the initial radiation-induced activation of the ErbB receptors approximately 0–10 minutes after exposure, it became evident that the ErbB receptors also were reactivated approximately 60–180+ minutes after irradiation. The primary mode of receptor activation at these later times occurred via a paracrine/autocrine mechanism (39,40). The initial activation of ErbB1 and the ERK1/2 pathway was directly responsible for the cleavage, release, and functional activation of presynthesized paracrine ligands, such as pro-transforming growth factor (TGF)-α, that fed back onto the irradiated tumor cell, and potentially in vivo onto unirradiated distant tumor cells, thereby re-energizing the signaling system (41). Several studies have independently argued that ERK1/2 and/or p38 MAPK signaling can enhance plasma membrane metalloprotease activities that promote cleavage of the pro-forms/zymogens of multiple growth factor ligands into their functionally activated states (42): this has led to the clinical development of protease inhibitors such as marimastat (43). Growth factors such as insulin-like growth factor (IGF)-1 can promote activation of ErbB1 by increasing the expression of ErbB1 paracrine ligands as well as promoting MAPK-dependent proteolytic processing of these ligands, for example HB-EGF (44). In irradiated HCT116 cells, the ErbB3/4 binding ligand heregulin, which in this cell type primarily interacts with ErbB3, can promote ErbB1, ErbB2 and AKT activation in a paracrine fashion 120–240 minutes after radiation exposure (45). Increasing the radiation dose from 2 Gy up to 10 Gy enhances both the amplitude and duration of the secondary activation of ErbB1 and the secondary activation of the intracellular signaling pathways, suggesting that radiation can promote a dose-dependent increase in the cleavage of pro-TGF-α that reaches a plateau at approximately 10 Gy (39,41). In contrast to the secondary receptor and pathway activations, primary receptor and signaling pathway activations appear to come to a plateau at 3–5 Gy.

The expression of paracrine factors in tumor cells can change in the short-term (hours) and in the long-term (weeks) after irradiation, as potentially can the expression of the growth factor receptors that bind the factors. For example, in the instances of RAS–ERK1/2 signaling and p53 transcriptional function, the activities of which can be increased shortly following radiation exposure, in a variety of cells, these proteins act to enhance the expression of autocrine factors such as HB-EGF and epiregulin (46). However, loss of p53 function can also alter ErbB1 expression; for example, in comparing HCT116 wild-type and HCT116 p53 –/– cells, ErbB1 expression is reduced, and both wild-type and mutant p53 proteins have been shown to regulate the ErbB1 promoter (47,48). In MCF7 mammary carcinoma cells exposed to multiple low doses of radiation, the expression of ErbB1 and TGF-α was noted to rise, and the expression of the estrogen receptor to decline (49). These findings argue that the activation by radiation of ErbB family receptors and downstream pathways has the potential to be influenced, in both the short- and long-term, by the amount of prior radiation exposure a cell has received and the mutational status of p53 and RAS proteins. Collectively, these observations argue that radiation generates ROS/RNS signals within tumor cells that promote activation of growth factor receptors and signaling pathways that in turn promote the release of paracrine ligands from cells, leading to the reactivation of receptors and intracellular signaling pathways.

Approaches to Radiosensitize Cells by Inhibition of Kinase Function

Signaling by ErbB family of receptors is, in general, believed to be pro-proliferative and cytoprotective, and inhibition of ErbB receptor function has been explored as a mode of cancer therapy (Table 2.1). Thus, when signaling from the ErbB family receptors is blocked, either by use of inhibitory antibodies or small-molecular-weight inhibitors of receptor TKs, tumor cell growth can be reduced and the sensitivity of these cells to being killed by noxious stresses increased (reviewed in 50–52). In vitro and xenograft tumor animal model studies have strongly argued that inhibition of ErbB receptor function using single drug/antibody dosing has radiosensitizing effects (53–55). In some animal studies, however, ErbB receptor inhibitors have not radiosensitized ErbB1-expressing tumors (56). Furthermore, as a collective group, clinical trials in which the modulation of ErbB receptor function was a primary goal for improved therapeutic outcomes have been considerably less successful in terms of tumor control than predicted based on in vitro studies (57,58).

Several possible explanations could exist as to why a drug effect observed in vitro or in animals did not translate into as profound an antitumor effect in patients:

- The required inhibitory concentration of the drug and the drug half-life are not achievable and are too short for a therapeutic effect, respectively, in patients.
- The relative dependency (addiction) of cultured tumor cell isolates on ErbB receptor signaling, including expression of hyperactive ErbB receptor mutants (e.g., ErbB1 L858R), when compared to actual tumors in patients, may be biased based on in vitro studies that use established cell lines. As well, the development of drug-resistant ErbB receptor mutants in patients after long-term exposure to ErbB inhibitors (e.g., ErbB1 T790M) may preclude drug actions.
- Exposure of tumor cells in vitro to kinase and other inhibitors, such as tamoxifen, has argued that compensatory activation of parallel growth factor receptors (such as the IGF-1 receptor and c-Kit) occurs to replace the loss of ErbB receptor signaling caused by drug exposure and acts to maintain tumor cell survival (59–61).
- The ErbB inhibitors that are often used in therapy only inhibit one ErbB family member, such as ErbB1, and, in a similar conceptual manner to the third point just listed, other ErbB family members, such as ErbB2, may provide compensatory survival signaling to overcome loss of survival signaling from the inhibited receptor.
- The development of other somatic mutations in survival signaling with the tumor cell, such as loss of PTEN (phosphatase and tensin homologue deleted in chromosome 10) function, which may be selected for in tumor cells undergoing ErbB receptor inhibitor therapy, will lead to the development of tumor cells that are more resistant in general to the inhibitors of growth factor receptors.

The role of RAS signaling in terms of regulating radiosensitivity directly downstream of plasma membrane receptor TKs has also been investigated by many groups, with comparative data using cells from diverse genetic backgrounds arguing that mutated active H-, K- and N-RAS proteins protect cells from the toxic effects of ionizing radiation by activating the PI3K pathway (62–68). In HCT116 colon cancer cells expressing activated K-RAS D13, radiosensitivity was linked to signaling by the ERK1/2 pathway (69). Studies by others have also demonstrated that HCT116 cells expressing active K-RAS use the ERK1/2 pathway as a primary signal to protect themselves from the toxic effect of radiation and, in these experiments, isogenic HCT116 cells expressing active H-RAS V12 (with expression of active K-RAS D13 deleted) were noted to use the PI3K pathway as a primary signal to protect themselves from radiation toxicity (70,71). This suggests different RAS family members, H-RAS and K-RAS, have the potential to generate qualitatively different radioprotective signals via activating different downstream signal transduction pathways.

As stated earlier, data from several groups have demonstrated that the PI3K pathway is a key radioprotective pathway downstream of receptors and RAS proteins (Table 2.1). Inhibition of PI3K pathway function by use of small-molecule inhibitors radiosensitizes tumor cells expressing mutant active RAS molecules or wild-type RAS molecules that are constitutively active due to upstream growth factor receptor signaling. It is possible that PI3K inhibitors may also exert a portion of their radiosensitizing properties by suppressing the function of proteins with PI3K-like kinase domains, such as ataxia-telangiectasia mutated (ATM), ataxia-telangiectasia- and rad3-related (ATR), and DNA protein kinase (DNA-PK). Expression of the constitutively active p110 PI3K molecule is able to partially recapitulate the expression of mutant (active) H-RAS proteins in protecting cells from radiation toxicity. In cell lines where PI3K regulates radiosensitivity, inhibition of the ERK1/2 pathway did not significantly alter the radiosensitivity of cells, in agreement with data from HCT116 cells. ERK1/2 signaling has often been stated to play no role in controlling radiosensitivity; in some cell lines, inhibition of ERK1/2 has been linked to *protection* from radiation toxicity (72,73).

In those cells in which radiosensitizing effects have been observed by blocking ERK1/2 activation, the abilities of MEK1/2 inhibitors to enhance cell killing by radiation was originally linked to a derangement of radiation-induced G2/M growth arrest and enhanced apoptosis (74,75). In DU145 human prostate cancer cells that express ErbB1 and the ligand TGF-α, ionizing radiation increases the release of TGF-α via ErbB1–ERK1/2 signaling. If radiation-induced ErbB1–ERK1/2 signaling is *transiently* blocked in DU145 cells either by the ErbB1 inhibitor AG1478 or a MEK1/2 inhibitor prior to and for 3 hours after irradiation, then radiation-induced cell killing is decreased (Table 2.1). Moreover, if ErbB1 is strongly activated by EGF or TGF-α immediately after

TABLE 2.1 Inhibitors of ErbB family receptors, signal transducers, and kinase proteins downstream of the growth factor receptors

Protein Target	Small Molecule Inhibitor	Antibody Inhibitor
ErbB1	AG1478, Erlotinib, Gefitinib, Lapatinib, EKB-569, HKI272, ZD6474, AEE788, Canertinib (CI-1033)	Cetuximab, Panitumumab, Matuzumab, Pertuzumab
ErbB2	Lapatinib, EKB-569, HKI272, Canertinib	Herceptin, Trastuzumab
ErbB3	Canertinib	—
H-RAS/K-RAS	Farnesyltransferase and Geranylgeranyl transferase inhibitors; statins	—
PI3K	LY294002, wortmannin, PX-866	—
PDK1	OSU-03012	—
AKT	SH-5, SH-6, AKT15B	—
RAF-1/B-RAF	Sorafenib	—
MEK1/2/5	PD98059, U0126, SL327	—
MEK1/2	PD184352, AZD6244	—

Effects on cell growth and cell viability will be cell type- and tumor origin-dependent.

irradiation, then cell killing is increased. Thus, the transient inhibition of radiation-induced ERK1/2 signaling or suprastimulation of ERK1/2 signaling at the time of irradiation radiosensitizes tumor cells. Removal of MEK1/2 inhibitor from the growth media 24 hours and 48 hours after irradiation results in a null effect on DU145 cell radiosensitivity, although the inhibition of MEK1/2 modestly enhanced radiation-induced apoptosis at these time points. Data in general agreement with this concept were also obtained in LNCaP, PC3, and in A431 squamous carcinoma cells (76). On the other hand, following irradiation, *prolonged* inhibition of ERK1/2 (> ~60–72 h) significantly increases the apoptotic response of DU145 and A431 cells and reduces clonogenic survival. Therefore, the interruption of ErbB1 and ERK1/2 signaling, depending on its timing and duration, can either enhance or degrade carcinoma cell survival after irradiation (41).

Downstream Targets of Radiation-induced Kinase Function

Growth factor–induced signaling from ErbB receptors through the PI3K/AKT and RAF-1/ERK1/2 pathways can increase expression of multiple antiapoptotic proteins, including BCL-$_{XL}$, MCL-1, and c-FLIP isoforms, as well as the phosphorylation and inactivation of proapoptotic proteins including BAD,

BIM, and pro-caspase 9 (77–82). Radiation-induced ERK1/2 activation has also been linked to increased expression of the DNA repair proteins ERCC1, XRCC1, and XPC (40,41). In contrast, radiation-induced activation of the c-Jun N-terminal (JNK) 1/2 pathway has been linked to activation of proapoptotic protein function, including those of BAX and BAK, and the promotion of mitochondrial dysfunction (83,84). Thus, as a general concept, activation of AKT and ERK1/2 will tend to suppress cell death processes, including those stimulated by activation of JNK1/2.

A downstream protein kinase effector of the ERK1/2 enzymes, $p90^{rsk}$, phosphorylates the transcription factors cAMP-response element-binding (CREB) and CCAAT/enhancer binding protein (C/EBP)-β, which can activate the promoters of several antiapoptotic proteins (85,86); recent studies have shown that radiation, via the ERK1/2 pathway, can enhance the DNA binding of CREB, which plays a causal role in radioresistance (87). Transcriptional regulation of the ERCC1, XRCC1, and XPC DNA repair genes after irradiation appears to be via AP-1 and Sp1 sites (41). ERK1/2 signaling has also been linked to enhanced expression of MDM2, which can suppress the expression of p53 and thus diminish the proapoptotic signaling effects of wild-type p53, as has been argued based on data from HCT116 cells (71). In contrast to potential radioprotective transcription factors downstream of ERK1/2, EGR-1 is an ERK1/2-dependent transcription factor that has been associated with enhanced cell killing following radiation exposure (88). The radiosensitizing effects of EGR-1 have been linked to increased TNF-α and PTEN expression, whereas the radioprotective effects of EGR-1 have been linked to TGF-β and enhanced growth arrest in the late G1 phase of the cell cycle (89). Thus, collectively, ERK1/2 may act to promote survival via increased activity of some transcription factors (CREB, C/EBPβ), decreased activity of others (p53), and may act in a cell-type dependent fashion to either promote survival or cell death through the activation of others (EGR-1, AP-1).

CONCLUSIONS

Ionizing radiation can activate multiple signaling pathways in cells and causes DNA damage. The ability of radiation to activate pathways depends upon the generation of ROS and RNS, the presence of DNA damage, alterations in the expression of many growth factor receptors and their cognate binding paracrine factors, and upon changes RAS mutational status. Thus, because a pathway is activated by radiation in one cell type does not mean that the same pathway will be activated in a different cell type. In some cell types, enhanced basal signaling by receptors such as ErbB1 or by oncogenes such as RAS proteins may provide a direct overriding radioprotective signal. In many cell types, this may be via PI3K signaling into AKT or mTOR–$p70^{S6K}$; in others, potentially by nuclear factor

(NF)-κB or ERK1/2. Radiation, however, causes the generation of ROS/RNS, which can stimulate the activities of pathways above the high basal levels caused by receptor overexpression or RAS mutation. The activation of signaling pathways occurs in waves and is dependent upon the dose of radiation exposure. Activation of pathways such as ERK1/2 and p38 can promote the cleavage, release, or activation of presynthesized paracrine ligands that can feed back onto irradiated and distant unirradiated tumor cells thereby reinitiating growth factor receptor signaling and reactivating intracellular signal transduction pathways and transcription. Thus, the signaling response of a low-dose irradiated tumor cell attempting to survive is in fact a very complicated series of cause-and-effect signals. Presumably, alterations in cell signaling function and transcriptional activity after this complicated signaling response will cause further ripple effects upon the long-term biologic behavior of tumor cells. With this in mind, it is noteworthy that repeated exposure of breast cancer cells can increase basal expression of survival signaling in ErbB family growth factor receptors.

Acknowledgments
This work was funded: to P.D. from PHS grants (R01-DK52825, P01-CA104177, R01-CA108520), Department of Defense Awards (BC980148, BC020338); to S.G. from PHS grants (R01-CA63753; R01-CA77141) and a Leukemia Society of America grant 6405-97. P.D. is the holder of the Universal Inc. Professorship in Signal Transduction Research. These studies were also supported by The Department of Radiation Oncology, Friede LLC, the Jim Valvano Foundation for Cancer Research, and by the Goodwin Foundation.

REFERENCES

1. Willers H, Held KD. Introduction to clinical radiation biology. *Hematol Oncol Clin North Am* 2006;1:1–24.
2. Bentzen SM, Atasoy BM, Daley FM, et al. Epidermal growth factor receptor expression in pretreatment biopsies from head and neck squamous cell carcinoma as a predictive factor for a benefit from accelerated radiation therapy in a randomized controlled trial. *J Clin Oncol* 2005;24:5560–5567.
3. Hammond EM, Giaccia AJ. The role of ATM and ATR in the cellular response to hypoxia and re-oxygenation. *DNA Repair* (Amst) 2004;3:1117–1122.
4. Barzilai A, Yamamoto K. DNA damage responses to oxidative stress. *DNA Repair* (Amst) 2004;3:1109–1115.
5. Abraham RT. Checkpoint signaling: Epigenetic events sound the DNA strand-breaks alarm to the ATM protein kinase. *Bioessays* 2003;25:627–630.
6. Amundson SA, Bittner M, Fornace AJ Jr. Functional genomics as a window on radiation stress signaling. *Oncogene* 2003;22:5828–5833.
7. Astsaturov I, Cohen RB, Harari P. Targeting epidermal growth factor receptor signaling in the treatment of head and neck cancer. *Expert Rev Anticancer Ther* 2006;6:1179–1193.
8. Chinnaiyan P, Allen GW, Harari PM. Radiation and new molecular agents, part II: Targeting HDAC, HSP90, IGF-1R, PI3K, and Ras. *Semin Radiat Oncol* 2006;16:59–64.

9. Kim DW, Huamani J, Fu A, Hallahan DE. Molecular strategies targeting the host component of cancer to enhance tumor response to radiation therapy. *Int J Radiat Oncol Biol Phys* 2006;64:38–46.
10. Brunner TB, Hahn SM, McKenna WG, Bernhard EJ. Radiation sensitization by inhibition of activated Ras. *Strahlenther Onkol* 2004;180:731–740.
11. Gulbins E, Kolesnick R. Raft ceramide in molecular medicine. *Oncogene* 2003;22:7070–7077.
12. Kavanagh BD, Lin PS, Chen P, et al. Radiation-induced enhanced proliferation of human squamous cancer cells in vitro: A release from inhibition by epidermal growth factor. *Clin Cancer Res* 1995;12:1557–1562.
13. Balaban N, Moni J, Shannon M, et al. The effect of ionizing radiation on signal transduction: Antibodies to EGF receptor sensitize A431 cells to radiation. *Biochim Biophys Acta* 1996;(1–2):147–156.
14. Goldkorn T, Balaban N, Shannon M, et al. EGF receptor phosphorylation is affected by ionizing radiation. *Biochim Biophys Acta* 1997;3:289–299.
15. Kavanagh BD, Dent P, Schmidt-Ullrich RK, et al. Calcium-dependent stimulation of mitogen-activated protein kinase activity in A431 cells by low doses of ionizing radiation. *Radiat Res* 1998;6:579–587.
16. Contessa JN, Reardon DB, Todd D, et al. The inducible expression of dominant-negative epidermal growth factor receptor-CD533 results in radiosensitization of human mammary carcinoma cells. *Clin Cancer Res* 1999;2:405–411.
17. Todd DG, Mikkelsen RB, Rorrer WK, et al. Ionizing radiation stimulates existing signal transduction pathways involving the activation of epidermal growth factor receptor and ErbB-3, and changes of intracellular calcium in A431 human squamous carcinoma cells. *J Recept Signal Transduct Res* 1999;6:885–908.
18. Meyer RG, Kupper JH, Kandolf R, et al. Early growth response-1 gene (Egr-1) promoter induction by ionizing radiation in U87 malignant glioma cells in vitro. *Eur J Biochem* 2002;1:337–346.
19. Bowers G, Reardon D, Hewitt T, et al. The relative role of ErbB1-4 receptor tyrosine kinases in radiation signal transduction responses of human carcinoma cells. *Oncogene* 2001;11:1388–1397.
20. Dent P, Reardon DB, Wood SL, et al. Inactivation of raf-1 by a protein-tyrosine phosphatase stimulated by GTP and reconstituted by Galphai/o subunits. *J Biol Chem* 1996;6:3119–3123.
21. Tonks NK. Protein tyrosine phosphatases and the control of cellular signaling responses. *Adv Pharmacol* 1996;36:91–119.
22. Van Montfort RL, Congreve M, Tisi D, et al. Oxidation state of the active-site cysteine in protein tyrosine phosphatase 1B. *Nature* 2003;423:773–777.
23. Mikkelsen RB, Wardman P. Biological chemistry of reactive oxygen and nitrogen and radiation-induced signal transduction mechanisms. *Oncogene* 2003;37:5734–5754.
24. Leach JK, Van Tuyle G, Lin PS, et al. Ionizing radiation-induced, mitochondria-dependent generation of reactive oxygen/nitrogen. *Cancer Res* 2001;10:3894–3901.
25. Sturla LM, Amorino G, Alexander MS, et al. Requirement of Tyr-992 and Tyr-1173 in phosphorylation of the epidermal growth factor receptor by ionizing radiation and modulation by SHP2. *J Biol Chem* 2005;15:14597–14604.
26. Barrett DM, Black SM, Todor H, et al. Inhibition of protein-tyrosine phosphatases by mild oxidative stresses is dependent on S-nitrosylation. *J Biol Chem* 2005;15:14453–14461.
27. Vega QC, Cochet C, Filhol O, et al. A site of tyrosine phosphorylation in the C terminus of the epidermal growth factor receptor is required to activate phospholipase C. *Mol Cell Biol* 1992;1:128–135.

28. Kasid U, Suy S, Dent P, et al. Activation of Raf by ionizing radiation. *Nature* 199;6594:813–816.
29. Kamata H, Honda S, Maeda S, et al. Reactive oxygen species promote TNFalpha-induced death and sustained JNK activation by inhibiting MAP kinase phosphatases. *Cell* 2005;120:649–661.
30. Nyati MK, Feng FY, Maheshwari D, et al. Ataxia telangiectasia mutated down-regulates phospho-extracellular signal-regulated kinase 1/2 via activation of MKP-1 in response to radiation. *Cancer Res* 2006;66:11554–11559.
31. Dent P, Yacoub A, Fisher PB, et al. MAPK pathways in radiation responses. *Oncogene* 2003;22:5885–5896.
32. Dent P, Han SI, Mitchell C, et al. Inhibition of insulin/IGF-1 receptor signaling enhances bile acid toxicity in primary hepatocytes. *Biochem Pharmacol* 2005;11:1685–1696.
33. Reinehr R, Becker S, Eberle A, et al. Involvement of NADPH oxidase isoforms and Src family kinases in CD95-dependent hepatocyte apoptosis. *J Biol Chem* 2005;29:27179–27194.
34. Fang Y, Han SI, Mitchell C, et al. Bile acids induce mitochondrial ROS, which promote activation of receptor tyrosine kinases and signaling pathways in rat hepatocytes. *Hepatology* 2004;4:961–971.
35. Reinehr R, Becker S, Keitel V, et al. Bile salt-induced apoptosis involves NADPH oxidase isoform activation. *Gastroenterology* 2005;6:2009–2031.
36. Han SI, Studer E, Gupta S, et al. Bile acids enhance the activity of the insulin receptor and glycogen synthase in primary rodent hepatocytes. *Hepatology* 2004;2:456–463.
37. Liu ZM, Huang HS. As2O3-induced c-Src/EGFR/ERK signaling is via Sp1 binding sites to stimulate p21WAF1/CIP1 expression in human epidermoid carcinoma A431 cells. *Cell Signal* 2006;2:244–255.
38. Khan EM, Heidinger JM, Levy M, et al. Epidermal growth factor receptor exposed to oxidative stress undergoes Src- and caveolin-1-dependent perinuclear trafficking. *J Biol Chem* 2006;20:14486–14493.
39. Dent P, Reardon DB, Park JS, et al. Radiation-induced release of transforming growth factor alpha activates the epidermal growth factor receptor and mitogen-activated protein kinase pathway in carcinoma cells, leading to increased proliferation and protection from radiation-induced cell death. *Mol Biol Cell* 1999;8:2493–2506.
40. Shvartsman SY, Hagan MP, Yacoub A, et al. Autocrine loops with positive feedback enable context-dependent cell signaling. *Am J Physiol Cell Physiol* 2002;3:C545–C559.
41. Hagan M, Yacoub A, Dent P. Ionizing radiation causes a dose-dependent release of transforming growth factor alpha in vitro from irradiated xenografts and during palliative treatment of hormone-refractory prostate carcinoma. *Clin Cancer Res* 2004;17:5724–5731.
42. O-Charoenrat P, Wongkajornsilp A, Rhys-Evans PH, et al. Signaling pathways required for matrix metalloproteinase-9 induction by betacellulin in head and neck squamous carcinoma cells. *Int J Cancer* 2004;2:174–183.
43. Zhang Q, Thomas SM, Xi S, et al. SRC family kinases mediate epidermal growth factor receptor ligand cleavage, proliferation, and invasion of head and neck cancer cells. *Cancer Res* 2004;17:6166–6173.
44. El-Shewy HM, Kelly FL, Barki-Harrington L, et al. Ectodomain shedding-dependent transactivation of epidermal growth factor receptors in response to insulin-like growth factor type I. *Mol Endocrinol* 2004;11:2727–2739.
45. Caron RW, Yacoub A, Zhu X, et al. H-RAS V12-induced radioresistance in HCT116 colon carcinoma cells is heregulin dependent. *Mol Cancer Ther* 2005;2:243–255.

46. Fang L, Li G, Liu G, et al. p53 induction of heparin-binding EGF-like growth factor counteracts p53 growth suppression through activation of MAPK and PI3K/Akt signaling cascades. *EMBO J* 2001;8:1931–1939.
47. Sheikh MS, Carrier F, Johnson AC, et al. Identification of an additional p53-responsive site in the human epidermal growth factor receptor gene promotor. *Oncogene* 1997;9:1095–1101.
48. Nishi H, Senoo M, Nishi KH, et al. p53 Homologue p63 represses epidermal growth factor receptor expression. *J Biol Chem* 2001;276:41717–41724.
49. Schmidt-Ullrich RK, Valerie K, Chan W, et al. Expression of oestrogen receptor and transforming growth factor-alpha in MCF-7 cells after exposure to fractionated irradiation. *Int J Radiat Biol* 1992;61:405–415.
50. Shelton JG, Steelman LS, Abrams SL, et al. The epidermal growth factor receptor gene family as a target for therapeutic intervention in numerous cancers: What's genetics got to do with it? *Expert Opin Ther Targets* 2005;5:1009–1030.
51. Baselga J, Arteaga CL. Critical update and emerging trends in epidermal growth factor receptor targeting in cancer. *J Clin Oncol* 2005;11:2445–2459.
52. Harari PM. Epidermal growth factor receptor inhibition strategies in oncology. *Endocr Relat Cancer* 2004;4:689–708.
53. Pino MS, Shrader M, Baker CH, et al. Transforming growth factor alpha expression drives constitutive epidermal growth factor receptor pathway activation and sensitivity to gefitinib (Iressa) in human pancreatic cancer cell lines. *Cancer Res* 2006;7:3802–3812.
54. Chinnaiyan P, Huang S, Vallabhaneni G, et al. Mechanisms of enhanced radiation response following epidermal growth factor receptor signaling inhibition by erlotinib (Tarceva). *Cancer Res* 2005;8:3328–3335.
55. Bianco C, Tortora G, Bianco R, et al. Enhancement of antitumor activity of ionizing radiation by combined treatment with the selective epidermal growth factor receptor-tyrosine kinase inhibitor ZD1839 (Iressa). *Clin Cancer Res* 2002;10:3250–3258.
56. Sarkaria JN, Carlson BL, Schroeder MA, et al. Use of an orthotopic xenograft model for assessing the effect of epidermal growth factor receptor amplification on glioblastoma radiation response. *Clin Cancer Res* 2006;7:2264–2271.
57. Raben D, Helfrich BA, Chan D, et al. ZD1839, a selective epidermal growth factor receptor tyrosine kinase inhibitor, alone and in combination with radiation and chemotherapy as a new therapeutic strategy in non-small cell lung cancer. *Semin Oncol* 2002;1:37–46.
58. Harari PM, Huang S. Radiation combined with EGFR signal inhibitors: Head and neck cancer focus. *Semin Radiat Oncol* 2006;1:38–44.
59. Kwak EL, Sordella R, Bell DW, et al. Irreversible inhibitors of the EGF receptor may circumvent acquired resistance to gefitinib. *Proc Natl Acad Sci USA* 2005;21:7665–7670.
60. Thomas RK, Greulich H, Yuza Y, et al. Detection of oncogenic mutations in the EGFR gene in lung adenocarcinoma with differential sensitivity to EGFR tyrosine kinase inhibitors. *Cold Spring Harbor Symp Quant Biol* 2005;70:73–81.
61. Jones HE, Gee JM, Barrow D, et al. Inhibition of insulin receptor isoform-A signalling restores sensitivity to gefitinib in previously de novo resistant colon cancer cells. *Br J Cancer* 2006;2:172–180.
62. Yacoub A, Park MA, Hanna D, et al. OSU-03012 promotes caspase-independent but PERK-, cathepsin B-, BID-, and AIF-dependent killing of transformed cells. *Mol Pharmacol* 2006;2:589–603.
63. Ihle NT, Paine-Murrieta G, Berggren MI, et al. The phosphatidylinositol-3-kinase inhibitor PX-866 overcomes resistance to the epidermal growth factor receptor inhibitor gefitinib in A-549 human non-small cell lung cancer xenografts. *Mol Cancer Ther* 2005;9:1349–1357.

64. Gupta AK, Bakanauskas VJ, Cerniglia GJ, et al. The Ras radiation resistance pathway. *Cancer Res* 2001;61:4278–4782.
65. Gupta AK, McKenna WG, Weber CN, et al. Local recurrence in head and neck cancer: Relationship to radiation resistance and signal transduction. *Clin Cancer Res* 2002;8:885–892.
66. Gupta AK, Bernhard EJ, Bakanauskas VJ, et al. RAS-mediated radiation resistance is not linked to MAP kinase activation in two bladder carcinoma cell lines. *Radiat Res* 2000;154:64–72.
67. Kim IA, Bae SS, Fernandes A, et al. Selective inhibition of Ras, phosphoinositide 3 kinase, and Akt isoforms increases the radiosensitivity of human carcinoma cell lines. *Cancer Res* 2005;17:7902–7910.
68. Brunner TB, Cengel KA, Hahn SM, et al. Pancreatic cancer cell radiation survival and prenyltransferase inhibition: The role of K-Ras. *Cancer Res* 2005;18:8433–8441.
69. Caron RW, Yacoub A, Li M, et al. Activated forms of H-RAS and K-RAS differentially regulate membrane association of PI3K, PDK-1, and AKT and the effect of therapeutic kinase inhibitors on cell survival. *Mol Cancer Ther* 2005;2:257–270.
70. Caron RW, Yacoub A, Mitchell C, et al. Radiation-stimulated ERK1/2 and JNK1/2 signaling can promote cell cycle progression in human colon cancer cells. *Cell Cycle* 2005;3:456–464.
71. Ries S, Biederer C, Woods D, et al. Opposing effects of Ras on p53: Transcriptional activation of mdm2 and induction of p19ARF. *Cell* 2000;2:321–330.
72. Shonai T, Adachi M, Sakata K, et al. MEK/ERK pathway protects ionizing radiation-induced loss of mitochondrial membrane potential and cell death in lymphocytic leukemia cells. *Cell Death Differ* 2002;9:963–971.
73. Lee YJ, Soh JW, Jeoung DI, et al. PKC epsilon-mediated ERK1/2 activation involved in radiation induced cell death in NIH3T3 cells. *Biochim Biophys Acta* 2003;3:219–229.
74. Abbott DW, Holt JT. Mitogen-activated protein kinase kinase 2 activation is essential for progression through the G2/M checkpoint arrest in cells exposed to ionizing radiation. *J Biol Chem* 1999;274:2732–2742.
75. Vrana JA, Grant S, Dent P. Inhibition of the MAPK pathway abrogates BCL2-mediated survival of leukemia cells after exposure to low-dose ionizing radiation. *Radiat Res* 1999;5:559–569.
76. Yacoub A, Hawkins W, Hanna D, et al. Human chorionic gonadotropin (hCG) modulates prostate cancer cell survival after irradiation or HMG CoA reductase inhibitor treatment. *Mol Pharmacol* 2007;71:259–275.
77. Jost M, Huggett TM, Kari C, et al. Epidermal growth factor receptor-dependent control of keratinocyte survival and Bcl-xL expression through a MEK-dependent pathway. *J Biol Chem* 2001;276:6320–6326.
78. Boucher MJ, Morisset J, Vachon PH, et al. MEK/ERK signaling pathway regulates the expression of Bcl-2, Bcl-X(L), and Mcl-1 and promotes survival of human pancreatic cancer cells. *J Cell Biochemistry* 2000;79:355–369.
79. Pardo OE, Arcaro A, Salerno G, et al. Seckl, Fibroblast growth factor-2 induces translational regulation of Bcl-XL and Bcl-2 via a MEK-dependent pathway: Correlation with resistance to etoposide-induced apoptosis. *J Biol Chem* 2002;277:12040–12046.
80. Reed JC, Doctor KS, Godzik A. The domains of apoptosis: A genomics perspective. *Sci STKE* 2004;239:re9.
81. Roth W, Reed JC. FLIP protein and TRAIL-induced apoptosis. *Vitam Horm* 2004;67:189–206.
82. Green DR. Apoptotic pathways: Ten minutes to dead. *Cell* 2005;5:671–674.

83. Kim BJ, Ryu SW, Song BJ. JNK- and p38 kinase-mediated phosphorylation of Bax leads to its activation and mitochondrial translocation and to apoptosis of human hepatoma HepG2 cells. *J Biol Chem* 2006;281:21256–21265.
84. Lei K, Nimnual A, Zong W-X, et al. The bax subfamily of Bcl2-related proteins is essential for apoptotic signal transduction by c-Jun NH2-terminal kinase. *Mol Cell Biol* 2002;22:4929–4942.
85. Amorino GP, Mikkelsen RB, Valerie K, et al. Dominant-negative cAMP-responsive element-binding protein inhibits proliferating cell nuclear antigen and DNA repair, leading to increased cellular radiosensitivity. *J Biol Chem* 2003;32:29394–29399.
86. Amorino GP, Hamilton VM, Valerie K, et al. Epidermal growth factor receptor dependence of radiation-induced transcription factor activation in human breast carcinoma cells. *Mol Biol Cell* 2002;7:2233–2244.
87. Virolle T, Adamson ED, Baron V, et al. The Egr-1 transcription factor directly activates PTEN during irradiation-induced signalling. *Nat Cell Biol* 2001;12:1124–1128.
88. Ahmed MM, Sells SF, Venkatasubbarao K, et al. Ionizing radiation-inducible apoptosis in the absence of p53 linked to transcription factor EGR-1. *J Biol Chem* 1997;52:33056–33061.
89. Criswell T, Beman M, Araki S, et al. Delayed activation of insulin-like growth factor-1 receptor/Src/MAPK/Egr-1 signaling regulates clusterin expression, a pro-survival factor. *J Biol Chem* 2005;14:14212–14221.

3 Vascular Epithelial Growth Factor (VEGF) Receptors

ANDREW N. FONTANELLA
YITING CAO
MARK W. DEWHIRST

In this chapter, we examine the relationships among hypoxia, angiogenesis, and tumor pathophysiology, and the roles that they play in the modulation of cytotoxic treatment efficacy. In order to gain a more thorough understanding of these highly interconnected aspects of tumor biology, we discuss the determinant factors of these processes and their significance in terms of clinical treatments.

The targeting of angiogenesis is a burgeoning field in cancer research, and a number of pioneering studies over the past few decades have yielded very promising options for the treatment of solid tumors. The anticipated potential of this field is reflected in the recent U.S. Food and Drug Administration (FDA) approval of antiangiogenic drugs for the treatment of various diseases. For cancer therapy, antiangiogenic agents are being explored largely in combination with cytotoxic therapies; by targeting the tumor vasculature, antiangiogenic agents may be able to potentiate these therapies through novel modalities that exploit changes in intertumoral oxygenation.

The ultimate aim of combinational strategies is to take advantage of vascular responses to antiangiogenic therapy or hypoxia-inducible factor (HIF)-1 blockade in order to indirectly improve the antitumor effect of radiotherapy or chemotherapy. By targeting the vasculature—the major biochemical regulator of any cellular system—physiologic responses can be modulated to produce an environment amenable to multiple antitumoral therapeutic modalities. In this chapter, we discuss factors that play a major role in the angiogenic process. We will also discuss how the functionality of these factors can be targeted for antiangiogenic strategies. The formulation of effective combinational therapies is dependent upon a thorough understanding of primary and metastatic tumor inception and progression, and so we will present an overview of the evolving model of tumor development. Finally, we will discuss current progress in the application of these therapies to the clinical setting and how ongoing research will ultimately lead to further advances in patient care.

■ THE TUMOR MICROENVIRONMENT

Hypoxia-inducible Factor and Hypoxia

Solid tumors are generally associated with a state of insufficient oxygen supply (1). The rapid proliferation of highly metabolic cells, combined with significant imbalances in angiogenesis regulation, inevitably leads to a failure of the vascular network to furnish an ideal environment for cellular growth and survival. The scarcity of important substrates contributes to the tumor's pathophysiologic response to its harsh environment. Through complex signal transduction pathways, tumors will initiate ameliorative adaptations to hypoxia that will contribute to resistance to many forms of treatment, including radiation (2), chemotherapy (3), and perhaps even targeted agents, such as growth factor receptor antagonists.

Hypoxia has been shown to have a negative effect on the management of many tumor types (4,5). Molecular oxygen is primarily needed to generate ion radicals and free radicals to break chemical bonds (6). In addition, molecular oxygen is known to inhibit DNA damage repair after radiation-induced damage (6). The absence of oxygen allows DNA damage to be corrected more effectively, causing hypoxic cells to be significantly more resistant to radiation than normally oxygenated cells. This decreased efficacy of radiation treatment is exacerbated by the tumor's selective adaptation to hypoxic conditions. For example, the tumor-suppressor protein p53 triggers apoptosis under oxygen-starvation; this leads to a selection for p53 mutated cells in which apoptosis is not stimulated by hypoxia, thus facilitating the survival and expansion of cells that have adopted dangerous mutations (7).

Hypoxia induces the expression of HIF-1 (of the family of *H*ypoxia *I*nducible *F*actors) (8). HIF-1 is a major transcription factor regulating cellular adaptation to low oxygen conditions (4). It is a heterodimer consisting of α and β subunits (9). Normally, HIF-1's α subunit is rapidly destroyed in the presence of oxygen by hydroxylation of proline residues in its oxygen-dependent degradation domain and proteosomal degradation, yielding a transcription factor that is significantly active primarily under hypoxic conditions (10–12). HIF-1 has also been shown to be stabilized following cytotoxic treatment-induced reoxygenation, implicating it in many post-treatment tumor responses (13).

Overexpression of HIF-1 has been observed in breast, cervix, lung, brain, ovarian, and prostate cancers (4). Many studies have shown that HIF-1 is an important transcription factor for angiogenesis, metabolic adaptation, apoptosis regulation, and metastasis—all of which are major aspects of tumorigenesis and tumor progression (14). Accordingly, blockade of HIF-1 activity can inhibit angiogenesis and even kill hypoxic cells by preventing their transition to an anaerobic metabolism (15). Although initially an elusive goal, emerging options for the direct inhibition of HIF-1 implore further investigation into the comparative benefits of targeting either HIF-1 or various downstream factors in the HIF-1 signal transduction pathways.

In targeting HIF-1 directly, the optimization of treatment schedules is a primary concern in ensuring the efficacy of this method. Pretreatment blockade of the factor is an obvious strategy for sensitizing the tumor to cytotoxic damage. However, it is important to consider that HIF-1 is also separately regulated by free radicals, even under aerobic conditions. Since cytotoxic therapies generate an abundance of free radicals, HIF-1 is often upregulated post cytotoxic treatment in a manner independent of hypoxia (13). The inhibition of HIF-1–induced angiogenesis after cytotoxic treatment may therefore confer a therapeutic advantage by sensitizing the tumor microvasculature to future cytotoxic damage (15).

Angiogenesis

Angiogenesis occurs through a process of *endothelial sprouting* in which new vessels branch from an existing vessel, and through *intussusception*, wherein endothelial cells within an existing vessel form a longitudinally dividing column that bifurcates the vessel (16). Vasculogenesis is also an important aspect of vascular expansion. Vasculogenesis involves the recruitment of bone marrow–derived endothelial-precursor cells into the vascular architecture (17). Whereas angiogenesis refers to endothelial cell proliferation and migration, vasculogenesis refers specifically to the de novo differentiation of endothelial cells from progenitor cells.

The formation of new blood vessels and the remodeling of existing ones must inevitably lead to instability of flow and distribution of red blood cells within the developing vascular network (18). The primary determinants of flow are the pressure gradient and flow resistance. Flow resistance is affected by microvessel diameter (it is dependent upon the fourth power of vessel radius) and the rheologic properties of the blood cells (19). Despite the flourishing angiogenic activity that hypoxia induces, oxygen diffusion is hindered by the erratic and inefficient structure of the newly formed vessels, and the hypoxic condition is not rectified, even at the earliest stages of growth (20).

Tumor growth and metastasis are dependent upon angiogenesis (21). It has generally been thought that, as tumor cells expand beyond the oxygen diffusion distance, the transcription factor HIF-1 is stabilized, and it begins to regulate downstream angiogenic factors (14). Recent results from our laboratory present a different paradigm, suggesting that angiogenesis initiation may not require hypoxia or HIF-1 activation, but that HIF-1 activation is strongly associated with angiogenesis acceleration (20).

■ ANGIOGENIC FACTORS

A History of Vascular Endothelial Growth Factor Discovery

For more than a century, cancer researchers have noted the abundant and uniquely structured vasculature of tumors and speculated on the significance of this finding. Indeed, the ubiquity of this observation led some researchers to propose that the pathology of malignant tumor growth involved a corresponding disorder of the vascular system (22). However, insight into the proper role and mechanism of vascular proliferation needed to wait until the early twentieth century and the emergence of in vivo imaging before its pathophysiologic significance could begin to be understood.

In 1928, a window chamber model for the optical imaging of living tissue in a rabbit ear was developed (23). The model was later incorporated into rabbit carcinoma studies by Gordon Ide, in 1939. Ide observed a strong correlation between vascular proliferation and tumor expansion. This and following optical studies showed that the capacity of the vascular endothelium to deliver oxygen and nutrients was a crucial rate-limiting step in tumor progression (22,24). It was now apparent that chemical growth factors must play some role in the recruitment of blood vessels by the expanding tumor. Further discovery was accelerated in 1943, when Glenn Algire pioneered the application of optical methods to mouse tumor models. A paper discussing a number of the window chambers he had developed was published in that year (25). The most important of these models would be the dorsal skin-flap chamber. Prior to this development, in vivo optical measurements were performed primarily in rabbits, dogs, and animals with ears large enough to facilitate a window chamber. With Algire's murine model, the optical observation of tumors within the biologic sciences' quintessential laboratory animal was developed.

In 1968, the interstitial diffusion of a proangiogenic growth factor was demonstrated in hamster carcinoma studies by Melvin Greenblatt and Philippe Shubik. They observed that the vascular response to a tumor transplanted into a hamster cheek pouch was not inhibited by a semipermeable filter that separated the tumor from the host tissue (26). It was thus assumed that the growth factor researchers were looking for could be characterized as an interstitial protein produced by tumor cells that induces radical modifications to an otherwise healthy vasculature. With the basic properties and mechanism of action established, work toward identifying the angiogenic factors began.

In 1983, Donald Senger and Harold Dvorak were able to identify a protein that induced vascular leakage. The protein was named vascular permeability factor, or VPF (27). A few years later, Napoleone Ferrara's group described vascular endothelial growth factor (VEGF), which was thought to be a major cytokine in the regulation of blood vessel growth (28). These molecules were later determined to be the same, proving that this single protein (thereafter referred to as VEGF) was responsible for the disparate functions of regulating vascular permeability and vascular expansion (29,30). Judah Folkman would also make invaluable contributions to the discovery of VEGF functionality, establishing VEGF as a mitogenic factor and a primary promoter of angiogenesis (29,31,32). Eventually, different isoforms of VEGF would be discovered, along with a number of related growth factors. Years of investigation would substantially broaden the known functions and targets of this family of growth factors, although a complete model of their complex signaling pathways is still being established.

The Vascular Endothelial Growth Factor Family

The VEGF family contains a number of isoforms and related proteins. The class of proteins associated with most tumor cells is commonly referred to as VEGF, although it is more precisely named VEGF-A. VEGF-A is known to have at least five splice variants consisting of 121, 145, 165, 189, and 206 amino acid residues, of which the 121, 165, and 189 variants are most commonly expressed. These are encoded by an approximately 14,000 base-pair gene with eight exons (33,34). The sixth and seventh exons encode a heparin-binding domain (34). VEGF-A_{121} lacks both heparin-binding domains and does not attach to the extracellular matrix or cell membrane (35,36). Conversely, VEGF-A_{189} binds to heparin with a high affinity and is found sequestered predominantly in the extracellular matrix and, to a small extent, on cell surfaces (36,37). Despite the fact that it becomes soluble with the cleaving of its carboxyl terminus, VEGF-A_{189} is not active in the signal transduction process to a significant degree (38). VEGF-A_{165} has a moderate affinity toward heparin. This splice variant lacks the heparin-binding domain encoded in the sixth exon, but retains that of seventh (28,39,40). About half of the 165-isoform growth factors that are produced will bind to the cell surface or extracellular matrix (37).

The heparin-binding ability of VEGF-A_{165} is significant in that, by binding to the heparan-sulfates of the extracellular matrix, VEGF-A_{165} is able to release angiogenic factors stored there. One such factor, basic fibroblast growth factor (bFGF), induces a strong angiogenic response, as it operates synergistically with VEGF (41,42). The heparin affinity of VEGF-A_{165} also assists in the amelioration of oxidative damage to the growth factor. Once oxidized, both VEGF-A_{165} and VEGF-A_{121} lose their ability to bind to the VEGF receptor VEGFR-2.

VEGF-A_{165}, however, is able to use heparan-sulfate proteoglycans as surrogate receptor-binding facilitators, compensating for this defect and significantly prolonging the bioactive lifetime of the growth factor (43,44).

The ubiquity and persistence of VEGF-A_{165} has led to a strong association of the isoform with angiogenesis. Historically, the diffusible heparin-binding protein that was revealed to be the archetypal angiogenic factor strongly corresponds to this particular isoform.

VEGF-B, has two isoforms, VEGF-B_{167} and VEGF-B_{186} (45,46). Both isoforms are most abundant in cardiac and skeletal muscles and bind to the VEGF receptors VEGFR-1 and neuropilin-1, but not to VEGFR-2 (47–49). VEGF-C and VEGF-D both bind to VEGFR-3, a receptor involved in lymphogenesis (50–55). They also bind to VEGFR-2, but generally do not display strong mitogenic effects in endothelial cells, as compared with VEGF-A (51,54). VEGF-E is a potent angiogenic factor (56). It binds to VEGFR-2 and is very similar in structure to VEGF-A, but its production is facilitated by the orf virus and it is not part of the human proteome (57). Although the B, C, D, and E families of VEGF serve important roles in angiogenesis and lymphogenesis, they are more specific than VEGF-A and play a lesser function in general tumor pathophysiology.

Various studies have shown a distinct spatial and temporal correlation between the expression of VEGF-A proteins and an increase in vascular permeability and endothelial cell mitosis (58–61). VEGF-A is distinct among the native VEGF proteins and related growth factors in that its expression is highly affected by hypoxia (62–65). An upstream hypoxia regulatory element that binds HIF-1 is a transcription enhancer, mobilizing VEGF-A as an adaptive response to oxygen starvation (66,67). Here, VEGF-A represents a critical component in the initiation of angiogenesis. It has been shown that VEGF-A is necessary for angiogenesis and vasculogenesis to occur, leading to a lethal embryonic vascular deficiency in animals with even a single nonfunctional VEGF-A allele (68,69). It is generally agreed that VEGF-A represents a critical bottleneck in angiogenic signal transduction. But, although this linchpin factor plays an indispensable role in vascular adaptation, it is by no means the only significant player.

The Vascular Endothelial Growth Factor Receptors

The various forms of VEGF bind to receptor tyrosine kinases (RTKs) (Fig. 3.1). Of primary importance to angiogenesis are VEGFR-1 and VEGFR-2 (alternatively named flt-1 and flk-1/KDR, respectively). The cell-bound form of these receptors consists of seven immunoglobulin-like domains in the extracellular region, a transmembrane segment, and a split tyrosine kinase (TK) domain in the intracellular region (70,71) (Fig. 3.2). The VEGF binding domains for

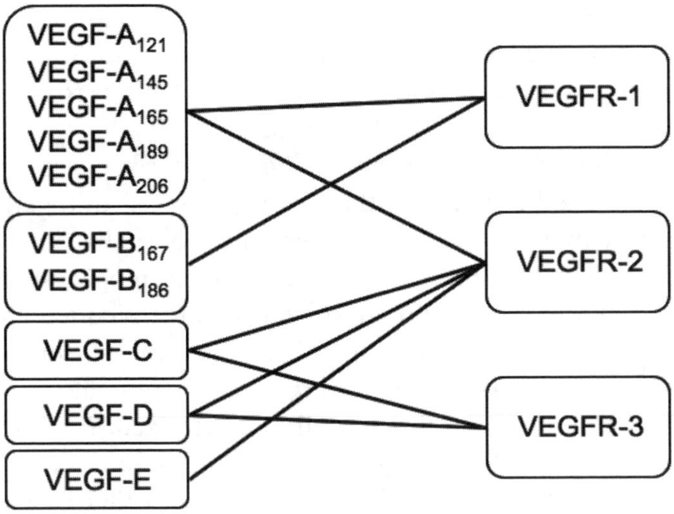

FIGURE 3.1 The VEGF variants and their respective receptors.

VEGFR-1 and VEGFR-2 occur at opposite ends of the VEGF monomer; two growth factor proteins will form disulfide bonds linking them in an antiparallel arrangement, such that the VEGFR-1 or VEGFR-2 binding domains of each monomer portion occur at opposite ends of the combined structure (72). The bound monomers thus contain a binding domain for both receptor types at both ends of the structure.

The VEGF binding site occurs at the second and third immunoglobin-like domains for both VEGFR-1 and VEGFR-2 (73). Upon binding to the receptors, the VEGF ligand will cause the fourth immunoglobin-like domains of two adjacent receptors to bind to each other (74). This domain is referred to as the

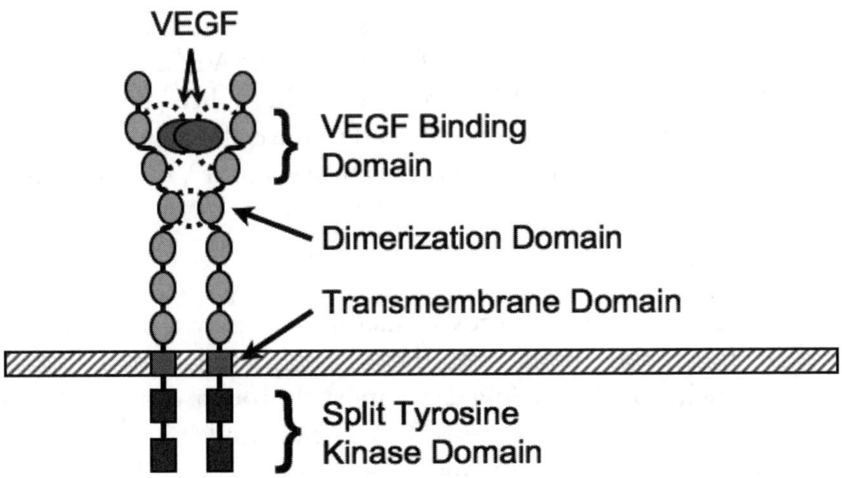

FIGURE 3.2 The VEGF receptor.

dimerization domain. Dimerization will induce a chemical cascade in which tyrosine phosphorylation facilitates the phosphorylation of intracellular proteins, thus initiating signal transduction (75). Once VEGF binds to its receptor, the complex is absorbed into the cell and digested.

VEGFR-2 is the primary receptor for the physiologic responses associated with VEGF (72,76). It has been shown that endothelial cell mitogenesis and vascular permeability enhancement are suppressed in the lethal knockout of VEGFR-2. Mice devoid of VEGFR-2 fail to undergo vasculogenesis and will die in utero at approximately 9 days post-fertilization due to inadequate blood supply to vital tissues (77). This suggests that VEGFR-2 plays a primary role in angiogenesis, vessel maintenance, and endothelial cell survival.

Although the function of VEGFR-2 is well characterized, the function of VEGFR-1 is not. Mice lacking VEGFR-1 also die in utero, but in this case the lethality is due to the extreme proliferation of angioblasts (78,79). Therefore, at least during the early developmental stage, VEGFR-1 seems to serve as a suppressor of VEGF vasculogenic signaling. In fact, it has been proposed that the primary function of VEGFR-1 is to serve as a decoy receptor for VEGF (80). By sequestering growth factors, VEGFR-1 moderates VEGFR-2 binding and thus serves as an inhibitor to angiogenesis even though it displays no overt antiangiogenic signaling properties (76,80). This theory is supported by the observation that a mutated form of VEGFR-1 that binds VEGF but lacks the TK domain is observed to cause no apparent deviation from normal vascular development (81). Other studies have shown that VEGFR-1 is able to facilitate monocyte chemotaxis and weak mitogenic signals, along with significant tissue-specific effects (81–83). So, although it is widely accepted that VEGFR-2 plays the major role in angiogenic signaling transduction, the function of VEGFR-1 seems to be more subtle and arrayed.

A third receptor, VEGFR-3 (flt-4), has been identified, although this receptor is primarily involved in lymphogenesis and plays little role in angiogenesis or vasculogenesis (84). Of the VEGF proteins, the VEGFR-3 receptor binds only VEGF-C and VEGF-D (51,52,54). A soluble splice variant of VEGFR-1 also exists. Since this receptor is not bound to the cell membrane, it cannot initiate signaling transduction and serves exclusively as a VEGF scavenger (85).

The Angiopoietins

The angiopoietins are protein growth factors that play a major role in maintaining the functional stability of the vasculature. Four angiopoietins are known, of which Ang-1 and Ang-2 are most thoroughly understood in terms of their contribution to angiogenesis (86). Both ligands bind to the TKR Tie-2 (*T*yrosine kinase receptors with *I*mmunoglobulin and *E*pidermal growth factor homology domains).

The Tie-2 receptor was first identified as an important component of the angiogenic process in 1997, when a soluble truncated form of the receptor was shown to stifle tumor growth and inhibit vascular proliferation (87,88). The antitumor effect elicited by the soluble receptor was shown to be primarily due to the limiting effect of vascular regression rather than any cell lethality, as viability was not altered in cultured tumor cells. This work firmly established the Tie-2 receptor and its ligands as important elements of angiogenic signal transduction.

Ang-1 is involved in the angiogenic process of pericyte recruitment (which provides structural support to the vasculature and defines the transition from immature to mature vessels) and the stabilization of the vasculature, although its ability to induce endothelial cell mitosis is not clearly defined (89–91). In fact, Ang-1 seems to play a complementary role to VEGF in the angiogenic process. Overexpression of VEGF produces a marked increase in vascular density by promoting the tortuous and branching expansion of immature vessels. On the other hand, Ang-1 overexpression causes an increase in vessel diameter (89). Under normal conditions, the constitutive expression of Ang-1 is necessary for the development, stabilization, and maintenance of a functional vascular network (92).

The action of Ang-2 is more complex. Ang-2 knockouts have shown that the absence of Ang-2 does not affect vasculogenesis; the prenatal vasculature develops normally in these animals (93). Ang-2 is normally upregulated at remodeling sites, and it is required for postnatal vascular reorganization (94). Accordingly, Ang-2 knockdown animals are unable to initiate angiogenic remodeling.

Whereas Ang-1 expression promotes vessel stabilization, Ang-2 has been shown to cause a destabilizing effect. It is upregulated in areas undergoing vascular restructuring, and whereas the Ang-2 ligand does not induce receptor kinase phosphorylation, it effectively blocks Ang-1 signaling by binding to their common Tie-2 receptor (94). This causes a degradation of the basement membrane and the detachment of vessel pericytes from the lumen (95,96). Hypoxia has been shown to increase the levels of both angiopoietins, although the induced amplification of Ang-2 is much greater than that of Ang-1 (64,97,98). Ang-2 is also observed in higher concentrations under increased VEGF expression, relative to Ang-1 (64,97). This suggests that the ratio of Ang-2 to Ang-1 is more important in predicting the dominant physiologic response than are absolute quantities (99). Ang-2's effects contribute to either angiogenic or antiangiogenic action depending on the context of its expression.

In the presence of VEGF signaling, the destabilization of mature vessels by Ang-2 is one of the first steps in the angiogenic process. The degradation of the basement membrane and the detachment of pericytes allow endothelial tubes to initiate budding and intussusception (the bifurcation and separation of a single vessel), hallmark features of angiogenesis and the primary features of proliferation (100). In the absence of VEGF signaling, the devolution of the vasculature initiated by Ang-2 will lead to vascular regression and an eventual depletion of the network—an antiangiogenic response (94) (Fig. 3.3).

The complex functionality of Ang-2 is emphasized in a recent paper that showed that when Ang-2 was systemically overexpressed, vascular regression was observed even in the absence of VEGF inhibition (96). Ang-2 overexpression also caused a transient exacerbation of hypoxia, with a return to an intertumoral oxygenation similar to the untreated control group with continued overexpression. Angiogenesis and tumor growth was inhibited, while the apoptotic response was enhanced. Interestingly, despite vascular regression and transient hypoxia, tumors showed an increased perfusion in the surviving vessels. After vascular regression, the remaining vessels became dilated due to the loss of pericytes. The overexpression of Ang-2 was shown to cause an inability of pericytes to remain attached to endothelial cells, although it did not directly lead to pericyte death.

Ang-2 overexpression, with or without VEGF inhibition, inhibits angiogenesis and promotes apoptosis; it has no apparent long-term effect upon hypoxia (96). Neither does it have an effect on cell proliferation, leading to the conclusion that the suppression of tumor growth caused by Ang-2 is attributed to enhanced tumor cell apoptosis (96). This suggests that the role Ang-2 plays as an adjunct to VEGF is dependent on a certain balance between the two ligands.

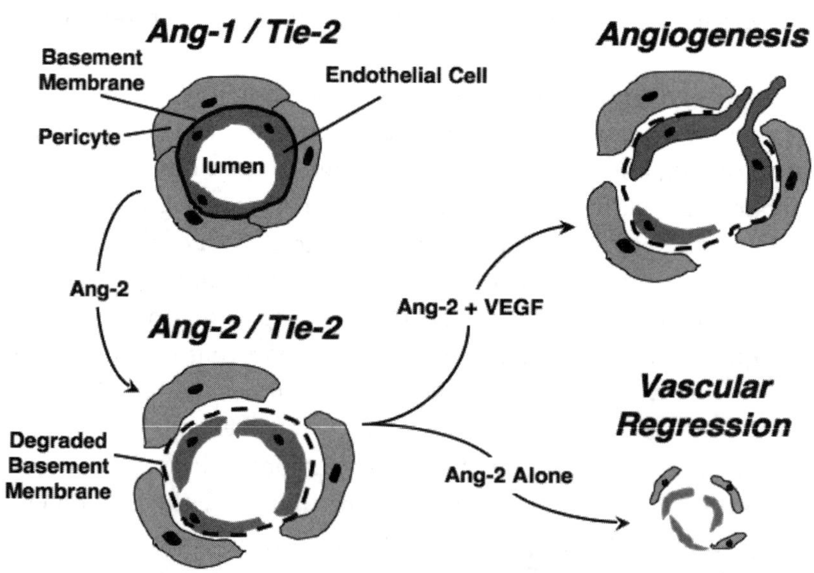

FIGURE 3.3 The physiologic effects of the angiopoietins: Ang-1 maintains vessel stability, whereas Ang-2 destabilizes vasculature. In the presence of VEGF, Ang-2 contributes to angiogenesis. In the absence of VEGF, Ang-2 causes vascular regression. (Figure courtesy of C. Kontos.)

It is not only the factors alone, but it is this balance that is the crucial aspect in the regulation of angiogenesis and blood vessel regression. In fact, it was shown that the blockade of the Tie-2 pathway by a soluble receptor significantly inhibits tumor growth and metastasis in murine mammary carcinoma and melanoma (101). These supplementary studies help to elucidate the angiogenic codependence of the VEGF and Tie-2 signal transduction components.

MODELS OF VASCULAR RESPONSE IN TUMORS

The VEGF variants, the angiopoietins, and their receptors— although among the most important components of an angiogenic response—are only a selection of the myriad of proteins capable of influencing vascular growth or regression. Yet, despite the sheer number of such factors, the vasculature of healthy tissue is maintained in a state of optimal balance through their precise regulation (102). Proangiogenic factors are upregulated in response to stimuli such as hypoxia (103). They initiate vascular expansion to the point at which the hypoxic condition is rectified or the cells undergo apoptosis (102). This healthy angiogenic response is uncommon during adult life and is typically limited to wound healing, physiologic organ growth, and female reproductive processes (104,105). In fact, the stability of adult vasculature is highlighted by the longevity of endothelial cells, which normally exhibit periods of turnover on the order of years (106).

The model of a balance between pro- and antiangiogenic factors readily lends itself to the concept of an "angiogenic switch." The angiogenic switch is the point at which the balanced regulation of angiogenic factors fails (102). For example, in healthy tissues, angiogenesis is initiated to assist in the process of reforming tissue that has been damaged by physical trauma. As the tissue repairs itself, angiogenic factors are downregulated again, and the vasculature returns to a static state. However, cancerous cells continue to proliferate and induce vessel expansion, thereby preventing a state of vascular stasis—the tumor becomes much like a "wound that never heals" (107). Although this model adequately explains the process of angiogenesis in well-established tumors, an accurate model of vascular adaptation in nascent tumors has only lately emerged.

Evidence for Hypoxia-independent Angiogenesis

The role of angiogenesis in incipient tumor growth is an important aspect of the tumorigenic process, although until recently, discovery in this area was obstructed by the technical difficulties of observing nascent tumor growth. In work done by our group, a small number of cancer cells engineered to express green fluorescent protein (GFP) were injected into a murine window chamber. The constitutive expression of GFP allowed the cells to be observed and tracked even while the burgeoning cancer was a collection of only a few cells. At the earliest stages of growth, the cells would preferentially divide in the direction of microvessels (108). The cells would take on a fibroblast-like form as they elongated and divided unidirectionally toward their nutrient supply (108) (Fig. 3.4). This chemotaxis-like feature is possibly due to oxygen, nutrient, growth factor, or other cytokine gradients emanating from the vasculature.

These observations may lend support to the model of vascular cooption that has been observed in a number of tumor types. Cooption was reported by Yancopoulos and Wiegand in brain tumor models (109) and by Pezzella and colleagues in primary and metastatic lung cancers (110). Rather than initiate new vessel growth, tumor cells will sustain themselves on oxygen and nutrients supplied by the existing vasculature for a period of time (109,110). The cancer will incorporate itself into the preexisting architecture of the primary or metastatic site before any expansive vascular remodeling occurs (109,110).

Yancopoulos reports that this relationship is short-lived, however, as Ang-2 expression is induced in the endothelium of coopted vessels not long after tu-

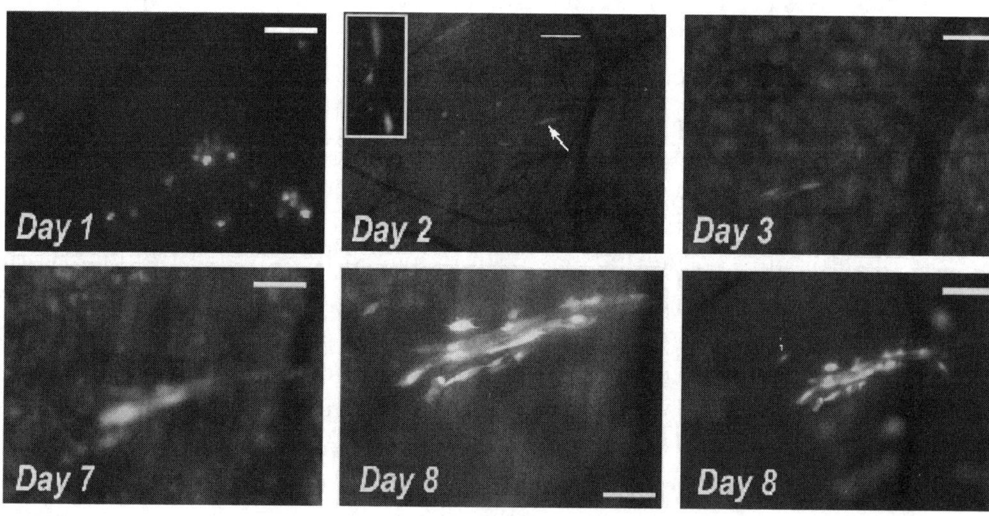

FIGURE 3.4 Approximately 20 tumor cells expressing a fluorescent protein were injected into a murine dorsal skin-fold window chamber on day one. Over the course of 8 days, some cells were observed to elongate and directionally divide toward the nearest preexisting vessel. The cells that failed to elongate underwent apoptosis. The arrow in the day two panel indicates an elongated cell, and the inset shows the apoptotic debris of a cell that failed to elongate. The panels representing day three, day seven, and day eight show a magnification of the region that contained the elongated cell noted in the day two panel. The preferential proliferation of the daughter cells toward the vessel is apparent. (Figure reproduced with permission from Li CY, Shan S, Huang Q, et al. Initial stages of tumor cell-induced angiogenesis: evaluation via skin window chambers in rodent models. *J Natl Cancer Instit* 2000;92(2):143–147.)

mor association, causing pericyte dissociation (109). It has been proposed that this response is part of an antitumor defense mechanism. In the absence of concurrent VEGF expression, this induces vascular regression and a hypoxic crisis that kills off most of the newly formed tumor. What's left of the viable mass initiates a survival reaction, upregulating VEGF expression. This facilitates the angiogenic response classically associated with tumor growth and saves the tumor. Although this is an interesting model for tumor angiogenesis initiation, Yancopoulus' group did not directly prove that a hypoxic crisis was necessary.

Recent work from our laboratory challenges the idea that hypoxia is responsible for the angiogenic switch. Two different tumor lines genetically engineered to express red fluorescent protein (RFP) and GFP as a reporter of HIF-1 activation were grown in skin-fold window chambers in mice. In both tumor models, angiogenesis preceded the first positive detection of hypoxia (through optical identification of green fluorescent cells) by a few days (20) (Fig. 3.5). To further prove that angiogenesis initiation was independent of hypoxia, the animals were treated with tirapazamine (a drug that selectively kills hypoxic cells). It was hypothesized that this treatment would delay the onset of ang-

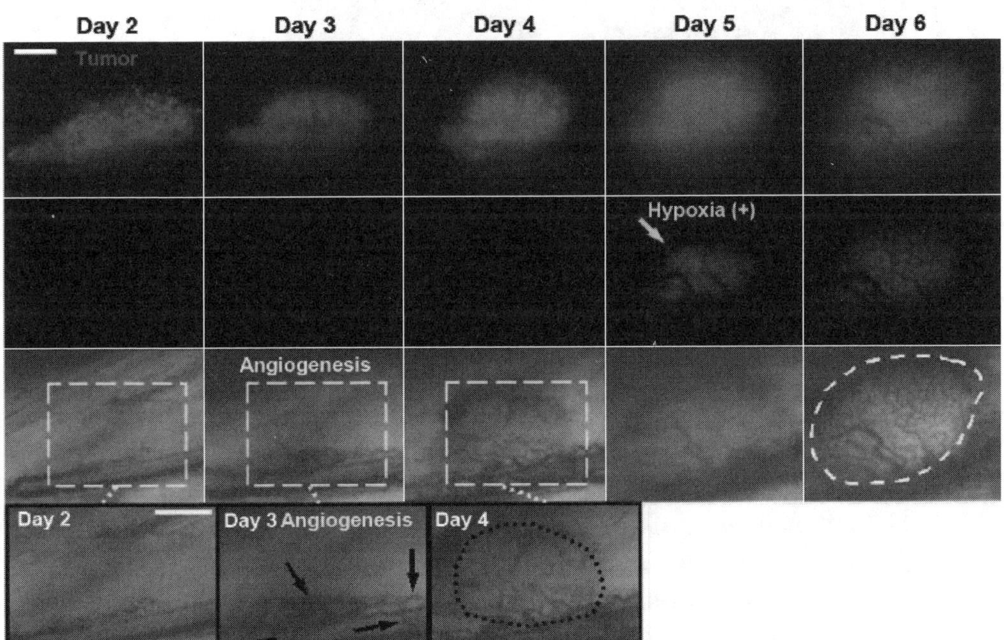

FIGURE 3.5 A tumor expressing a constitutively active fluorescent protein (top row) shows clear signs of angiogenesis 4 days after transplant (lower panels). Another fluorescent protein controlled by HIF-1 was expressed following the detection of angiogenesis (second row). Data were obtained from a skin-fold window chamber in a mouse. (Figure reproduced with permission from Cao Y, Li CY, Moeller BJ, et al. Observation of incipient tumor angiogenesis that is independent of hypoxia and hypoxia inducible factor-1 activation. *Cancer Res* 2005;65(13):5498–5505.)

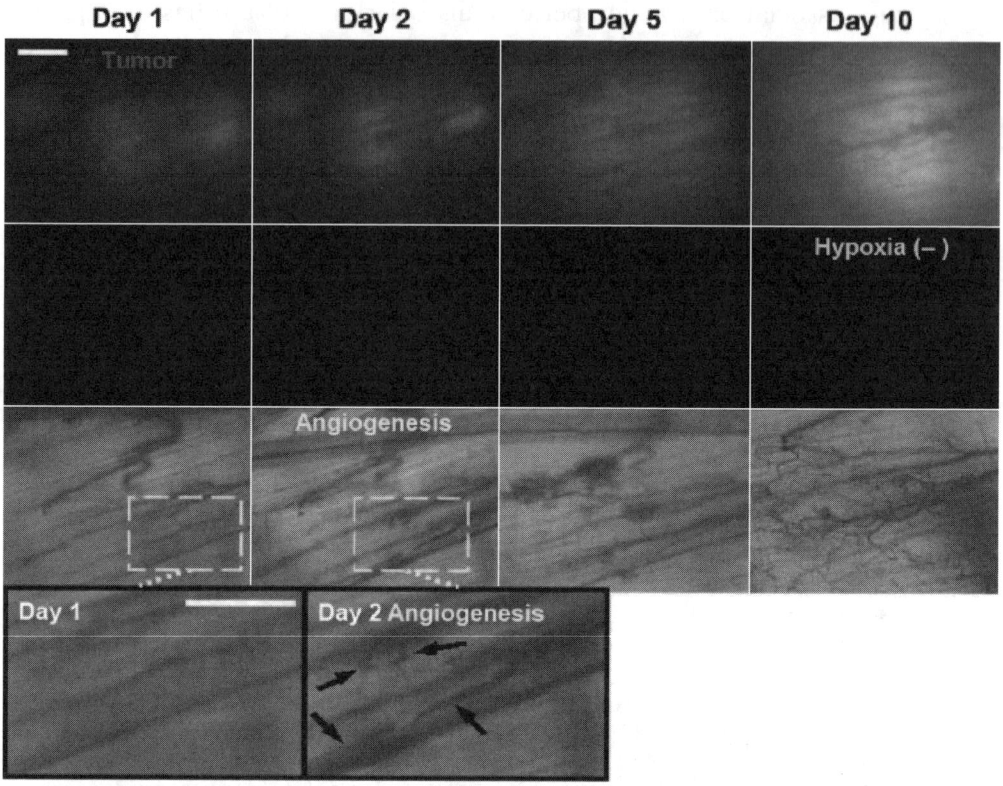

FIGURE 3.6 The same tumor model as shown Figure 3.5 was treated with tirapazamine (which selectively kills hypoxic cells). This inhibited HIF-1 fluorescent reporter-protein expression through day ten, although signs of vascular remodeling appear as early as day two, and angiogenesis is clearly observed at day ten. (Figure reproduced with permission Cao Y, Li CY, Moeller BJ, et al. Observation of incipient tumor angiogenesis that is independent of hypoxia and hypoxia inducible factor-1 activation. *Cancer Res* 2005;65(13):5498–5505.)

iogenesis if hypoxia were required for angiogenesis initiation. The results did not validate this hypothesis: tirapazamine delayed the detection of hypoxic, HIF-1+ cells, but had no effect on the initiation of angiogenesis (20) (Fig. 3.6). These results do not support Yancopoulus' theory. Both cell lines were shown to express low levels of VEGF under aerobic conditions, which likely explains the independence of angiogenesis initiation from hypoxia.

Our group also examined the role of VEGF in the early phases of tumor angiogenesis by adding soluble VEGF receptor protein to window chambers at the time of tumor cell transplant. When the soluble receptor was added, tumor growth was suppressed before any signs of angiogenesis were manifest (108). Conversely, the control group displayed vascular tortuosity and budding at even a few hundred cells, and newly formed vasculature filled the tumor by 20 days post-injection (108). This indicates that angiogenesis or angiogenic signaling plays a critical role in tumor survival and progression long before the tumor reaches a critical vascular perfusion limit and the onset of hypoxia.

The study also reported that the chemotactic signaling of endothelial cells induced an epithelial–mesenchymal transformation of tumor cells. After the tumor cells migrated to the vasculature, they did not grow randomly, but aligned themselves longitudinally along the direction of the nearby vessels, further indicating the presence of a signaling agent secreted by the endothelium (108). The ability of the earliest tumor cells to communicate with the vasculature through mutual signaling is likely a crucial aspect of tumorigenesis, as tumors cells that failed to show the epithelial–mesenchymal transition died after a few days (108). Folkman has expressed strong support for this model of cosignaling; he has further suggested that the angiogenic signals released by the cancer cells not only prepare the endothelium for remodeling, but also elicit the release of chemoattractants that guide the burgeoning tumor to the vasculature (111).

A paper by Raleigh and colleagues questions the assumption that hypoxia is a prerequisite for VEGF induction by using a drug that binds preferentially to hypoxic tissues. Employing immunohistochemistry techniques in a number of human tumor types, they were able to find no spatial correlation between hypoxia and VEGF abundance (112).

These studies establish an interesting model for VEGF functionality beyond the scope of angiogenesis. They suggest a new model of tumorigenesis that challenges the longstanding paradigm in which tumors grow as an avascular mass to a state of vascular deficiency and chronic hypoxia (1–2 mm diameter) before angiogenesis is induced. They force a reevaluation of the classical relationship between hypoxia and angiogenesis. A relationship that was once generally causal in nature has been shown to be much more complex and interdependent than previously believed. Accordingly, this new insight into the interaction between hypoxia and angiogenesis forces a paradigm shift in the modeling and appropriate antiangiogenic treatment of tumors in all stages of growth, with major implications for patients undergoing combinational therapies.

The Rationale for Antiangiogenic Treatment

The untreated tumor vasculature is malformed and marginally effective (102). Its physical structure is in a constant state of flux (102). The imbalance between pro- and antiangiogenic factors leads to excessive endothelial cell proliferation and pericyte detachment (102). Vessels become tortuous and hyperpermeable, leading to longitudinal variations in nutrient concentrations (18). Tumors are also prone to pathologically high interstitial pressure, due to microvessel hyperpermeability, the lack of a functional lymphatic system, and the solid stress of confined growth (113,114). This solid stress increases interstitial and intravascular pressure, inhibiting the ability of the vasculature to maintain a cross-sectional gradient sufficient for adequate perfusion (114).

Vascular remodeling and constant angiogenic signaling in tumors ultimately lead to spatial and temporal heterogeneity in oxygenation (18). Despite this severe environment, many tumor cells manage to subsist on what oxygen they receive and increasingly incorporate more plentiful substrates into their metabolic cycle (115). The hypoxic environment promotes a number of pathologic adaptations, including antiapoptosis (4,7), metastasis (116,117), and further angiogenic signaling. To yield the tumor environment less conducive to aggressive growth, many cancer treatments thus focus on breaking the vicious cycle of angiogenesis.

Antiangiogenesis was first considered as a treatment option based upon the hope that it would destroy tumor vasculature to the point at which the tumor regressed under severe oxygen starvation (118). Treatments that employed antiangiogenic agents alone showed some benefits; however, significant gains in overall survival were not realized (119,120). At high dosages, antiangiogenic agents begin to adversely affect healthy vasculature, as evidenced by the increased risk of arterial thromboembolisms and congestive heart failure associated with the antiangiogenic drug bevacizumab (121). Therefore, clinical doses are more moderate and probably incapable of causing total vascular regression. It is important to note, however, that because of the abnormality and instability of the tumor vasculature, tumor vessels are usually more sensitive to antiangiogenic therapies than are normal vessels. The optimization of clinical doses is therefore a highly faceted problem requiring extensive clinical assessment.

As opposed to lone administration, evidence suggests that when antiangiogenic agents are combined with cytotoxic treatment, the antitumor effect is heightened (122). Such responses were predicted by Beverly Teicher, who proposed that, by using combinational treatments, disparate aspects of tumor pathophysiology could be targeted; cytotoxic treatments would destroy the tumor cells directly, while antiangiogenic agents would destroy the vasculature that provides nutritional support to the growing tumor (122).

However, if antiangiogenic treatment caused vascular regression through an indiscriminate destruction of vessels, one would expect that this would lead to increased hypoxia and cell starvation. Destroying the vasculature would destroy the delivery route of the tumor's oxygen and nutrients. Concurrent antiangiogenesis would therefore be expected to decrease the efficacy of cytotoxic therapy. The synergistic effect of combined therapy observed in preclinical studies is thus at odds with the established antiangiogenic model.

Vascular Normalization

Rakesh Jain would later suggest an explanation for this in terms of a new model of antiangiogenic activity that emphasizes a process of vascular "normalization." Although the precise mechanism of this process is not well understood, it would involve the ordered pruning and reorganization of vessels, such that the vasculature develops a structure more similar to normal tissue, increasing its oxygen and drug transport capacity (123).

It is likely that potent and continued antiangiogenic induction will result in a severe depletion of the vasculature and inadequate supply. However, Jain suggests that with proper dosage and scheduling of antiangiogenic agents, there may develop a critical window en route to vascular regression in which vessels become "normalized" (123). During this transient time frame, the vasculature takes on a structure more similar to that found in normal tissues than the tortuous and inefficient architecture that is characteristic of tumors (123). As the inhibition of angiogenic factors induces vascular regression, immature vessels are preferentially pruned (124). These immature vessels contribute most predominantly to the inefficiencies of an excessive architecture. The degree of vascular pericyte coverage (which defines vessel maturity) is a major factor in determining the fate of vessels exposed to antiangiogenic factors (96,125). Thus, blocking angiogenic factors would have a different effect on the pruning of microvessels, depending on the degree of maturation.

The inhibition of VEGF leads to an overall reduction in vessel diameter. Vascular endothelial growth factor induces the production of nitric oxide, which causes vessels to dilate (126). In the absence of VEGF, these vessels shrink in diameter. Since excessively large vessels dominate flow through the tumor because they have the lowest flow resistance, smaller vessels are prone to weak or static blood flow. With the inhibition of VEGF, vascular diameter becomes more uniform, and blood flows more evenly throughout the vascular network (127) (Fig. 3.7).

With the temporary transition to a somewhat normalized structure, oxygenation is improved (123). Blockade of VEGF signaling reduces vascular permeability and interstitial fluid pressure, allowing nutrients to perfuse more freely (123). Although hypoxia is reduced and nutrient delivery is improved during the normalization window, a number of clinical and preclinical trials have shown that this does not have an accelerating effect on tumor growth (123).

The effect of antiangiogenesis on perfusion was recently observed in a rectal carcinoma trial in which patients underwent combined antiangiogenic, radiation, and chemotherapy treatments prior to surgery. At 12 days after the first antiangiogenic (bevacizumab) treatment, functional computed tomography showed significant decreases in tumor blood perfusion and blood volume (128,129). Interstitial fluid pressure and vascular density were also reduced. However, despite vascular regression, these tumors showed no decrease in the uptake of fluorodeoxyglucose, a radioactive glucose analog, as measured by positron emission tomography (128,129). Despite vascular regression, the tumors showed no signs of impaired transport, suggesting a normalization effect was induced. At the lower of two investigated bevacizumab doses, all six patients showed a marked response to therapy in the analysis of the surgical

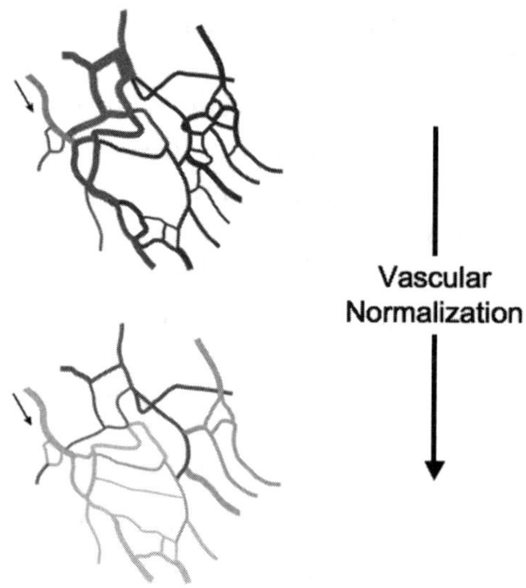

FIGURE 3.7 Antiangiogenic agents cause vessel diameters to decrease due to the inhibition of VEGF-stimulated nitric oxide production. Since flow resistance decreases with the fourth power of vessel diameter, flow is largely confined to a few dilated vessels, and blood flow in smaller vessels is relatively low or absent (high-flow vessels are represented by lighter shades of gray in this diagram, whereas darker shaded vessels represent regions of lower flow). Antiangiogenic agents cause the vasculature to become more uniform in diameter, leading to more homogenous flow throughout the tumor. Along with the pruning of immature vessels, this vascular normalization effect may produce better overall oxygenation. (Figure reproduced with permission from Dewhirst MW, Navia IC, Brizel DM, et al. Multiple etiologies of tumor hypoxia require multifaceted solutions. *Clin Cancer Res* 2007;13(2 Pt 1):375–377.)

specimen (128). Furthermore, at the higher dose, combinational treatment induced two complete pathologic responses out of five patients (129).

In a later study, Batchelor and Jain presented evidence for normalization in human glioblastoma patients (130). These patients, who all failed under conventional treatment, underwent antiangiogenic monotherapy. Using an array of magnetic resonance imaging techniques, it was shown that the treatment achieved a reduction in edema, which is consistent with a reduction in hyperpermeability. A simultaneous drop in vessel diameter suggested an improvement in pericyte coverage. These normalization responses accompanied a decrease in the rate of tumor growth (130).

Jain proposed that future studies that incorporate combinational treatments would show increased survival statistics over antiangiogenic monotherapy. With improved oxygenation and perfusion during the normalization window, it is reasonable to assume the tumor will become more susceptible to cytotoxicity. Studies such as this, which examine induced normalization effects, are therefore critical in establishing a combinational treatment time line for eliciting a maximal cytotoxin-induced antitumor effect.

■ ANTIANGIOGENIC AGENTS

Unique Targets

There are a number of ways by which an inhibition of angiogenesis can be achieved. VEGF signaling is currently a primary target pursued in antiangiogenic research. Clinical agents may depend on an antibody response to VEGF or its VEGFR-2 receptor, such as seen with the VEGF antibody effect of bevacizumab (131). Many drugs exploit proteins and small molecules that achieve an antiangiogenic effect by inhibiting endothelial cell proliferation and migration or prevent vascular expansion by preventing the breakdown of the basement membrane or extracellular matrix proteins, such as collagens. Clinical trials are also exploring the use of small-molecule inhibitors that suppress kinase activities required in angiogenic signaling pathways. Some of these drugs are further discussed in the final section of this chapter. In recent animal studies, VEGF inhibition was achieved through the use of an adenoviral vector encoding soluble VEGFR-1 (96). Since this method eliminates off-target effects, it is a very useful tool in preclinical investigations.

Because of its preeminent role in the process, it is tempting to focus on eliciting an antiangiogenic effect through the inhibition of VEGF signaling. Although VEGF plays a principal role in angiogenesis, it is important that treatments targeting other key molecules in alternative signal transduction pathways be established. For example, in an early phase III combinational treatment trial, bevacizumab failed to prolong breast cancer patient survival (131). This could possibly be attributed to a decreased tumor dependence on VEGF signaling and an increased reliance on other angiogenic factors in later stages of growth (131). These results stress the importance of establishing an array of drugs with unique functionalities. As targeting agents continue to be developed, however, it is important to establish their characteristics in terms of the disparate effects they produce, in order to optimize clinical treatments.

The Disparate Effects of Antiangiogenic Agents

Investigations into various antiangiogenic agents have shown unique scheduling efficacy characteristics. For example, when combined with cyclophosphamide in animal liver-tumor models, the antiangiogenic agent thalidomide induced a significantly potentiated antitumor response only when administered on both of the 2 days prior to cytotoxic treatment (132). This was likely due to the observed simultaneous peak in intertumoral Po_2 levels at between 2 and 3 days post thalidomide treatment, indicating a normalization effect. A similar normalization time frame was observed in fibrosarcoma models (133). Interestingly, when the drug was delivered at the same dose for 4 consecutive days prior to treatment, no significant antitumor response was observed, suggesting the normalization window had already passed (132). In highly contrasting AZD2171-treated glioblastoma clinical trials, normalization was induced within 24 hours and sustained for at least 28 days with daily treatment at a properly chosen dose (130). Although it is questionable whether meaningful comparisons can be drawn between such clinical and preclinical data, this further highlights the sheer disparity of antiangiogenic effects as a function of all aspects of their application.

Cao's previously discussed Ang-2 paper early emphasizes this point. Earlier studies had highlighted the clinical significance of the angiopoietins by showing that high Ang-2 levels in the absence of VEGF overexpression correspond to an improved long-term prognosis in non-small cell lung (NSCL) cancer (134) and acute myelogenous leukemia (135). But, in exploiting Ang-2, or different components of the angiogenesis in general, it is imperative that thorough investigations into the treatment strategies' elicited effects be made, as not all antiangiogenic treatments achieve the same physiologic response. Cao's results demonstrate that the transient increase in hypoxia induced by Ang-2 overexpression (as opposed to VEGF inhibition) implies unique vascular normalization windows between the two therapies, if indeed Ang-2 induces any normalization effect at all.

Comparisons of the same drugs have also shown contrasting results depending on the dosing and scheduling of administration. When the antiangiogenic agent TNP-470 was combined with radiation therapy, significant growth delays were observed in animal tumor models (122). On the other hand, another group showed that the same drug administered along with fractionated radiation schedules actually elicited a poorer growth delay than did radiation alone (136). The group acknowledged that their results were likely the consequence of counteracting effects brought on by improper scheduling (136). It is proposed that antagonism between radiation and antiangiogenic therapies is a potential consequence of applying cytotoxic agents outside the normalization window, or when the antiangiogenic effect is brought on too strong; that is, when the tumor is in a poorly oxygenated state and more resistant to treatment (137). Thus, in terms of combinational treatment efficacy, it is important that antiangiogenic agents be fully characterized in terms of the physiologic responses they induce. As any normalization window they create will be a transient effect, determining the optimal therapeutic window of combinational therapies is of great importance. To this end, imaging techniques that are capable of tracking changes in intratumoral oxygenation are critically important to the success of such studies.

ANTIANGIOGENIC TREATMENT IN COMBINATION WITH RADIOTHERAPY

Optimizing Combinational Approaches

Pioneering research by Beverly Teicher strongly advocated the use of antiangiogenesis as a supplement to radiation treatment. In an early Lewis lung carcinoma animal study, Teicher was able to show that the combination of antiangiogenic and radiation treatment achieved a significant tumor growth delay over either therapy alone (138). Combined therapies were also shown to be effective in other preclinical models (139–142). Results from human colorectal cancer trails (143) and other clinical trials have showed that this is indeed a promising treatment combination.

Before Jain's normalization theory emerged as a likely explanation for the efficacy of combined treatment, some studies hinted at a physiologically induced mechanism for the potentiation of radiation treatment. In 1999, a paper by Gorski and colleagues presented evidence that VEGF inhibition prior to radiation treatment caused a more than additive antitumor effect in Lewis lung carcinoma xenografts (144). This supported the hypothesis that radiation-induced VEGF upregulation serves to protect the vasculature from radiation-mediated apoptosis, thus protecting the tumor against vascular destruction.

When considering antiangiogenic treatment in terms of a vascular normalization model, the appropriate dosage of antiangiogenic treatment with radiation is a fragile balance. Excessive inhibition of angiogenic factors will cause the vasculature to quickly degrade to a point of inadequate oxygenation in addition to causing debilitating effects on non–tumor associated vasculature (123,145). Additionally, the time line of administration is critically important. Application of radiation outside the normalization window will result in decreased efficacy, as the tumor will not be optimally oxygenated and the combined treatments will operate antagonistically (136). Oxygen helps to facilitate cellular radiation damage through free radical action (6). Since the majority of radiation does not directly damage DNA, the production of free radicals by ionizing radiation is a critical factor in producing a destructive effect (6). Therefore, exploiting normalization-induced oxygenation to potentiate radiation treatment is an obvious strategy.

Although it is tempting to focus solely on this approach, it is important to consider that, despite strong evidence for its existence, vascular normalization has not been established as a general characteristic of an antiangiogenic response. There is no widespread consensus on the mechanism of action by which combinational therapy enhances antitumor effect. It is possible that there exist more efficacious treatment schedules wherein an antiangiogenic treatment is administered at different physiologic time points in the radiotherapeutic response.

Further, radiation therapy has been shown to affect tumor angiogenesis and radioresistance in unpredictable ways. For example, it has been suggested that HIF-1 inhibition may be a useful tool in cancer therapy, as it is a nearly universally expressed promoter of malignant behavior across tumor types (14,146). Radiation is likely to promote an angiogenic response through modified HIF-1 activity that could indirectly promote tumor recurrence (13). Further investigation into the impact HIF-1 has on the radiosensitivity of tumors has revealed other interesting effects, however. It has been established that HIF-1 helps to promote energy metabolism, proliferation, and p53 activation—effects that contribute to radiosensitizing benefits (15). On the other hand, the blockade of HIF-1 kills hypoxic cells, whereas HIF-1 promotes endothelial cell survival through VEGF upregulation, which indirectly contributes to tumor radioresistance (144). Furthermore, the effects of HIF-1 blockade are modulated by the relative timing of radiation treatment (15). The role HIF-1 plays in relation to radiotherapy is highly complex, and it is not clear how HIF-1 should best be exploited to maximize antitumor effects.

Although the optimization of antiangiogenic dosing and scheduling is a daunting task, extensive testing has achieved promising strides toward maximizing the efficacy of these agents. Clinical trials have achieved expanded treatment options for a number of specific tumor types thanks to the incorporation of these drugs. This has led to the FDA approval of a number of antiangiogenic drugs in recent years.

Clinical Trials and Approved Antiangiogenic Drugs

The FDA-approved antiangiogenic drugs are broadly categorized as monoclonal antibodies or small-molecule TK inhibitors. The monoclonal antibodies include bevacizumab (147), cetuximab (148), panitumumab (149), and trastuzumab (150). The small-molecule TK inhibitors include erlotinib (151), sorafenib (152), and sunitinib (153). Bortezomib and thalidomide are believed to have antiangiogenic effects, but their method of action is not clearly understood (154). Information regarding these approved drugs is summarized in Table 3.1.

In 2004, bevacizumab, a monoclonal antibody against VEGF, was the first antiangiogenic agent approved by the FDA for clinical use (147). Since then, it has become one of the most widely explored antiangiogenic agents in combined therapies. Its application is presently emerging as a promising treatment option for a number of cancer types. It is currently approved for the combinational treatment of metastatic colorectal cancer and nonresectable, locally advanced, recurrent, or metastatic, nonsquamous, NSCL cancer (147). Clinical trials are exploring its efficacy in multitreatment combinations employing radiotherapy for NSCL cancer, rectal cancer, prostate cancer, head and neck cancer, gallbladder cancer, pancreatic cancer, and sarcomas (155). Other drugs are also being explored in combination with radiation, such as thalidomide, which has shown positive results in phase II clinical glioma studies (156).

Cetuximab is approved for administration with radiation therapy. It is presently the only drug approved for use in combination with radiation. Although it does not target VEGF directly, cetuximab inhibits epidermal growth factor receptor (EGFR), which leads to an indirect inhibition of VEGF. Cetuximab re-

TABLE 3.1 A brief overview of FDA-approved antiangiogenic drugs

Drug	Method of Action	Cancer Type	Concurrent Treatment
	VEGF and VEGFR Targeting Drugs		
Bevacizumab	Monoclonal antibody against VEGF	Metastatic Colorectal Cancer	5-FU
		Non-Small Cell Lung Cancer	Carboplatin and Paclitaxel
Sorafenib Tosylate	A multikinase inhibitor which blocks signal transduction in a number of receptors, including VEGFR-2	Renal Cell Carcinoma	Monotherapy
Sunitinib Malate	A multikinase inhibitor which blocks signal trasduction in a number of receptors, including the VEGFRs	Renal Cell Carcinoma	Monotherapy
		Gastrointestinal Stromal Tumor	Monotherapy
	Indirect Inhibitors of VEGF†		
Cetuximab	Monoclonal antibody against the epidermal growth factor receptor (EGFR)	Metastatic Colorectal Cancer	Irinotecan/ Monotherapy
		Head and Neck Cancer	Radiation/ Monotherapy
Erlotinib Hydrochloride	Binds to the catalytic tyrosine kinase domain of EGFR, blocking signal transduction	Non-Small Cell Lung Cancer	Monotherapy
		Pancreatic Cancer	Gemcitabine
Panitumumab	Monoclonal antibody against EGFR	Metastatic Colorectal Cancer	Monotherapy
Trastuzumab	A monoclonal antibody against Human Epidermal Growth Factor Receptor-2 (HER-2)—HER-2 is structurally and functionally similar to EGFR and is overexpressed in approximately 25% of primary breast cancers	Breast Cancer	Doxorubicin, Cyclophos-phamide, and Paclitaxel/ Paclitaxel/ Monotherapy
	Other Anti-angiogenic Agents		
Bortezomib§	Inhibits activity of the 26S proteasome, which is involved in many signaling pathways, affecting the regulation of associated proteins—may affect the production of certain angiogenic proteins	Multiple Myeloma	Monotherapy
		Mantle Cell Lymphona	Monotherapy
Thalidomide	Unknown	Multiple Myeloma	Dexamethasone

† EGFR activation has been shown to stimulate VEGF production in tumors.
§ The anti-angiogenic activity of this drugs has not been definitively established.

ceived FDA approval for the treatment of locally or regionally advanced squamous cell carcinoma of the head and neck in March of 2006 (157). Compared with radiation alone, combined cetuximab-radiation treatment has shown a significant improvement in patient survival and local control. In a multinational, randomized study that helped lead to the drug's approval, the median overall survival time for combined treatment was 49 months, compared to 29.3 months for monotherapy (158). The median duration of local control was 24.4 and 14.9 months for combined therapy and radiation monotherapy, respectively (158). Patients who had previously failed under platinum-based therapy received cetuximab alone; the objective response rate of this cohort was 12.6%, with a median response duration of 5.8 months (158). The compared treatments showed no significant difference in metastatic control, however (158). Neither were the benefits of combined treatment evenly distributed across cancer subtypes. Patients with oropharyngeal cancer (more than half the patients in the study) responded well, whereas patients with laryngeal and hypopharyngeal cancer showed no significant improvement in survival (158). It remains to be seen how these results compare to combined radiotherapy and cisplatin chemotherapy, which remains the most common standard for patients who are able to tolerate it.

■ CONCLUSIONS

Overall, a paucity of information is available concerning the efficacy of radiation treatment with antiangiogenic agents. Clinical trials are only beginning to shed light on the potential of this treatment combination, as is evident from its approved use in only one particular cancer type. Currently, the focus of clinical investigation tends toward chemotherapy-antiangiogenesis combinations. Results from the cetuximab study and current clinical and preclinical trials will likely encourage more encompassing research into antiangiogenesis as a modulator of radiotherapy. The combination presents a promising therapeutic strategy for targeting both endothelial cells and tumor cells. However, researchers must be careful to consider the subtle aspects of dosing and scheduling for each therapy when developing treatment strategies. Although it is tempting to model the cancerous cells and the vasculature as separate aspects of tumor pathology, it is important to remember that these are interdependent systems. The proliferating tumor cells cannot survive without the vessel network, and the extensive vasculature is maintained through constant angiogenic stimulators.

Although early combinational therapies achieved a serendipitous degree of success, it was for reasons that are only presently becoming clearer. The emergence of the vascular normalization model was an important step in the process of developing combined strategies, but this was only the beginning. Many more studies must be done in order to establish optimal agents, doses, and treatment timelines. Further preclinical and clinical trials will undoubtedly provide invaluable information for developing and optimizing novel therapeutic modalities of combined ionizing radiation and antiangiogenic treatment.

Acknowledgments
The authors thank Melanie Wergin, Theis Schröder, and Katharina Fleckenstein for their invaluable assistance in the research and composition of this chapter. This work was supported by grant CA40355 from the NIH/NCI.

REFERENCES

1. Vaupel P, Harrison L. Tumor hypoxia: Causative factors, compensatory mechanisms, and cellular response. *Oncologist* 2004;9(Suppl 5):4–9.
2. Gray LH, Conger AD, Ebert M, et al. The concentration of oxygen dissolved in tissues at the time of irradiation as a factor in radiotherapy. *Br J Radiol* 1953;26(312):638–648.
3. Teicher BA. Hypoxia and drug resistance. *Cancer Metastasis Rev* 1994;13(2):139–168.
4. Moon EJ, Brizel DM, Chi JT, Dewhirst MW. The potential role of intrinsic hypoxia markers as prognostic variables in cancer. *Antioxid Redox Signal* 2007;9(8):1237–1294.
5. Hockel M, Vorndran B, Schlenger K, et al. Tumor oxygenation: a new predictive parameter in locally advanced cancer of the uterine cervix. *Gynecol Oncol* 1993;51(2):141–149.
6. McBride W, Withers H. Biological basis of radiation therapy. In: Perez C, Brady L, Halperin E, Schmidt-Ullrich R, eds. *Principles and Practice of Radiation Oncology*. 4th ed. Philadelphia: Lippincott, Williams, and Wilkins; 2004:110.
7. Graeber TG, Osmanian C, Jacks T, et al. Hypoxia-mediated selection of cells with diminished apoptotic potential in solid tumours. *Nature* 1996;379(6560):88–91.
8. Semenza GL, Wang GL. A nuclear factor induced by hypoxia via de novo protein synthesis binds to the human erythropoietin gene enhancer at a site required for transcriptional activation. *Mol Cell Biol* 1992;12(12):5447–5454.
9. Wang GL, Jiang BH, Rue EA, Semenza GL. Hypoxia-inducible factor 1 is a basic-helix-loop-helix-PAS heterodimer regulated by cellular O2 tension. *Proc Natl Acad Sci USA* 1995;92(12):5510–5514.
10. Huang LE, Arany Z, Livingston DM, Bunn HF. Activation of hypoxia-inducible transcription factor depends primarily upon redox-sensitive stabilization of its alpha subunit. *J Biol Chem* 1996;271(50):32253–32259.
11. Sutter CH, Laughner E, Semenza GL. Hypoxia-inducible factor 1alpha protein expression is controlled by oxygen-regulated ubiquitination that is disrupted by deletions and missense mutations. *Proc Natl Acad Sci USA* 2000;97(9):4748–4753.
12. Cockman ME, Masson N, Mole DR, et al. Hypoxia inducible factor-alpha binding and ubiquitination by the von Hippel-Lindau tumor suppressor protein. *J Biol Chem* 2000;275(33):25733–25741.
13. Moeller BJ, Cao Y, Li CY, Dewhirst MW. Radiation activates HIF-1 to regulate vascular radiosensitivity in tumors: Role of reoxygenation, free radicals, and stress granules. *Cancer Cell* 2004;5(5):429–441.
14. Semenza GL. Targeting HIF-1 for cancer therapy. *Nat Rev Cancer* 2003;3(10):721–732.
15. Moeller BJ, Dreher MR, Rabbani ZN, et al. Pleiotropic effects of HIF-1 blockade on tumor radiosensitivity. *Cancer Cell* 2005;8(2):99–110.

16. Burri PH, Tarek MR. A novel mechanism of capillary growth in the rat pulmonary microcirculation. *Anat Rec* 1990;228(1):35–45.
17. Lyden D, Hattori K, Dias S, et al. Impaired recruitment of bone-marrow-derived endothelial and hematopoietic precursor cells blocks tumor angiogenesis and growth. *Nat Med* 2001;7(11):1194–1201.
18. Dewhirst MW, Richardson R, Cardenas-Navia I, Cao Y. The relationship between the tumor physiologic microenvironment and angiogenesis. *Hematol Oncol Clin North Am* 2004;18(5):973–990, vii.
19. Haroon Z, Peters K, Greenberg C, Dewhirst M. Angiogenesis and oxygen transport in solid tumors. In: Teicher BA, ed. *Antiangiogenic Agents in Cancer Therapy*. Totowa, NJ: Humana Press Inc.;1999:3–21.
20. Cao Y, Li CY, Moeller BJ, et al. Observation of incipient tumor angiogenesis that is independent of hypoxia and hypoxia inducible factor-1 activation. *Cancer Res* 2005;65(13):5498–5505.
21. Folkman J. Tumor angiogenesis: Therapeutic implications. *N Engl J Med* 1971;285(21): 1182–1186.
22. Algire GH, Chalkley HW, Earle WE, et al. Vascular reactions of normal and malignant tissues in vivo. III. Vascular reactions of mice to fibroblasts treated in vitro with methylcholanthrene. *J Natl Cancer Inst* 1950;11(3):555–580.
23. Sandison JC. Observations on growth of blood vessels as seen in transparent chamber introduced into rabbit's ear. *Am J Anat* 1928;41:475–496.
24. Ide AG, Warren SL. Vascularization of the Brown Pearce rabbit epithelioma transplant as seen in the transparent ear chamber. *Am J Roentgenol* 1939;42:891–89.
25. Algire GH. An adaptation of the transparent chamber technique to the mouse. *J Natl Cancer Inst* 1943;4:1–10.
26. Greenblatt M, Shubi P. Tumor angiogenesis: Transfilter diffusion studies in the hamster by the transparent chamber technique. *J Natl Cancer Inst* 1968;41(1):111–124.
27. Senger DR, Galli SJ, Dvorak AM, et al. Tumor cells secrete a vascular permeability factor that promotes accumulation of ascites fluid. *Science (New York, NY)* 1983;219(4587):983–985.
28. Ferrara N, Henzel WJ. Pituitary follicular cells secrete a novel heparin-binding growth factor specific for vascular endothelial cells. *Biochem Biophys Res Commun* 1989;161(2):851–858.
29. Leung DW, Cachianes G, Kuang WJ, et al. Vascular endothelial growth factor is a secreted angiogenic mitogen. *Science (New York, NY)* 1989;246(4935):1306–1309.
30. Keck PJ, Hauser SD, Krivi G, et al. Vascular permeability factor, an endothelial cell mitogen related to PDGF. *Science (New York, NY)* 1989;246(4935):1309–1312.
31. Folkman J, Haudenschild CC, Zetter BR. Long-term culture of capillary endothelial cells. *Proc Natl Acad Sci USA* 1979;76(10):5217–5221.
32. Folkman J, Klagsbrun M. Angiogenic factors. *Science (New York, NY)* 1987;235(4787):442–447.
33. Houck KA, Ferrara N, Winer J, et al. The vascular endothelial growth factor family: Identification of a fourth molecular species and characterization of alternative splicing of RNA. *Mol Endocrinol* 1991;5(12):1806–1814.
34. Tischer E, Mitchell R, Hartman T, et al. The human gene for vascular endothelial growth factor. Multiple protein forms are encoded through alternative exon splicing. *J Biol Chem* 1991;266(18):11947–11954.
35. Cohen T, Gitay-Goren H, Sharon R, et al. VEGF121, a vascular endothelial growth factor (VEGF) isoform lacking heparin binding ability, requires cell-surface heparan sul-

fates for efficient binding to the VEGF receptors of human melanoma cells. *J Biol Chem* 1995;270(19):11322–11326.

36. Park JE, Keller GA, Ferrara N. The vascular endothelial growth factor (VEGF) isoforms: Differential deposition into the subepithelial extracellular matrix and bioactivity of extracellular matrix-bound VEGF. *Mol Biol Cell* 1993;4(12):1317–1326.
37. Houck KA, Leung DW, Rowland AM, et al. Dual regulation of vascular endothelial growth factor bioavailability by genetic and proteolytic mechanisms. *J Biol Chem* 1992;267(36):26031–26037.
38. Plouet J, Moro F, Bertagnolli S, et al. Extracellular cleavage of the vascular endothelial growth factor 189-amino acid form by urokinase is required for its mitogenic effect. *J Biol Chem* 1997;272(20):13390–13396.
39. Plouet J, Schilling J, Gospodarowicz D. Isolation and characterization of a newly identified endothelial cell mitogen produced by AtT-20 cells. *EMBO J* 1989;8(12):3801–3806.
40. Gospodarowicz D, Abraham JA, Schilling J. Isolation and characterization of a vascular endothelial cell mitogen produced by pituitary-derived folliculo stellate cells. *Proc Natl Acad Sci USA* 1989;86(19):7311–7315.
41. Asahara T, Bauters C, Zheng LP, et al. Synergistic effect of vascular endothelial growth factor and basic fibroblast growth factor on angiogenesis in vivo. *Circulation* 1995;92(Suppl 9):II365–II371.
42. Jonca F, Ortega N, Gleizes PE, et al. Cell release of bioactive fibroblast growth factor 2 by exon 6-encoded sequence of vascular endothelial growth factor. *J Biol Chem* 1997;272(39):24203–24209.
43. Gitay-Goren H, Cohen T, Tessler S, et al. Selective binding of VEGF121 to one of the three vascular endothelial growth factor receptors of vascular endothelial cells. *J Biol Chem* 1996;271(10):5519–5523.
44. Gengrinovitch S, Berman B, David G, et al. Glypican-1 is a VEGF165 binding proteoglycan that acts as an extracellular chaperone for VEGF165. *J Biol Chem* 1999;274(16):10816–10822.
45. Grimmond S, Lagercrantz J, Drinkwater C, et al. Cloning and characterization of a novel human gene related to vascular endothelial growth factor. *Genome Res* 1996;6(2):124–131.
46. Olofsson B, Pajusola K, von Euler G, et al. Genomic organization of the mouse and human genes for vascular endothelial growth factor B (VEGF-B) and characterization of a second splice isoform. *J Biol Chem* 1996;271(32):19310–19317.
47. Makinen T, Olofsson B, Karpanen T, et al. Differential binding of vascular endothelial growth factor B splice and proteolytic isoforms to neuropilin-1. *J Biol Chem* 1999;274(30):21217–21222.
48. Olofsson B, Korpelainen E, Pepper MS, et al. Vascular endothelial growth factor B (VEGF-B) binds to VEGF receptor-1 and regulates plasminogen activator activity in endothelial cells. *Proc Natl Acad Sci USA* 1998;95(20):11709–11714.
49. Olofsson B, Pajusola K, Kaipainen A, et al. Vascular endothelial growth factor B, a novel growth factor for endothelial cells. *Proc Natl Acad Sci USA* 1996;93(6):2576–2581.
50. Jeltsch M, Kaipainen A, Joukov V, et al. Hyperplasia of lymphatic vessels in VEGF-C transgenic mice. *Science (New York, NY)* 1997;276(5317):1423–1425.
51. Achen MG, Jeltsch M, Kukk E, et al. Vascular endothelial growth factor D (VEGF-D) is a ligand for the tyrosine kinases VEGF receptor 2 (Flk1) and VEGF receptor 3 (Flt4). *Proc Natl Acad Sci USA* 1998;95(2):548–553.
52. Lee J, Gray A, Yuan J, et al. Vascular endothelial growth factor-related protein: A ligand and specific activator of the tyrosine kinase receptor Flt4. *Proc Natl Acad Sci USA* 1996;93(5):1988–1992.

53. Karkkainen MJ, Makinen T, Alitalo K. Lymphatic endothelium: A new frontier of metastasis research. *Nat Cell Biol* 2002;4(1):E2–E5.
54. Joukov V, Pajusola K, Kaipainen A, et al. A novel vascular endothelial growth factor, VEGF-C, is a ligand for the Flt4 (VEGFR-3) and KDR (VEGFR-2) receptor tyrosine kinases. *EMBO J* 1996;15(2):290–298.
55. Kukk E, Lymboussaki A, Taira S, et al. VEGF-C receptor binding and pattern of expression with VEGFR-3 suggests a role in lymphatic vascular development. *Development* 1996;122(12):3829–3837.
56. Ogawa S, Oku A, Sawano A, et al. A novel type of vascular endothelial growth factor, VEGF-E (NZ-7 VEGF), preferentially utilizes KDR/Flk-1 receptor and carries a potent mitotic activity without heparin-binding domain. *J Biol Chem* 1998;273(47):31273–31282.
57. Lyttle DJ, Fraser KM, Fleming SB, et al. Homologs of vascular endothelial growth factor are encoded by the poxvirus orf virus. *J Virol* 1994;68(1):84–92.
58. Phillips HS, Hains J, Leung DW, Ferrara N. Vascular endothelial growth factor is expressed in rat corpus luteum. *Endocrinology* 1990;127(2):965–967.
59. Jakeman LB, Armanini M, Phillips HS, Ferrara N. Developmental expression of binding sites and messenger ribonucleic acid for vascular endothelial growth factor suggests a role for this protein in vasculogenesis and angiogenesis. *Endocrinology* 1993;133(2):848–859.
60. Shweiki D, Itin A, Neufeld G, et al. Patterns of expression of vascular endothelial growth factor (VEGF) and VEGF receptors in mice suggest a role in hormonally regulated angiogenesis. *J Clin Invest* 1993;91(5):2235–2243.
61. Miller JW, Adamis AP, Shima DT, et al. Vascular endothelial growth factor/vascular permeability factor is temporally and spatially correlated with ocular angiogenesis in a primate model. *Am J Pathol* 1994;145(3):574–584.
62. Shweiki D, Itin A, Soffer D, Keshet E. Vascular endothelial growth factor induced by hypoxia may mediate hypoxia-initiated angiogenesis. *Nature* 1992;359(6398):843–845.
63. Minchenko A, Bauer T, Salceda S, Caro J. Hypoxic stimulation of vascular endothelial growth factor expression in vitro and in vivo. *Lab Invest* 1994;71(3):374–379.
64. Enholm B, Paavonen K, Ristimaki A, et al. Comparison of VEGF, VEGF-B, VEGF-C and Ang-1 mRNA regulation by serum, growth factors, oncoproteins and hypoxia. *Oncogene* 1997;14(20):2475–2483.
65. Brogi E, Wu T, Namiki A, Isner JM. Indirect angiogenic cytokines upregulate VEGF and bFGF gene expression in vascular smooth muscle cells, whereas hypoxia upregulates VEGF expression only. *Circulation* 1994;90(2):649–652.
66. Levy AP, Levy NS, Wegner S, Goldberg MA. Transcriptional regulation of the rat vascular endothelial growth factor gene by hypoxia. *J Biol Chem* 1995;270(22):13333–13340.
67. Liu Y, Cox SR, Morita T, Kourembanas S. Hypoxia regulates vascular endothelial growth factor gene expression in endothelial cells. Identification of a 5' enhancer. *Circ Res* 1995;77(3):638–643.
68. Carmeliet P, Ferreira V, Breier G, et al. Abnormal blood vessel development and lethality in embryos lacking a single VEGF allele. *Nature* 1996;380(6573):435–439.
69. Ferrara N, Carver-Moore K, Chen H, et al. Heterozygous embryonic lethality induced by targeted inactivation of the VEGF gene. *Nature* 1996;380(6573):439–442.
70. Shibuya M, Yamaguchi S, Yamane A, et al. Nucleotide sequence and expression of a novel human receptor-type tyrosine kinase gene (flt) closely related to the fms family. *Oncogene* 1990;5(4):519–524.
71. Terman BI, Carrion ME, Kovacs E, et al. Identification of a new endothelial cell growth factor receptor tyrosine kinase. *Oncogene* 1991;6(9):1677–1683.

72. Keyt BA, Nguyen HV, Berleau LT, et al. Identification of vascular endothelial growth factor determinants for binding KDR and FLT-1 receptors. Generation of receptor-selective VEGF variants by site-directed mutagenesis. *J Biol Chem* 1996;271(10):5638–5646.
73. Wiesmann C, Fuh G, Christinger HW, et al. Crystal structure at 1.7 A resolution of VEGF in complex with domain 2 of the Flt-1 receptor. *Cell* 1997;91(5):695–704.
74. Barleon B, Totzke F, Herzog C, et al. Mapping of the sites for ligand binding and receptor dimerization at the extracellular domain of the vascular endothelial growth factor receptor FLT-1. *J Biol Chem* 1997;272(16):10382–10388.
75. Guo D, Jia Q, Song HY, et al. Vascular endothelial cell growth factor promotes tyrosine phosphorylation of mediators of signal transduction that contain SH2 domains. Association with endothelial cell proliferation. *J Biol Chem* 1995;270(12):6729–6733.
76. Waltenberger J, Claesson-Welsh L, Siegbahn A, et al. Different signal transduction properties of KDR and Flt1, two receptors for vascular endothelial growth factor. *J Biol Chem* 1994;269(43):26988–26995.
77. Shalaby F, Rossant J, Yamaguchi TP, et al. Failure of blood-island formation and vasculogenesis in Flk-1-deficient mice. *Nature* 1995;376(6535):62–66.
78. Fong GH, Rossant J, Gertsenstein M, Breitman ML. Role of the Flt-1 receptor tyrosine kinase in regulating the assembly of vascular endothelium. *Nature* 1995;376(6535):66–70.
79. Fong GH, Zhang L, Bryce DM, Peng J. Increased hemangioblast commitment, not vascular disorganization, is the primary defect in flt-1 knock-out mice. *Development* 1999; 126(13):3015–3025.
80. Park JE, Chen HH, Winer J, et al. Placenta growth factor. Potentiation of vascular endothelial growth factor bioactivity, in vitro and in vivo, and high affinity binding to Flt-1 but not to Flk-1/KDR. *J Biol Chem* 1994;269(41):25646–25654.
81. Hiratsuka S, Minowa O, Kuno J, et al. Flt-1 lacking the tyrosine kinase domain is sufficient for normal development and angiogenesis in mice. *Proc Natl Acad Sci USA* 1998;95(16): 9349–9354.
82. Barleon B, Sozzani S, Zhou D, et al. Migration of human monocytes in response to vascular endothelial growth factor (VEGF) is mediated via the VEGF receptor flt-1. *Blood* 1996;87(8):3336–3343.
83. Clauss M, Weich H, Breier G, et al. The vascular endothelial growth factor receptor Flt-1 mediates biological activities. Implications for a functional role of placenta growth factor in monocyte activation and chemotaxis. *J Biol Chem* 1996;271(30):17629–17634.
84. Kaipainen A, Korhonen J, Mustonen T, et al. Expression of the fms-like tyrosine kinase 4 gene becomes restricted to lymphatic endothelium during development. *Proc Natl Acad Sci USA* 1995;92(8):3566–3570.
85. Kendall RL, Wang G, Thomas KA. Identification of a natural soluble form of the vascular endothelial growth factor receptor, FLT-1, and its heterodimerization with KDR. *Biochem Biophys Res Commun* 1996;226(2):324–328.
86. Jones N, Iljin K, Dumont DJ, Alitalo K. Tie receptors: New modulators of angiogenic and lymphangiogenic responses. *Nature Rev* 2001;2(4):257–267.
87. Wood JM, Bold G, Buchdunger E, et al. PTK787/ZK 222584, a novel and potent inhibitor of vascular endothelial growth factor receptor tyrosine kinases, impairs vascular endothelial growth factor-induced responses and tumor growth after oral administration. *Cancer Res* 2000;60(8):2178–2189.
88. Lin P, Polverini P, Dewhirst M, et al. Inhibition of tumor angiogenesis using a soluble receptor establishes a role for Tie2 in pathologic vascular growth. *J Clin Invest* 1997;100(8): 2072–2078.

89. Thurston G, Suri C, Smith K, et al. Leakage-resistant blood vessels in mice transgenically overexpressing angiopoietin-1. *Science (New York, NY)* 1999;286(5449):2511–2514.
90. Davis S, Aldrich TH, Jones PF, et al. Isolation of angiopoietin-1, a ligand for the TIE2 receptor, by secretion-trap expression cloning. *Cell* 1996;87(7):1161–1169.
91. Kanda S, Miyata Y, Mochizuki Y, et al. Angiopoietin 1 is mitogenic for cultured endothelial cells. *Cancer Res* 2005;65(15):6820–6827.
92. Suri C, Jones PF, Patan S, et al. Requisite role of angiopoietin-1, a ligand for the TIE2 receptor, during embryonic angiogenesis. *Cell* 1996;87(7):1171–1180.
93. Gale NW, Thurston G, Hackett SF, et al. Angiopoietin-2 is required for postnatal angiogenesis and lymphatic patterning, and only the latter role is rescued by Angiopoietin-1. *Dev Cell* 2002;3(3):411–423.
94. Maisonpierre PC, Suri C, Jones PF, et al. Angiopoietin-2, a natural antagonist for Tie2 that disrupts in vivo angiogenesis. *Science (New York, NY)* 1997;277(5322):55–60.
95. Hammes HP, Lin J, Wagner P, et al. Angiopoietin-2 causes pericyte dropout in the normal retina: Evidence for involvement in diabetic retinopathy. *Diabetes* 2004;53(4):1104–1110.
96. Cao Y, Sonveaux P, Liu S, et al. Systemic overexpression of angiopoietin-2 promotes tumor microvessel regression and inhibits angiogenesis and tumor growth. *Cancer Res* 2007;67(8):3835–3844.
97. Oh H, Takagi H, Suzuma K, et al. Hypoxia and vascular endothelial growth factor selectively up-regulate angiopoietin-2 in bovine microvascular endothelial cells. *J Biol Chem* 1999;274(22):15732–15739.
98. Currie MJ, Gunningham SP, Turner K, et al. Expression of the angiopoietins and their receptor Tie2 in human renal clear cell carcinomas; Regulation by the von Hippel-Lindau gene and hypoxia. *J Pathol* 2002;198(4):502–510.
99. Tait CR, Jones PF. Angiopoietins in tumours: The angiogenic switch. *J Pathol* 2004;204(1):1–10.
100. Lobov IB, Brooks PC, Lang RA. Angiopoietin-2 displays VEGF-dependent modulation of capillary structure and endothelial cell survival in vivo. *Proc Natl Acad Sci USA* 2002;99(17):11205–11210.
101. Lin P, Buxton JA, Acheson A, et al. Antiangiogenic gene therapy targeting the endothelium-specific receptor tyrosine kinase Tie2. *Proc Natl Acad Sci USA* 1998;95(15):8829–8834.
102. Bergers G, Benjamin LE. Tumorigenesis and the angiogenic switch. *Nat Rev Cancer* 2003;3(6):401–410.
103. Dor Y, Porat R, Keshet E. Vascular endothelial growth factor and vascular adjustments to perturbations in oxygen homeostasis. *Am J Physiol* 2001;280(6):C1367–C1374.
104. Folkman J. Angiogenesis in cancer, vascular, rheumatoid and other disease. *Nat Med* 1995;1(1):27–31.
105. Hanahan D, Folkman J. Patterns and emerging mechanisms of the angiogenic switch during tumorigenesis. *Cell* 1996;86(3):353–364.
106. Hobson B, Denekamp J. Endothelial proliferation in tumours and normal tissues: continuous labelling studies. *Br J Cancer* 1984;49(4):405–413.
107. Dvorak HF. Tumors: Wounds that do not heal. Similarities between tumor stroma generation and wound healing. *N Engl J Med* 1986;315(26):1650–1659.
108. Li CY, Shan S, Huang Q, et al. Initial stages of tumor cell-induced angiogenesis: Evaluation via skin window chambers in rodent models. *J Natl Cancer Inst* 2000;92(2):143–147.
109. Holash J, Maisonpierre PC, Compton D, et al. Vessel cooption, regression, and growth in tumors mediated by angiopoietins and VEGF. *Science (New York, NY)* 1999;284(5422):1994–1998.

110. Pezzella F, Di Bacco A, Andreola S, et al. Angiogenesis in primary lung cancer and lung secondaries. *Eur J Cancer* 1996;32A(14):2494–2500.
111. Folkman J. Incipient angiogenesis. *J Natl Cancer Inst* 2000;92(2):94–95.
112. Raleigh JA, Calkins-Adams DP, Rinker LH, et al. Hypoxia and vascular endothelial growth factor expression in human squamous cell carcinomas using pimonidazole as a hypoxia marker. *Cancer Res* 1998;58(17):3765–3768.
113. Padera TP, Stoll BR, Tooredman JB, et al. Pathology: cancer cells compress intratumour vessels. *Nature* 2004;427(6976):695.
114. Griffon-Etienne G, Boucher Y, Brekken C, et al. Taxane-induced apoptosis decompresses blood vessels and lowers interstitial fluid pressure in solid tumors: Clinical implications. *Cancer Res* 1999;59(15):3776–3782.
115. Warburg O, Wind F, Negelein E. The metabolism of tumors in the body. *J Gen Physiol* 1927;8(6):519–530.
116. Brizel DM, Scully SP, Harrelson JM, et al. Tumor oxygenation predicts for the likelihood of distant metastases in human soft tissue sarcoma. *Cancer Res* 1996;56(5):941–943.
117. Hockel M, Schlenger K, Aral B, et al. Association between tumor hypoxia and malignant progression in advanced cancer of the uterine cervix. *Cancer Res* 1996;56(19):4509–4515.
118. Kerbel R, Folkman J. Clinical translation of angiogenesis inhibitors. *Nat Rev Cancer* 2002;2(10):727–739.
119. Yang JC, Haworth L, Sherry RM, et al. A randomized trial of bevacizumab, an anti-vascular endothelial growth factor antibody, for metastatic renal cancer. *N Engl J Med* 2003;349(5):427–434.
120. Mayer RJ. Two steps forward in the treatment of colorectal cancer. *N Engl J Med* 2004;350(23):2406–2408.
121. Skillings JR, Johnson DH, Miller K, Kabbinavar F. Arterial thromboembolic events (ATEs) in a pooled analysis of 5 randomized, controlled trials (RCTs) of bevacizumab (BV) with chemotherapy. *J Clin Oncol* 2005;23(16S).
122. Teicher BA. A systems approach to cancer therapy. (Antioncogenics + standard cytotoxics mechanism(s) of interaction). *Cancer Metastasis Rev* 1996;15(2):247–272.
123. Jain RK. Normalization of tumor vasculature: An emerging concept in antiangiogenic therapy. *Science (New York, NY)* 2005;307(5706):58–62.
124. Tong RT, Boucher Y, Kozin SV, et al. Vascular normalization by vascular endothelial growth factor receptor 2 blockade induces a pressure gradient across the vasculature and improves drug penetration in tumors. *Cancer Res* 2004;64(11):3731–3736.
125. Shih SC, Ju M, Liu N, et al. Transforming growth factor beta1 induction of vascular endothelial growth factor receptor 1: Mechanism of pericyte-induced vascular survival in vivo. *Proc Natl Acad Sci USA* 2003;100(26):15859–15864.
126. Ku DD, Zaleski JK, Liu S, Brock TA. Vascular endothelial growth factor induces EDRF-dependent relaxation in coronary arteries. *Am J Physiol* 1993;265(2 Pt 2):H586–H592.
127. Dewhirst MW, Navia IC, Brizel DM, et al. Multiple etiologies of tumor hypoxia require multifaceted solutions. *Clin Cancer Res* 2007;13(2 Pt 1):375–377.
128. Willett CG, Boucher Y, di Tomaso E, et al. Direct evidence that the VEGF-specific antibody bevacizumab has antivascular effects in human rectal cancer. *Nat Med* 2004;10(2):145–147.
129. Willett CG, Boucher Y, Duda DG, et al. Surrogate markers for antiangiogenic therapy and dose-limiting toxicities for bevacizumab with radiation and chemotherapy: Continued experience of a phase I trial in rectal cancer patients. *J Clin Oncol* 2005;23(31):8136–8139.

130. Batchelor TT, Sorensen AG, di Tomaso E, et al. AZD2171, a pan-VEGF receptor tyrosine kinase inhibitor, normalizes tumor vasculature and alleviates edema in glioblastoma patients. *Cancer Cell* 2007;11(1):83–95.
131. Miller KD, Chap LI, Holmes FA, et al. Randomized phase III trial of capecitabine compared with bevacizumab plus capecitabine in patients with previously treated metastatic breast cancer. *J Clin Oncol* 2005;23(4):792–799.
132. Segers J, Fazio VD, Ansiaux R, et al. Potentiation of cyclophosphamide chemotherapy using the anti-angiogenic drug thalidomide: Importance of optimal scheduling to exploit the "normalization" window of the tumor vasculature. *Cancer Lett* 2006;244(1):129–135.
133. Ansiaux R, Baudelet C, Jordan BF, et al. Thalidomide radiosensitizes tumors through early changes in the tumor microenvironment. *Clin Cancer Res* 2005;11(2 Pt 1):743–750.
134. Tanaka F, Ishikawa S, Yanagihara K, et al. Expression of angiopoietins and its clinical significance in non-small cell lung cancer. *Cancer Res* 2002;62(23):7124–7129.
135. Loges S, Heil G, Bruweleit M, et al. Analysis of concerted expression of angiogenic growth factors in acute myeloid leukemia: Expression of angiopoietin-2 represents an independent prognostic factor for overall survival. *J Clin Oncol* 2005;23(6):1109–1117.
136. Murata R, Nishimura Y, Hiraoka M. An antiangiogenic agent (TNP-470) inhibited reoxygenation during fractionated radiotherapy of murine mammary carcinoma. *Int J Radiat Oncol Biol Phys* 1997;37(5):1107–1113.
137. Jain RK. Normalizing tumor vasculature with anti-angiogenic therapy: A new paradigm for combination therapy. *Nat Med* 2001;7(9):987–989.
138. Teicher BA, Sotomayor EA, Huang ZD. Antiangiogenic agents potentiate cytotoxic cancer therapies against primary and metastatic disease. *Cancer Res* 1992;52(23):6702–6704.
139. Horsman MR, Murata R. Vascular targeting effects of ZD6126 in a C3H mouse mammary carcinoma and the enhancement of radiation response. *Int J Radiat Oncol Biol Phys* 2003;57(4):1047–1055.
140. Lee CG, Heijn M, di Tomaso E, et al. Anti-vascular endothelial growth factor treatment augments tumor radiation response under normoxic or hypoxic conditions. *Cancer Res* 2000;60(19):5565–5570.
141. Hess C, Vuong V, Hegyi I, et al. Effect of VEGF receptor inhibitor PTK787/ZK222584 [correction of ZK222548] combined with ionizing radiation on endothelial cells and tumour growth. *Br J Cancer* 2001;85(12):2010–2016.
142. Li J, Huang S, Armstrong EA, et al. Angiogenesis and radiation response modulation after vascular endothelial growth factor receptor-2 (VEGFR2) blockade. *Int J Radiat Oncol Biol Phys* 2005;62(5):1477–1485.
143. Hurwitz H, Fehrenbacher L, Novotny W, et al. Bevacizumab plus irinotecan, fluorouracil, and leucovorin for metastatic colorectal cancer. *N Engl J Med* 2004;350(23):2335–2342.
144. Gorski DH, Beckett MA, Jaskowiak NT, et al. Blockage of the vascular endothelial growth factor stress response increases the antitumor effects of ionizing radiation. *Cancer Res* 1999;59(14):3374–3378.
145. Carmeliet P, Jain RK. Angiogenesis in cancer and other diseases. *Nature* 2000;407(6801):249–257.
146. Giaccia A, Siim BG, Johnson RS. HIF-1 as a target for drug development. *Nat Rev Drug Discov* 2003;2(10):803–811.
147. Cohen MH, Gootenberg J, Keegan P, Pazdur R. FDA drug approval summary: Bevacizumab (Avastin) plus Carboplatin and Paclitaxel as first-line treatment of advanced/metastatic recurrent nonsquamous non-small cell lung cancer. *Oncologist* 2007;12(6):713–718.
148. Goldberg RM. Cetuximab. *Nat Rev Drug Discov* 2005;(Suppl):S10–S11.

149. Giusti RM, Shastri KA, Cohen MH, et al. FDA drug approval summary: Panitumumab (Vectibix). *Oncologist* 2007;12(5):577–583.
150. Lin A, Rugo HS. The role of trastuzumab in early stage breast cancer: Current data and treatment recommendations. *Curr Treat Options Oncol* 2007;8(1):47–60.
151. Cohen MH, Johnson JR, Chen YF, et al. FDA drug approval summary: Erlotinib (Tarceva) tablets. *Oncologist* 2005;10(7):461–466.
152. Wilhelm S, Carter C, Lynch M, et al. Discovery and development of sorafenib: A multikinase inhibitor for treating cancer. *Nat Rev Drug Discov* 2006;5(10):835–844.
153. Rock EP, Goodman V, Jiang JX, et al. Food and Drug Administration drug approval summary: Sunitinib malate for the treatment of gastrointestinal stromal tumor and advanced renal cell carcinoma. *Oncologist* 2007;12(1):107–113.
154. Richardson PG, Mitsiades C, Schlossman R, et al. New drugs for myeloma. *Oncologist* 2007;12(6): 664–689.
155. National Cancer Institute Clinical Trial Database. Available at: http://www.cancer.gov/Search/SearchClinicalTrialsAdvanced.aspx. Accessed January 5, 2008.
156. Turner CD, Chi S, Marcus KJ, et al. Phase II study of thalidomide and radiation in children with newly diagnosed brain stem gliomas and glioblastoma multiforme. *J Neurooncol* 2007;82(1):95–101.
157. Altaha R, Abraham J. Epidermal growth factor receptor as a target for cancer therapy. *Expert Rev Anticancer Ther* 2007;7(1):1–3.
158. Bonner JA, Harari PM, Giralt J, et al. Radiotherapy plus cetuximab for squamous-cell carcinoma of the head and neck. *N Engl J Med* 2006;354(6):567–578.

4 Dermatologic Manifestations of Targeted Therapies

MARIO E. LACOUTURE

BHARAT B. MITTAL

MARK AGULNIK

■ BACKGROUND ON CUTANEOUS REACTIONS TO TARGETED AGENTS AND RADIATION

Dermatologic side effects to targeted agents have received considerable attention, because of their high incidence, occurring in 75–87% of patients (1), negative impact on psychosocial function (2), and detrimental effect on consistent therapy, with drug dose modification or discontinuation needed in 4–17% of patients (3,4). Most publications on untoward dermatologic events have been based on data from their use in the absence of concurrent radiation (5); thus, extrapolation of their effects in the setting of radiation therapy should be made with caution. Importantly, the frequency and severity of dermatologic toxicities to targeted therapies will differ in patients with concurrent or prior radiation, due to the fact that the duration of therapy with targeted agents may vary, typically being shorter when radiation is being administered; the combined effect of pathway inhibition and ionizing radiation in skin will result in greater toxicity; and, in patients with prior radiation, long-term sequelae in cutaneous structures will lead to a decreased severity in clinical presentation of dermatologic side effects.

■ USE OF CONCURRENT TARGETED AGENTS AND RADIATION THERAPY

An emerging strategy to improve outcomes in patients with solid tumor malignancies is to incorporate newer, biologically active, targeted agents into their treatment programs. Molecular targeted agents offer attractive therapeutic options by restoring normal control to oncogenic processes. Aberrant activity of the epidermal growth factor receptor (EGFR) due to overexpression or activating mutations has been correlated with a poor prognosis and decreased survival in a variety of solid tumors (6). The use of monoclonal antibodies or small molecules that block ligand binding or intracytoplasmic domain phosphorylation, respectively, have shown prolonged survival times in advanced colorectal, head and neck, pancreatic, and non-small cell lung cancer (7). The higher specificity of these drugs is associated with lower systemic and hematopoietic side effects when compared to conventional chemotherapy (8). The goal of combining these agents with radiation therapy is to reduce radioresistance and consequently improve upon the therapeutic index.

In no other setting has this become more apparent than in the treatment of patients with squamous cell carcinoma of the head and neck (SCCHN). Over the last several decades, the treatment of locally advanced SCCHN has evolved from surgery to radiation therapy to concurrent chemotherapy and radiation. Most recently, a role for concurrent cetuximab, an IgG_1 monoclonal antibody against the ligand-binding domain of the EGFR, with radiation therapy has emerged (3,9–11). To date, the phase III clinical trial published by Bonner and colleagues of radiation plus cetuximab for SCCHN is the only published phase III data to support the use of concurrent radiation and a targeted agent, and confirms the safety of this combination (Table 4.1) (3). This study marks the complete evolution and proof of concept that was first tested in preclinical models (12–18) and has now established a U.S. Food and Drug Administration (FDA)-approved indication for the concurrent use of cetuximab and radiation therapy in SCCHN (*www.fda.gov*).

With the emergence of this FDA-approved indication, further studies are currently underway to expand upon the use of targeted agents and radiation therapy, as well as to integrate targeted agents into concurrent chemoradiation protocols. Knowledge of the dermatologic side effects and treatment of these effects will become integral for the ability to maintain the dose intensity of these regimens.

DERMATOLOGIC TOXICITIES TO TARGETED THERAPIES

Despite a more beneficial side effect profile, EGFR inhibitors frequently lead to dermatologic (45%–100%) and ocular (12%) toxicities (3,4,19,20) (Fig. 4.1). A papulopustular reaction is the more frequent manifestation, affecting 87% of patients receiving monoclonal antibodies (3), and occurring in the face and upper trunk within the first few days to weeks of therapy. The rash is considered to be mechanistically related to EGFR inhibition in epidermal keratinocytes (21). Clinical and experimental data suggest that the papulopustules are a consequence of the blockade of EGFR-mediated signaling pathways, which affect keratinocytes by inducing growth arrest and apoptosis, decreas-

TABLE 4.1 Nonhematologic adverse events reported in the Phase III trial of radiotherapy and cetuximab for squamous cell carcinoma of the head and neck

	Radiation Alone		Radiation plus Cetuximab	
Adverse Event	**All Grades**	**Grade 3–5**	**All Grades**	**Grade 3–5**
Mucositis	94	52	93	56
Acneiform rash	10	1	87	17
Radiation dermatitis	90	18	86	23
Weight loss	72	7	84	11
Xerostomia	71	3	72	5
Dysphagia	63	30	65	26
Asthenia	49	5	56	4
Nausea	37	2	49	2
Constipation	30	5	35	5
Taste perversion	28	0	29	0
Vomiting	23	4	29	2
Pain	28	7	28	6
Anorexia	23	2	27	2
Fever	13	1	26	1
Pharyngitis	19	4	26	3
Dehydration	19	8	25	6
Oral candidiasis	22	0	20	0
Coughing	19	0	20	<1
Voice alteration	22	0	19	2
Diarrhea	13	1	19	2
Headache	8	<1	19	<1
Pruritus	4	0	16	0
Infusion reaction	2	0	15	3
Insomnia	14	0	15	0
Dyspepsia	9	1	14	0
Increased sputum	15	1	13	<1
Infection	9	1	13	1
Anxiety	9	1	11	<1
Chills	5	0	11	0

All values reported as a percent of patients.

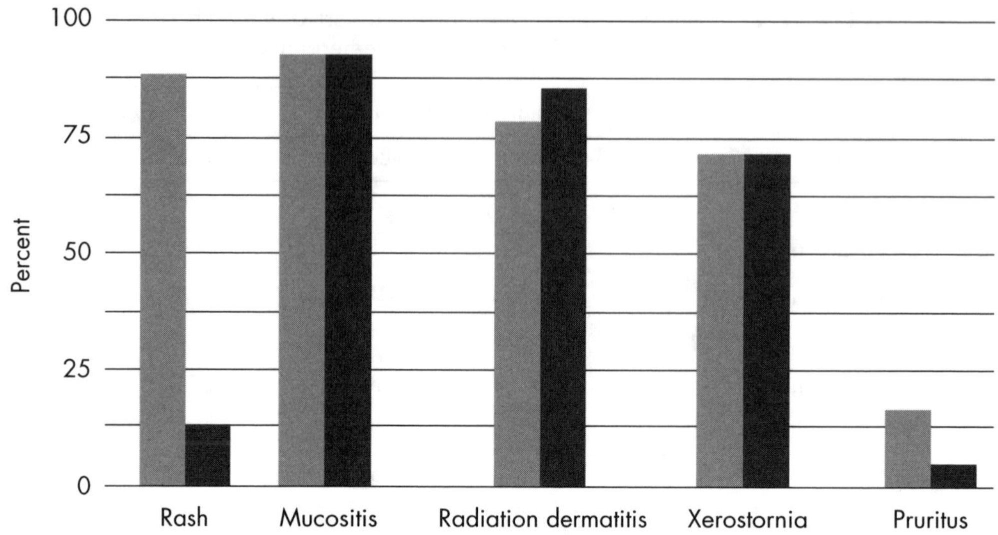

FIGURE 4.1 Dermatologic toxicities (all grades) in patients with advanced locoregional head and neck squamous cell carcinoma treated with radiotherapy (dark gray bars) (n = 212) or radiotherapy plus cetuximab (light gray bars) (n = 208). (Figure reproduced with permission from Bonner JA, Harari PM, Giralt J, et al. Radiotherapy plus cetuximab for squamous-cell carcinoma of the head and neck. *N Engl J Med* 2006;354:567–578.) (Bonner et al., 2006)

ing cell migration, increasing cell attachment and differentiation, and stimulating inflammation, all of which result in distinctive cutaneous manifestations (22). The acute effects of ionizing radiation in epidermal keratinocytes include apoptosis, synthesis of chemokines, and dermal and perivascular inflammation (23). As with SCCHN cell lines (24), it is hypothesized that combined radiation and anti-EGFR therapy would lead to greater keratinocyte radiosensitivity and radiation-induced apoptosis. This notion was not supported by the Bonner trial, in which dermatitis at the radiation site was not significantly greater in patients treated with cetuximab plus radiation when compared to those treated with radiation alone. Factors contributing to this unexpected result include inconsistencies between investigators due to the use of the National Cancer Institute's Common Terminology Criteria for Adverse Events (*http://ctep.cancer.gov*) (Table 4.2), which does not adequately measure these toxicities, as well as other side effects recorded during these trials that may have taken precedence.

In patients with SCCHN treated with radiation and cetuximab, dermatologic reactions required dose modification in 17% and discontinuation in 3.8% of treated patients (3), both of which may decrease quality of life and affect clinical outcome. A noteworthy correlation has been demonstrated across a variety of solid tumors treated with EGFR inhibitors, in which the severity of the papulopustular reaction parallels the antitumor efficacy (1). This finding supports the notion that skin toxicities should be managed effectively and

TABLE 4.2 Description and grading of rash as per the common terminology criteria for adverse events v3.0 (CTCAE) (www.ctep.cancer.gov)

Adverse Event	Short Name	Grade				
		1	2	3	4	5
Rash/desquamation	Rash	Macular or papular eruption or erythema without associated symptoms	Macular or papular eruption or erythema with pruritus or other associated symptoms; localized desquamation or other lesions covering <50% BSA	Severe, generalized erythroderma or macular, papular or vesicular eruption; desquamation covering ≥50% BSA	Generalized exfoliative, ulcerative, or bolus dermatitis	Death
Rash: Acne/ acneiform	Acne	Intervention not indicated	Intervention indicated	Associated with pain, disfigurement, ulceration, or desquamation		Death
Rash: Dermatitis associated with radiation *Select:* i) Chemoradiation ii) Radiation	Dermatitis–*Select*	Faint erythema or dry desquamation	Moderate to brisk erythema; patchy moist desquamation, mostly confined to skin folds and creases; moderate edema	Moist desquamation other than skin folds and creases; bleeding induced by minor trauma or abrasion	Skin necrosis or ulceration of full thickness dermis; spontaneous bleeding from involved site	Death

Abbreviations: BSA- body surface area

patients should be maintained on the regimen, as patients who could benefit the most are those most likely to necessitate modifications in drug dose. The lack of management guidelines and poor understanding of these toxicities has prompted the establishment of interdisciplinary efforts among oncologists, dermatologists, and ophthalmologists such as the SERIES (*S*kin and *E*ye *R*eactions to *I*nhibitors of the *E*GFR and kinase*S*) clinic, a clinical program dedicated to the understanding and management of side effects to these novel anticancer therapies (25).

Later events of EGFR inhibitor therapy, which usually occur after 4–8 weeks, include periungual reactions (inflammation in tissues surrounding the nails), which develop in 12–16% of patients; hair abnormalities, which include a rapidly developing, diffuse, nonscarring alopecia frequently associated with pruritus; trichomegaly (enlargement) and curling of the eyelashes; and hypertrichosis (increased hair growth) of the face in up to 16% of patients (26). Dry skin (xerosis) occurs in 7–35% of patients and is frequently associated with pruritus (4,19,26). All of these effects are likely not to appear as frequently in patients treated in current radiation-anti-EGFRI protocols for SCCHN, because of the shorter duration of therapy (Fig. 4.2).

■ DERMATOLOGIC TOXICITIES TO COMBINED EPIDERMAL GROWTH FACTOR RECEPTOR INHIBITION AND RADIATION THERAPY

Abundant clinical and experimental data show the additive or synergistic inhibitory effect on tumor growth when radiation is combined with EGFR inhib-

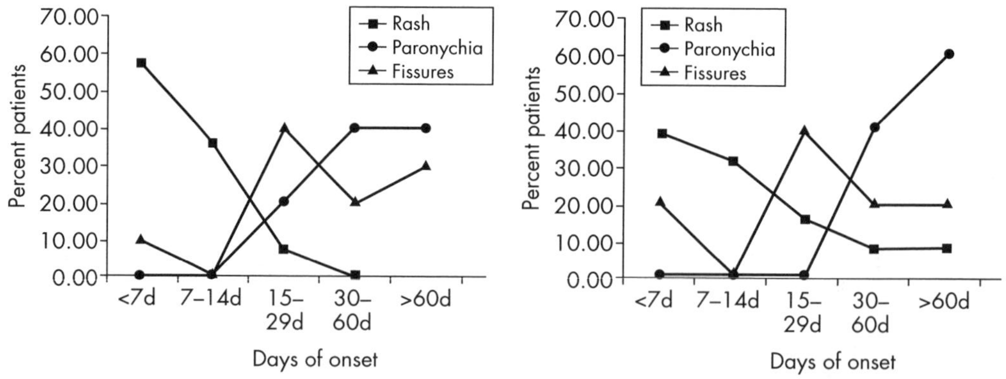

FIGURE 4.2 Chronologic appearance of dermatologic toxicities to cetuximab and erlotinib (n = 30). (Figure reproduced with permission from Roe E, Garcia-Muret MP, Marcuello E et al. Description and management of cutaneous side effects during cetuximab or erlotinib treatments: A prospective study of 30 patients. *J Am Acad Dermatol* 2006;55:429–437. (Roe et al., 2006).

itors (27). The tumor radiosensitizing effect of EGFR inhibitors, which is used advantageously in the clinic, will also lead to increased toxicity in skin and appendages overlying irradiated sites. Exposure of human and mouse epidermal keratinocytes incubated in vitro with anti-EGFR antibodies to ionizing radiation will result in increased expression of functional EGFR (28) and receptor phosphorylation (29), respectively. Similarly, growth inhibition of non-small cell lung (NSCL) cancer xenografts implanted onto nude mice by the anti-EGFR monoclonal antibody cetuximab will be greater when combined with radiation or chemotherapy. Skin from patients subjected to radiation will also show increased levels of EGFR expression (28). Taken as a whole, these events suggest that ionizing radiation leads to a stress response in keratinocytes, in which increased EGFR activity would play a protective role in repopulating affected sites.

In the pivotal study for SCCHN, hypersensitivity reactions led to cetuximab discontinuation in four of 211 patients, and the most common cause for dose modification or interruption was the papulopustular (incorrectly referred to as acneiform) rash. Grades 1 or 2 papulopustular rash were seen in 70% of patients, whereas grades 3 or 4 were documented in 17% of patients, which led to dose modification in 17% and discontinuation in 3.8% of patients. Moreover, concurrent administration of cetuximab did not lead to an increase in other radiotherapy-induced effects, such as mucositis and xerostomia (Fig. 4.1). The rate of grades 3–5 mucositis was 52% and 56% in patients receiving radiotherapy alone and radiotherapy with cetuximab, respectively. Severe (grades 3–5) radiation dermatitis rates were similar in both arms of the study: 18% for patients receiving radiation alone versus 23% for patients with radiotherapy plus cetuximab.

Importantly, prior radiation (3–68 months) with doses ranging from 36 to 70 Gy has been shown to result in skin areas unable to develop the papulopustular reaction to cetuximab (30). This phenomenon may be a result of late consequences of irradiated skin, which include dermal fibrosis, depletion of antigen-presenting Langerhans cells (31), and epidermal hyperproliferation and abnormal differentiation (32) (Fig. 4.3). This may result in altered microvasculature that precludes sufficient amounts of drug reaching the area, altered antigen-presenting capacity, or biochemical alterations at the keratinocyte molecular level—all of which lead to decreased sensitivity to EGFR inhibitors. Conversely, concurrent administration of cetuximab results in a more confluent area of papulopustules (Fig. 4.3). Histologic analysis of these areas showed the characteristic changes of EGFR inhibitor–induced papulopustular reaction (not radiation dermatitis), suggesting that, in addition to tumors, cetuximab will also sensitize skin to the effects of ionizing radiation (33,34).

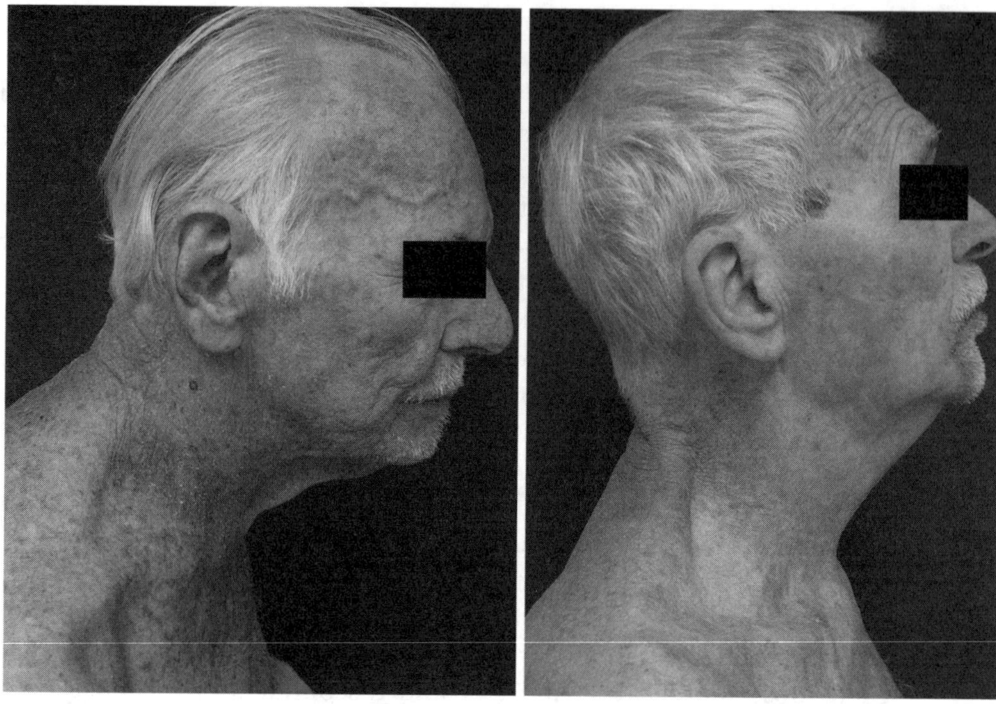

FIGURE 4.3 Effect of concurrent versus delayed administration of EGFR inhibitor on the development of papulopustular reaction. Simultaneous (left panel) and 1-year delayed administration of cetuximab will lead to aggravation and sparing of rash in overlying skin, respectively.

MANAGEMENT OF SKIN TOXICITIES

The papulopustular reaction is the earliest occurring toxicity, and usually the most clinically significant. Randomized trials for the management of this toxicity are underway, and uncontrolled reports and experience from a referral center for the management of such events (22,35) suggest that the use of topical corticosteroids and oral tetracycline antibiotics may be of value. An algorithm for the management of such reactions has been employed (Fig. 4.4). Corticosteroids have also been effective in the management of radiation dermatitis (36,37) and semisynthetic tetracyclines (i.e. doxycycline or minocycline) have shown anti-inflammatory activity (38), which makes them effective against other skin diseases in which infection does not play a major role, such as acne and rosacea. As demonstrated by Oishi and colleagues in SCCHN, management of erlotinib-induced grade 1 rash will result in greater complete responses (described as downgrading of the rash), when compared to patients with grade 2/3 rash, in which seven of nine had a partial response (in this subset, four patients required erlotinib dose modification), thus suggesting that interventions when rash is of lower grade may lead to better results and minimize the need for anticancer drug modification. Additional recommendations for pruritus and xerosis are described in Table 4.3.

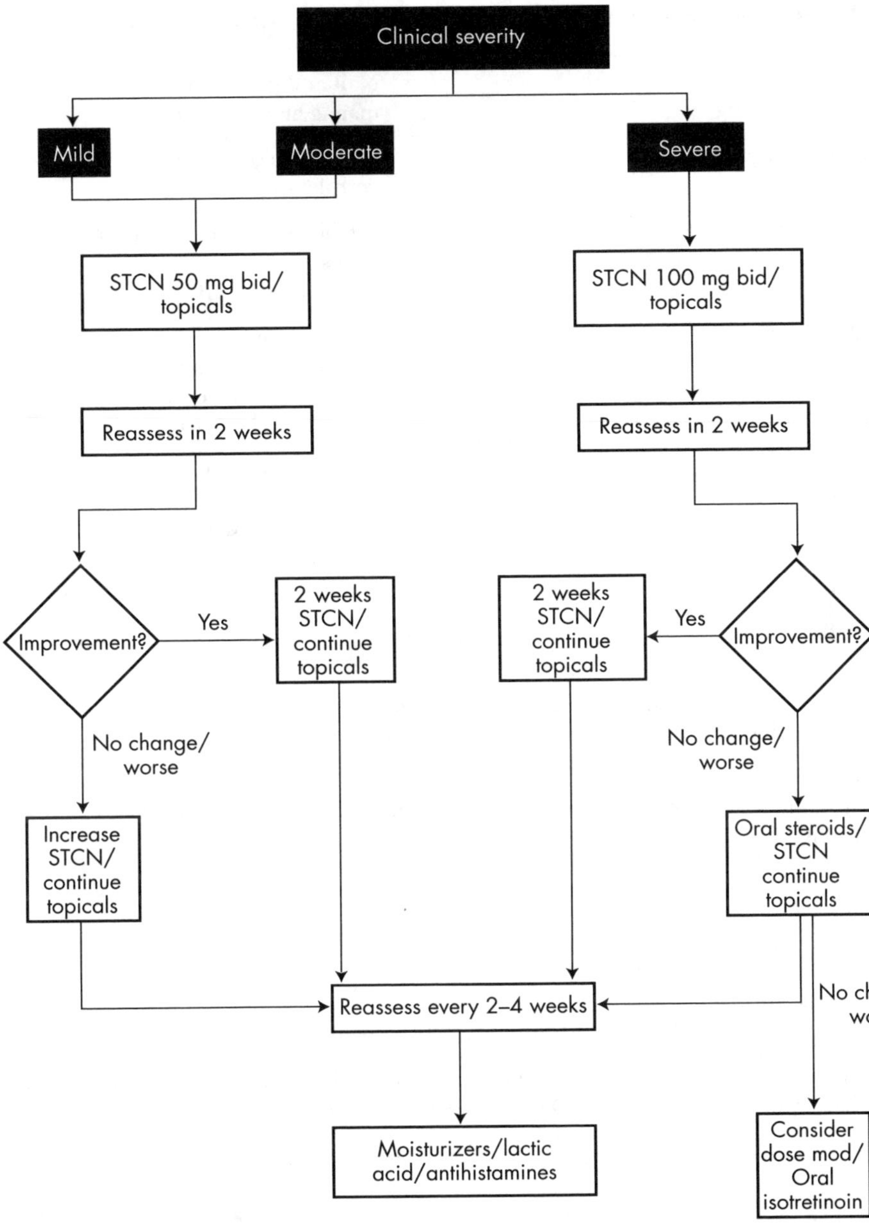

FIGURE 4.4 SERIES management algorithm for papulopustular reactions to EGFR inhibitors. Severity of papulopustular reaction is graded based on clinical findings and symptoms (mild/moderate, severe). SERIES, Skin and Eye Reactions to Inhibitors of EGFR and kinaseS; EGFR, epidermal growth factor receptor inhibitor; STCN, semisynthetic tetracyclines (doxycycline); topicals (steroids or calcineurin inhibitors); dose mod, EGFR inhibitor dose reduction or interruption; isotretinoin, low doses (10–20 mg/day) isotretinoin. (Figure reproduced with permission from Lacouture ME, Basti S, Patel J, Benson A, 3rd. (2006). The SERIES clinic: an interdisciplinary approach to the management of toxicities of EGFR inhibitors. *J Support Oncol* 2006;4:236–238.) (from Lacouture et al., *J Supportive Oncol*, with permission) (Lacouture et al., 2006)

TABLE 4.3 Management recommendations for nail and periungual toxicities, pruritus, and xerosis

Treatment setting	Nail and periungual toxicity management options
Prophylactic care	Avoidance of irritants Petroleum jelly emolliation
Local care	Petroleum jelly emolliation Soaks Cushioning of affected areas
Mild/moderate	Disinfectants Topical or systemic antibiotics Topical corticosteroids Intralesional corticosteroids
Severe	Electrodesiccation Cryosurgery Surgical debridement Nail plate avulsion EGFR inhibitor dose modification

Pruritus

Topicals
Body: Sarna ultra® cream, Regenecare® gel as needed
Scalp: Fluocinonide 0.05% shampoo, clobetasol foam daily

Orals
Antihistamines: (diphenhydramine 25–50 mg b.i.d., cetirizine 10–20 mg/day) and pregabalin 75–100 mg b.i.d.

Xerosis

Emollients
Vanicream®, Eucerin®, Aquaphor®

Exfoliants (for scaly areas)
Ammonium lactate 12% for body and urea 20% cream for palms and soles and fissures

Adapted with permission from Fox LP (2006). Pathology and management of dermatologic toxicities associated with anti-EGFR therapy. *Oncology* 2006;20:26–34.

■ CONCLUSIONS

In all, dermatologic toxicities represent an obstacle toward the optimal use of combined radiation-EGFR inhibitor regimens. Grading systems and management guidelines should be tailored to the use of both modalities, as the use of those derived from targeted therapies alone would not be representative. Thus, multidisciplinary clinical programs including radiation oncologists, dermatologists, and medical oncologists would typify an ideal approach toward the improved identification, reporting, and management of these events. Increased attention to dermatologic toxicities is anticipated with the expanding use of radiation to currently established targeted-therapy regimens and with longer survival times and increased emphasis on survivorship issues.

REFERENCES

1. Perez-Soler R, Saltz L. Cutaneous adverse effects with HER1/EGFR-targeted agents: Is there a silver lining? *J Clin Oncol* 2005;23:5235–5246.
2. Molinari E, De Quatrebarbes J, Andre T, Aractingi S. Cetuximab-induced acne. *Dermatology* 2005;211:330–333.
3. Bonner JA, Harari PM, Giralt J, et al. Radiotherapy plus cetuximab for squamous-cell carcinoma of the head and neck. *N Engl J Med* 2006;354:567–578.
4. Cunningham D, Humblet Y, Siena S, et al. Cetuximab monotherapy and cetuximab plus irinotecan in irinotecan-refractory metastatic colorectal cancer. *N Engl J Med* 2004;351:337–345.
5. Robert C, Soria JC, Spatz A, et al. Cutaneous side-effects of kinase inhibitors and blocking antibodies. *Lancet Oncol* 2005;6:491–500.
6. Hynes NE, Lane HA. ErbB receptors and cancer: The complexity of targeted inhibitors. *Nat Rev Cancer* 2005;5:341–354.
7. Imai K, Takaoka A. Comparing antibody and small-molecule therapies for cancer. *Nat Rev Cancer* 2006;6:714–727.
8. Dancey J, Sausville EA. Issues and progress with protein kinase inhibitors for cancer treatment. *Nat Rev Drug Discov* 2003;2:296–313.
9. Brizel DM, Albers ME, Fisher SR, et al. Hyperfractionated irradiation with or without concurrent chemotherapy for locally advanced head and neck cancer. *N Engl J Med* 1998;338:1798–1804.
10. Kramer S, Gelber RD, Snow JB, et al. Combined radiation therapy and surgery in the management of advanced head and neck cancer: Final report of study 73-03 of the Radiation Therapy Oncology Group. *Head Neck Surg* 1987;10:19–30.
11. Pignon JP, Bourhis J, Domenge C, Designe L. Chemotherapy added to locoregional treatment for head and neck squamous-cell carcinoma: Three meta-analyses of updated individual data. MACH-NC Collaborative Group. Meta-analysis of Chemotherapy on Head and Neck Cancer. *Lancet* 2000;355;949–955.
12. Milas L, Mason K, Hunter N, et al. In vivo enhancement of tumor radioresponse by C225 antiepidermal growth factor receptor antibody. *Clin Cancer Res* 2000;6:701–708.
13. Nasu S, Ang KK, Fan Z, Milas L. C225 antiepidermal growth factor receptor antibody enhances tumor radiocurability. *Int J Radiat Oncol Biol Phys* 2001;51:474–477.
14. Pietras RJ, Poen JC, Gallardo D, et al. Monoclonal antibody to HER-2/neureceptor modulates repair of radiation-induced DNA damage and enhances radiosensitivity of human breast cancer cells overexpressing this oncogene. *Cancer Res* 1999;59:1347–1355.
15. Rao GS, Murray S, Ethier SP. Radiosensitization of human breast cancer cells by a novel ErbB family receptor tyrosine kinase inhibitor. *Int J Radiat Oncol Biol Phys* 2000;48:1519–1528.
16. Saleh MN, Raisch KP, Stackhouse MA, et al. Combined modality therapy of A431 human epidermoid cancer using anti-EGFr antibody C225 and radiation. *Cancer Biother Radiopharm* 1999;14:451–463.
17. Williams KJ, Telfer BA, Stratford IJ, Wedge SR. ZD1839 ("Iressa"), a specific oral epidermal growth factor receptor-tyrosine kinase inhibitor, potentiates radiotherapy in a human colorectal cancer xenograft model. *Br J Cancer* 2002;86:1157–1161.

18. Wollman R, Yahalom J, Maxy R, et al. Effect of epidermal growth factor on the growth and radiation sensitivity of human breast cancer cells in vitro. *Int J Radiat Oncol Biol Phys* 1994;30:91–98.
19. Shepherd FA, Rodrigues Pereira J, Ciuleanu T, et al. Erlotinib in previously treated non-small-cell lung cancer. *N Engl J Med* 2005;353:123–132.
20. Tullo AB, Esmaeli B, Murray PI, et al. Ocular findings in patients with solid tumours treated with the epidermal growth factor receptor tyrosine kinase inhibitor gefitinib ("Iressa", ZD1839) in Phase I and II clinical trials. *Eye* 2005;19:729–738.
21. Kari C, Chan TO, Rocha de Quadros M, Rodeck U. Targeting the epidermal growth factor receptor in cancer: Apoptosis takes center stage. *Cancer Res* 2003;63:1–5.
22. Lacouture ME. Mechanisms of cutaneous toxicities to EGFR inhibitors. *Nat Rev Cancer* 2006;6:803–812.
23. Hymes SR, Strom EA, Fife C. Radiation dermatitis: Clinical presentation, pathophysiology, and treatment. *J Am Acad Dermatol* 2006;54:28–46.
24. Huang SM, Bock JM, Harari PM. Epidermal growth factor receptor blockade with C225 modulates proliferation, apoptosis, and radiosensitivity in squamous cell carcinomas of the head and neck. *Cancer Res* 1999;59:1935–1940.
25. Lacouture ME, Basti S, Patel J, Benson A 3rd. The SERIES clinic: An interdisciplinary approach to the management of toxicities of EGFR inhibitors. *J Support Oncol* 2006;4:236–238.
26. Roe E, Garcia Muret MP, Marcuello E, et al. Description and management of cutaneous side effects during cetuximab or erlotinib treatments: A prospective study of 30 patients. *J Am Acad Dermatol* 2006;55:429–437.
27. Raben D, Helfrich B, Chan DC, et al. The effects of cetuximab alone and in combination with radiation and/or chemotherapy in lung cancer. *Clin Cancer Res* 2005;11:795–805.
28. Peter RU, Beetz A, Ried C, et al. Increased expression of the epidermal growth factor receptor in human epidermal keratinocytes after exposure to ionizing radiation. *Radiat Res* 1993;136:65–70.
29. Song HJ, Kim TH, Cho CK, et al. Increased expression of ornithine decarboxylase by gamma-ray in mouse epidermal cells: relationship with protein kinase C signaling pathway. *J Radiat Res (Tokyo)* 1998;39:175–184.
30. Bossi P, Liberatoscioli C, Bergamini C, et al. Previously irradiated areas spared from skin toxicity induced by cetuximab in six patients: Implications for the administration of EGFR inhibitors in previously irradiated patients. *Ann Oncol* 2007;18:601–602.
31. Cole S. Long-term effects of local ionizing radiation treatment on Langerhans cells in mouse footpad epidermis. *J Invest Dermatol* 1986;87:608–612.
32. Sivan V, Vozenin-Brotons MC, Tricaud Y, et al. Altered proliferation and differentiation of human epidermis in cases of skin fibrosis after radiotherapy. *Int J Radiat Oncol Biol Phys* 2002;53:385–393.
33. Harari PM, Huang SM. Epidermal growth factor receptor modulation of radiation response: Preclinical and clinical development. *Semin Radiat Oncol* 2002;12:21–26.
34. Lacouture ME, Hwang C, Patel J, et al. Temporal dependence of the effect of radiation on erlotinib-induced skin rash. *J Clin Oncol* 2007;25:2140.
35. Oishi KJ, Garey JS, Burke BJ, et al. Managing cutaneous side effects associated with erlotinib in head and neck cancer (HNC) and non-small cell lung cancer (NSCLC) patients (pts). ASCO Annual Meeting Proceedings. *J Clin Oncol* 2006;24:18538.
36. Bostrom A, Lindman H, Swartling C, et al. Potent corticosteroid cream (mometasone furoate) significantly reduces acute radiation dermatitis: Results from a double-blind, randomized study. *Radiother Oncol* 2001;59:257–265.

37. Schmuth M, Wimmer MA, Hofer S, et al. Topical corticosteroid therapy for acute radiation dermatitis: A prospective, randomized, double-blind study. *Br J Dermatol* 2002;146:983–991.
38. Sapadin AN, Fleischmajer R. Tetracyclines: nonantibiotic properties and their clinical implications. *J Am Acad Dermatol* 2006;54:258–265.
39. Fox LP. Pathology and management of dermatologic toxicities associated with anti-EGFR therapy. *Oncology (Williston Park)* 2006;20:26–34.

5 Radiolabeled Monoclonal Antibody Therapies

LANEA M. M. KELLER
ANTONIO MARTIN JIMENEZ
WILLIAM SMALL, JR.
LEO I. GORDON

Over the past decade the US Food and Drug Administration (FDA) has approved several monoclonal antibodies (mAbs) for the treatment of specific cancers. Presently, mAbs are the most widely used form of cancer immunotherapy, a passive form of therapy utilizing these biologic agents to target to specific antigens. Much attention has been focused in the direction of conjugated mAbs: mAbs joined with drugs, toxins, or radionuclides in efforts to exploit the specific targeting of mAb to deliver cytotoxic moieties directly to cancerous cells and the surrounding area. Mylotarg (gemtuzumab ozogamicin) is a calicheamicin-conjugated antibody with specificity for CD33; calicheamicin's exquisite cytotoxicity precludes systemic administration. Mylotarg has proven effective in the treatment of acute myeloid leukemia (AML), and it gained FDA approval in 2000. Another exciting area of research in conjugated mAb therapeutics lies with radioimmunotherapy (RIT), with the laudable goal of delivering a radiation payload at a specific site of disease. Radioimmunotherapy carries the added benefit of irradiating a localized area and, while not to imply that RIT is not subject to resistance, RIT is not subject to the same multidrug-resistant pathways as some chemotherapeutics. Zevalin (ibritumomab tiuxetan) and Bexxar (Tositumomab and ^{131}I Tositumomab), are both murine anti-CD20 mAbs armed with ^{90}Y and ^{131}I, respectively. They are the only two FDA-approved radionuclide-bearing mAbs and are indicated for the treatment of non-Hodgkin's lymphoma (NHL). The field of RIT is very much in its infancy, as the most successful results have been obtained in the filed of hematopoietic malignancies, with sluggish progress noted beyond early phase II solid tumor studies. Today, the field of oncology is poised to define a real role for RIT with respect to solid tumor therapy. This chapter presents the general background and critical considerations with respect to RIT as well as the promising clinical results realized to date.

■ BACKGROUND

At the birth of the twentieth century, the German pathologist Paul Ehrlich proposed the use of antibodies as "magic bullets" in efforts to eradicate disease; the first evidence that a radionuclide could be conjugated to an antibody was reported in the mid-1950s (1,2). However, the first real progress toward the clinical application of antibodies was realized in 1975, with the Nobel Prize-winning advent of the hybridoma. The technique described in Kohler and Milstein's seminal work described the fusion of murine splenic B cells with a plasmacytoma. Pioneering studies with radiolabeled anticarcinoembryonic antigen (CEA) by Goldenberg and Mach in the mid-1970s provided proof of principle for *in vivo* RIT (3,4). Interest was dedicated throughout the 1980s to the development of mAbs against and identification of specific tumor-associated antigens (TAAs). In the following decades, many TAAs, such as CEA, the membrane-bound glycosylated phosphoprotein Mucin-1 (Muc-1), prostate-specific membrane antigen (PSMA), pancarcinoma antigen (TAG-72), and epidermal growth factor receptor (EGFR) were subsequently discovered and characterized. Ideally, a targeted antigen is present only on neoplastic tissue, is highly overexpressed and readily accessible on the cellular surface, and is not secreted. Numerous preclinical studies supported the utility of mAbs in trafficking to specific TAAs but also revealed limitations that required attention if any clinical success was to be realized. The most obvious limitation to therapeutic efficacy was the production of human antimurine immunoglobulin antibodies (HAMA) after one to three exposures to the murine mAb (5). In general, exposure to foreign proteins (murine mAb) elicits an immunologic response (HAMA) that results in the rapid clearance of the foreign biologic from the circulation. While acutely this may manifest as an allergic-type reaction, overall, the efficacy of the mAb is severely diminished upon the presence of HAMA due to this fundamental alteration in biodistribution and pharmacokinetics. Other constraints include insufficient activation of effector functions, slow clearance from the central vasculature, low affinity and avidity, and trafficking through and even targeting of normal organs (5). Genetic engineering techniques have addressed most of these challenges and have been applied to eliminating HAMA by fusing the variable region of the murine antibody with the constant region of a human antibody to produce chimeric mAbs. The complementarity-determining region (CDR) is then grafted onto the human protein scaffold, thereby producing a humanized mAb (6). Fully human mAbs have also been generated (7). With each advance, a compromise is usually observed; for example, humanized mAbs tend to remain in circulation longer, effectively decreasing the relative tumor residence time and, when considering radiolabeled mAbs, increasing hematologic toxicity as bone marrow has a dose limit of 50–200 cGy (8).

Advances in the understanding of tumor biology and biologic engineering techniques, coupled with the numerous lessons learned from previous preclinical and clinical studies, have advanced the field to the point at which RIT's potential can be fully defined. With the ongoing successes of RIT in the treatment of NHL, coupled with a better understanding of the inherent limitations of RIT, several radiolabeled mAbs are currently being evaluated in clinical trials. The groundbreaking FDA approval of Zevalin and Bexxar has certainly fueled interest and efforts in developing additional targeted radiation therapy therapeutics (9).

■ MONOCLONAL ANTIBODIES

Monoclonal antibodies that have shown efficacy in clinical trials and have gained FDA approval include rituximab (Rituxan), trastuzumab (Herceptin), alemtuzumab (Campath), cetuximab (Erbitux), bevacizumab (Avastin), and panitumumab (Vectibix) (Table 5.1). Monoclonal nomenclature specifically identifies the biologic agent's species of origin, with -umab referring to human, -omab referring to murine, -ximab referring to chimeric, and -zumab referring to humanized forms. Intact immunoglobulin (IgG) antibodies are approximately 150-kDa in size, with half-lives of approximately 3 weeks; their metabolism is through the reticuloendothelial system. As size is an important factor vis á vis the time in circulation, recent efforts has been directed toward engineering mAbs into various "abbreviated forms," such as monovalent single-chain fragments (scFv) and divalent moieties (Fab), in attempts to speed clearance from the blood to the tumor. As an example, the renally excreted scFv is approximately 25-kDa and has a blood clearance time of less than 10 hours (8). It has been noted that these smaller fragments generally show faster tumor localization. However, they also exhibit faster washout and a shorter overall residence time. Despite the advances in genetic engineering techniques, the FDA-approved radiolabeled antibodies Bexxar and Zevalin are both fully sized murine IgG antibodies.

Radioimmunotherapies use the given mAb in subtherapeutic concentrations; however, its contribution to therapeutic efficacy itself should not be discounted. Indeed, the mAb can have a direct cytotoxic effect by both antibody-dependent cell cytotoxicity (ADCC) and complement-dependent cytotoxicity (CDC). Successes with unconjugated mAbs, such as rituximab, demonstrate the clinical importance of the ADCC pathway. When an Fcγ receptor on an effector cell (T-lymphocytes, mononuclear phagocytes, and natural killer cells) engages the Fc region on the terminal potion of an antibody, cell death pro-

TABLE 5.1 FDA-approved mAbs with associated target and clinical indications

Commerical Name	Generic Name	Target	Indications
Rituxan	rituximab	CD20	Treatment of relpased or refractory, low grade or follicular, CD20 positive B cell, non-Hodgkin lymphoma
Herceptin	trastuzumab	HER-2/neu	Adjuvant treatment of HER-2-overexpressing, node-positive breast cancer with a treatment regimen containing doxorubicin, cyclophosphamide, and paclitaxel
			Single-agent treatment of metastatic breast cancer that overexpresses HER-2, which has previously been treated with one or more regimens
			Treatment of metastatic breast cancer that overexpresses HER-2, combined with paclitaxol in those chemotherapeautically niave
Campath	alemtuzumab	CD52	Single agent treatment of B-cell chronic lymphocytic leukemia previously treated with alkylating agents and failure on fludarabine
Erbitux	cetuximab	EGFR	Treatment with irinotecan of EGFR-expressing metastatic colorectal carcinoma refractory to irinotecan alone
			Single-agent treatment of EGFR expressing metastatic colorectal carcinoma after failing both irinotecan- and oxaliplatin-based regimens
			First line treatment of locally or regionally advanced squamous cell carcinoma of the head and neck (SCCHN) in combination with radiation therapy (RT)
			Single agent in recurrent or metastatic SCCHN where prior platinum-based chemotherapy has failed
Avastin	bevacizumab	VEGF	First- or second-line treatment of metastatic carcinoma of the colon or rectum in combination with intravenous 5-fluorouracil based chemotherapy
			First-line treatment of unresectable, locally advanced, recurrent or metastatic nonsquamous, non-small cell lung cancer in combination with carboplatin and paclitaxel.
Vectibix	panitumumab	EGFR	EGFR-expressing metastatic colorectal cancer with disease progression on or despite treatment with fluoropyrimidine, oxliplatin, or irinotecan-based chemotherapeautic regimens

ceeds through an effector cell–dependent mechanism. Most mAbs that mediate ADCC also activate the more primitive complement system. When the complement protein C1q binds to the Fc region of an engaged antibody, the CDC pathway is initiated, culminating in the formation of the cytolytic membrane attack complex and tumor cell death in an effector cell–independent manner. Preclinical studies have demonstrated the therapeutic importance of the Fc region of the mAb. For example, trastuzumab and rituximab, lacking the Fc region, showed decreased therapeutic effects against breast cancer and lymphoma, respectively (10,11).

In a mechanism independent of the immune system, natural ligands are blocked from the cell by the mAb. Cellular proliferation, migration, and cell-to-cell communications are only a few vital functions mediated through the interactions of various extracellular proteins and growth factors. Binding of membrane receptors by antibodies can induce either cell growth through the activation of mitogenic growth pathways or may lead to programmed cellular death (12,13). Rituximab, the chimeric anti-CD20 mAb used in numerous NHL treatment protocols, invokes a series of signaling events including increased phosphorylation, phospholipase Cγ activation, c-myc upregulation, and apoptosis in normal and malignant B lymphocytes (14–16). Trastuzumab (Herceptin), the humanized mAb with specificity for the extracellular domain of the protein kinase HER-2, which can be overexpressed in breast cancer and some adenocarcinomas, works by downregulating the extracellular tyrosine kinase (TK) receptor. This prevents receptor dimerization, blocks receptor–ligand interactions, and thereby inhibits growth signals to the malignant cell (17,18). Daclizumab (anti-Tac), with specificity for the α-chain of the interleukin (IL)-2 receptor, inhibits T-lymphocyte proliferation by blocking the interaction of the IL-2 cytokine with its growth factor receptor (19). It was approved in 1997 for the prevention of renal allograft rejection and has since shown efficacy in select T-cell malignancies and some inflammatory autoimmune disorders (20).

When used in conjunction with chemotherapy or conventional external beam radiation, the addition of a mAb has resulted in a greater therapeutic effect in numerous settings. Preclinical studies in animal models have served to confirm this, as anti-HER-2 mAbs in combination with external beam radiation have resulted in therapeutic efficacy where radiation or mAb alone had minimal effect on tumor xenografts (21). In patients with advanced breast cancer, trastuzumab combined with paclitaxel or doxorubicin enhanced both rates of response and duration of response (22). As mAbs are further investigated with respect to standard chemotherapeutic and radiation regimens, a better understanding of their utility will emerge.

THERAPEUTIC RADIOISOTOPES

Disease burden is a critical consideration when considering the most appropriate radionuclide for RIT treatment, and no single radionuclide can address every therapeutic need. In general, targeting micrometastatic or a minimal disease volume appears to hold the most promise for successful RIT of the less radiosensitive, heterogeneous solid tumors. Fractionation of RIT is currently being investigated, and work has suggested that fractionated RIT may also improve therapeutic responses (23). As the limitations of the radiolabeled mAb in terms of biodistribution and pharmacokinetics become more clearly defined, a rational plan for future clinical trials will ultimately follow. One must consider the important physical properties such as emission type, energy and range of emission, and the radionuclide half-life when choosing a therapeutic radionuclide. A diverse library of radionuclides is available (Table 5.2). Particulate emissions include particulate α particles (helium nuclei), β^- particles (negative electrons), positrons (positive electrons, β^+ particles), and Auger electrons. Historically, β^- emitters have received the greatest attention, and the use of β^- emitters continues to dominate preclinical and clinical trials; Zevalin and Bexxar are both armed with β^- emitters, although their physical properties are very different indeed (vide infra).

The emission path lengths of β^- emitters are long, with a maximum range of 500–600 nm and average range of 275 nm (for ^{90}Y) (24,25). The path lengths associated with a given radionuclide are determined by the spectrum (not a defined value) of its β^- emission energy, and the ability to target an entire lesion

TABLE 5.2 Physical properties of select radionuclides utilized for RIT (Kocher 1981; Milenic et al 2004)

Radionuclide	Emisson Type	Emisson Energy (keV)	Average Emission Range (mm)	Half Life (hr)
90Y	β-	935 (β)	3.78	64.08
131I	γ / β-	182 (β)	0.36	192.96
177Lu	γ / β-	133 (β)	0.22	161.04
67Cu	γ / β-	141 (β)	0.24	61.92
212Bi	α / β- / γ	6090 (α)	0.04–0.1	1.01
213Bi	α / β-	5870 (α)	0.04–0.1	0.76
211At	α	5867 (α)	0.04–0.1	7.21
149Tb	α	3967 (α)	0.04–0.1	4.12
125I	γ / Auger	35.49 (γ)	<0.02	1443.4
111In	γ / Auger	171.3 (γ)	<0.02	67.31

becomes possible when the particle emission range exceeds the radius of the lesion (26). In general, β^- emitters travel long distances before dissipating their kinetic energy, and this low linear energy transfer (LET) results in energy deposition that takes place at a distance from the actual decay event. Thus, a degree of irradiation occurs in neighboring receptor-negative tumor and normal cells (27). This therapeutic benefit is referred to as "crossfire," where the targeted cell is not necessarily the effective target of the decay event. The ability to bypass tumor antigen heterogeneity through the differential penetration of the labeled mAb is the great advantage of β^- emitters. On the other hand, one important limitation is that β^- emitters cannot adequately treat micrometastatic disease as their dose is distributed elsewhere (27). Comparing the radionuclides found in Zevalin and Bexxar, ^{90}Y has a pure β^- emission that delivers a more energetic tumor–killing β^- emission of 935 keV versus 182 keV of ^{131}I. ^{90}Y also has a longer average emission range (3.78 mm) as compared to ^{131}I (0.36 mm), and the majority its decay energy is deposited in targets with a diameter of at least 1 cm (24). The longer emission range associated with ^{90}Y may result in a significant degree of irradiation of normal surrounding tissue, and myelosuppression is a consistent dose-limiting toxicity (28). Unlike ^{90}Y, ^{131}I has a γ emission which, while useful for imaging, also contributes to normal tissue toxicity, thus serving to further illustrate the desires and compromises that must be balanced in the schema of RIT. The lower-energy β-emitters, ^{177}Lu and ^{67}Cu, provide the distinct advantage of treating smaller lesions as they possess shorter emission ranges. ^{177}Lu and ^{67}Cu have both been evaluated in clinical trials for therapeutic efficacy (29,30). Both radionuclides possess imageable γ emissions, permitting determination of disease extent, calculation and prediction of dosimetry, and monitoring of therapeutic efficacy. Tumor sizes have been analyzed in computational models for therapeutic efficacy with respect to the various available particle ranges, with optimal diameters ranging from less than 1 mm for short-range emitters and up to several centimeters for long-range emitters such as ^{90}Y (26). Other investigations are focusing on β-particle combinations in efforts to uniformly target lesions, and a successful ^{177}Lu/^{90}Y combination has been reported (31).

α-particles are large, with high energies of several million electron volts (MeV) that travel short distances of less than 100 μm (32). The very dense emission path lengths and dose rates of 1 cGy/hr make the high LET α-emitters exquisitely cytotoxic (33). Additionally, the relative biologic effectiveness (RBE) of high-LET radiation is not dependent on dose rate or oxygenation of the environment. A very low number (one to three) of nuclear traversals are all that is required to inflict irreparable double-strand DNA breaks with an α-emitter (34). Compared with β-emitters, the LET is approximately 400 times greater (~100 versus 0.2 keV/μm) with energy deposition taking place immediately at the tumor site and not within the surrounding normal tissue (27). The short emission range limits their use to micrometastatic disease, with efficacy resulting from the direct emission of the α-particle at the targeted cell and immediate neighboring cells. The short physical half-life and emission path length has generally been thought to limit the use of α-emitters to leukemias, highly vascularized tumors, and occult disease, all in efforts to optimize access, targeting time, and appropriate disease converge. Half-life constraints make the list of α-emitting radionuclides available for RIT short. Currently ^{212}Bi, ^{213}Bi, ^{211}At, and ^{149}Tb are actively being studied (35–37). The bismuth radioisotopes ^{212}Bi and ^{213}Bi are achieved from generators based on the parent isotopes ^{212}Pb or ^{225}Ac, respectively. The isotopes decay via branched pathways, resulting in both α- and β-emissions (38). ^{212}Bi is generally considered a more attractive candidate for RIT as 32% of ^{212}Bi decay is high-energy γ emissions, whereas ^{213}Bi decay lacks γ emission (39). The use of α-emitters in the treatment of hematologic cancers, myeloablative protocols prior to bone marrow transplant, or in the setting of disease present at the surface of cavities, such as intraperitoneal carcinomatosis, may ultimately prove beneficial (36,40,41).

Auger electrons are extremely low-energy atomic orbital electrons emitted as an alternative to x-ray emission following electron capture, a form of β^- decay (42,43). This emission is a useful strategy for specific tumor cell kill on a subcellular (nm) level and highly localized energy deposition (10^6–10^9 cGy) in an extremely small volume (several nm^3) around the decay site (44). Auger electron emitters produce an array of reactive radicals (e.g., OH·, H·, e^-_{aq},) similar to the high-LET α-emitters. Auger emitters have received the least attention with respect to RIT due to the fact that their emissions must occur within the cell nucleus (45–47). The estimated absorbed dose rate at the center of a cell delivered by ^{99m}Tc, ^{123}I, ^{111}In, ^{67}Ga, and ^{201}Tl is 94, 21, 18, 74, and 76 times higher, respectively, if the radioactivity is localized within the nucleus as opposed to on the cell membrane (48). Compared to standard β-emitters, the auger emitters ^{125}I and ^{111}In have shown better therapeutic results when conjugated with internalizing mAbs (49). Current work is attempting to bypass the nuclear localization requirement of auger electron emitters by utilizing nuclear localization peptides (50,51).

CONJUGATION: JOINING THE RADIONUCLIDE TO THE MONOCLONAL ANTIBODY

Monoclonal antibodies are joined to radionuclides through protocols based on the chemical characteristics of the radionuclide itself. The overall goal of any radiolabeling procedure is to create a stable radiolabeled product without affecting the immunoreactivity of the mAb. However, the process must also be sufficiently affordable, reproducible, and efficient. All metallic radionuclides require chelation chemistry for attachment to a mAb. By contrast, halogens such as ^{131}I, ^{125}I, ^{124}I, and ^{123}I are routinely introduced by direct radioiodination of tyrosine moieties of the mAb. The mAb in Bexxar, tositumomab, is radiolabeled with ^{131}I by direct halogenation. The ease and familiarity of direct radioiodination comes at the cost of lysosomal degradation to mono- or di-iodotyrosine species, which are released from cells. This phenomenon is bypassed when a radiometal is chemically conjugated to the mAb, as the radiometals are residualized intracellularly if the mAb is internalized. Better therapeutic results with radiometals as compared to radioiodine have also been demonstrated (49,52). Metallic radionuclides, such as ^{111}In or ^{90}Y, require a bifunctional chelator for conjugation to the mAb. Bifunctional chelating agents (BCA) are chemical moieties possessing specific functional groups that permit the conjugation of the mAb to stable metallic radionuclide complexes. This chelating agent frequently targets *N*-terminal and ε-amines of lysine residues (53). For example, ^{90}Y is chelated by tiuxetan, which is covalently linked to lysine residues of the IgG ibritumomab by thiourea bonds. While the actual radiolabeling protocols are beyond the scope of this text, numerous chemical criteria must be considered in the choice of the BCA with respect to the characteristics of the radionuclide (namely half-life), thermodynamic stability, and formation kinetics (54). There are a number of BCA agents, including cyclic and acyclic forms, which have been studied with numerous radionuclides under various conditions in preclinical studies.

CLINICAL RESULTS: NON-HODGKIN'S LYMPHOMA

Bexxar (^{131}I-tositumab) and Zevalin (^{90}Y-ibritumomab tiuxetan) are both murine antibodies directed against the CD20 antigen present on more than 90% of malignant B lymphocytes (55) and normal B cells. Currently, they are the only radiolabeled antibodies that have consistently shown efficacy in clinical studies and have gained FDA approved for the treatment of low-grade (follicular) NHL, with or without transformation. Studies in pretreated, chemotherapy-resistant patients with low-grade follicular and transformed NHL revealed a response rate of 65% versus 28% for the last chemotherapy and a complete response of 30% for Bexxar (56). In clinical trials investigating patients with recurring or refractory NHL, Zevalin has shown an overall response rate between 73% and 83% (57–60). Bexxar is composed of the labeled IgG_{2a} tositumab antibody, and Zevalin contains the labeled IgG1 chimeric Rituxan (rituximab); both preparations utilize a pretreatment infusion of the naked mAb in efforts to saturate CD20 sites on normal B lymphocytes, which improves the biodistribution of the radiolabeled moiety (61,62). These agents have demonstrated higher and more durable responses with a combination of the labeled and unlabeled, as compared to either treatment alone, suggesting that the unlabeled antibody contributes to the antitumor response of the labeled form (63). Prior to Bexxar administration, thyroid blockade is required due to the systemic release of ^{131}I, and pretreatment dosimetry is utilized. Zevalin is administered on a body weight basis without prerequisite dosimetry.

Dose-limiting toxicity is myelosuppression, which is usually supportable and reversible. Utilizing myeloablative doses of Bexxar combined with peripheral blood stem cell (PBSC) support, investigators observed complete responses in 79% of patients with an overall objective response rate of 86% (64,65). Notably, 39% of patients survived free of recurrence and not requiring further therapy for 5–10 years (65). Reported long-term toxicities associated with RIT include hypothyroidism (Bexxar), myelodysplasia (MDS), and secondary malignancy including acute myelogenous leukemia (AML). However, a multivariate cohort analysis of relapsed follicular NHL patients revealed a 0.076 probability of developing MDS/AML at 8 years after treatment with myeloablative dose of ^{131}I anti-CD20 IgG, as compared to 0.086 at 7 years for those receiving high-dose chemotherapy (66). This suggests that the overall risk of developing MDS/AML is no higher than the risk associated with conventional high-dose chemotherapeutic regimens. In patients previously treated with chemotherapy, the HAMA response is blunted, but it can be significant in those who are chemotherapy naïve, as seen in approximately 60% of those treated with Bexxar (67). Notably, a phase II trial of Bexxar in untreated low-grade or transformed NHL showed a 63% complete response with an overall objective response rate of 97%, suggesting that those without a significant pretreatment history respond well to Bexxar without late toxicity (67).

In general, both preparations have been studied as a single cycle therapy; however, there are several reports of retreatment in patients previously treated with other forms of RIT (68–70). Additionally, Ansell and associates reported standard doses of chemotherapy safely administered to patients previously treated with nonmyeloablative doses of RIT, without an increase in the number or severity of side effects (71). Conversely, Press and associates reported a phase II trial in which Bexxar was administered 4–6 weeks after standard CHOP chemotherapy and noted that reversible myelosuppression was the main adverse event, which was more severe during chemotherapy than following radioimmunotherapy (72). Other investigations have sought to establish the safety of combining RIT with existing chemotherapy regimens. When myeloablative doses of Bexxar were studied in combination with etoposide and cyclophosphamine, followed by autologous stem cell transplantation, a 68% and 83% progression-free survival rate and overall survival rate, respectively, was observed at 2 years (73). Notably, the control group, which received total body irradiation, had a 36% and 53% progression-free survival rate and overall survival rate, respectively. These results and those of ongoing studies may establish a feasible, well-tolerated, and efficacious regimen consisting of multiple cycles and/or combinations of RIT with established chemotherapy with the overall goal of improving response and overall outcomes.

CLINICAL RESULTS: THE SOLID TUMORS

Whereas RIT of low-grade follicular lymphoma is quickly becoming an established and valid treatment modality, solid tumor studies to date have yielded modest results, with most favorable terms described as partial, short-lived responses. Perhaps some of the disappointing results can be attributed to the specifics of the patient population studied, as most phase I/II clinical trials investigate safety and efficacy in patients with advanced or bulky disease and in those who have failed other therapies. Indeed it is becoming recognized that the future of RIT with respect to solid tumors lies in very specific settings, such as in the setting of low-burden and occult disease or as an adjuvant therapy within other established chemotherapeutic regimens, or in the context of easily compartmentalized disease (cranial, peritoneal, etc.). Despite the fact that solid tumor–to-blood ratios as high as 30:1 have been reported, radiation-absorbed doses are generally far less than that needed for therapeutic efficacy, with tumor doses often <1,500 cGy (8). Specific constraints with respect to tumor biology that may explain insufficient tumor response include a higher radioresistance of solid tumors; inherent barriers of macromolecular entry into solid tumors with resulting slow uptake, such as heterogeneity of receptor expression; and varying levels of vascularity within the tumor itself. These constraints equate to longer blood circulation times and narrowing of the therapeutic index. Despite lackluster results of numerous clinical trials, solid tumor RIT has had some promising results and its utility will be more clearly defined in the near future. A brief review of some of the notable RIT studies in colorectal cancer, medullary thyroid cancer, lung cancer, gliomas, and breast cancer will briefly be described.

Colorectal Cancer

Goldenberg and colleagues first used ^{131}I-labeled polyclonal anti-CEA Abs in efforts to treat patients with recurrent CEA-positive adenocarcinomas. Since then, a number of phase I and phase II clinical trials have investigated the role of RIT in the treatment of colorectal cancer. Targeted epitopes include the transmembrane glycoprotein A33, CEA, and TAG-72. Perhaps the most promising RIT results have been obtained following salvage resection of hepatic metastasis. Complete resection of liver metastases is considered the gold standard of care for patients with hepatic involvement. In a recent report, 23 patients received a single treatment of ^{131}I-labetuzumab (a humanized mAb targeting CEA), after undergoing resection of hepatic colorectal cancer metastases (74). From the time of the first liver resection, patients in the RIT arm had a median overall survival time of 68.0 months with a median disease-free survival of 18.0 months. Notably, the 5-year survival rate was 51.3% for adjuvant RIT, as compared to 33% for those patients who underwent complete resection of hepatic metastasis alone. Radioimmunotherapy benefited patients independently of bilobar involvement, size and number metastasis, and resection margins. Transient myelosuppression was the major reported side effect. Compared to the expected outcomes of partial hepatectomy alone, these results are promising but require further investigation in multicenter, randomized trials.

Medullary Thyroid Cancer

The expression of CEA on metastatic medullary thyroid carcinoma (MTC) cells has led to several RIT investigations. In a notable early study, two different types of ^{131}I-labeled murine anti-CEA antibodies, NP-4 and MN-14 F(ab)2, were given to a total of 18 patients with advanced MTC, resulting in 50% of the patients showing evidence of antitumor effects lasting up to 26 months (75). Recent investigations have focused on the development of radiolabeled anti-CEA bispecific mAbs (BsmAbs) for RIT under a pretargeted schema. In general, pretargeting involves the sequential delivery of the BsmAb to the tumor followed by administration of a radiolabeled hapten, which specifically binds to the tumor-targeted BsmAb. In a recent clinical trial, 29 patients with advanced, progressive MTC, characterized by short serum calcitonin doubling times, received an anti-CEA/anti-diethylenetriamine pentaacetic acid (DTPA)-indium BsmAb, followed by a ^{131}I-labeled bivalent hapten (76). As compared to the untreated MTC population, overall survival was significantly longer in the RIT treated group, with a median time of 110 versus 61 months, respectively. Patients with bone marrow involvement had a 10-year overall survival of 83%, significantly longer than that observed in patients without marrow involvement (10-year overall survival, 14%). A biologic response, defined as a serum calcitonin doubling time increase of more than 100%, was noted in 47% of the RIT patients. Interestingly, this subset of patients experienced considerably longer survival as opposed to the nonbiologic responders, with a median overall survival over 159 versus 109 months, respectively, or as compared to the non-RIT treated patients who experienced a median overall survival of 61 months. Additionally, in the subset of patients with calcitonin doubling times of less than 2 years, as compared with similarly high-risk untreated patients, improved overall survival and long-term disease stabilization was noted. Toxicity was primarily hematologic suppression. Results of this study have suggested the importance of calcitonin doubling times and bone-marrow involvement as prognostic indicators in MTC patients undergoing RIT.

Lung Carcinoma

^{131}I-labeled tumor necrosis treatment (TNT), a recombinant chimeric murine mAb that targets a universal, intracellular antigen exposed in the necrotic core of malignant solid tumors, has been reported in the successful management of a number of solid lung tumors. These results were noted to be independent of the location or type of malignancy studied. In a recent multicenter study, 107 patients with advanced or refractory lung carcinoma were treated with systemic or direct intratumoral injections of ^{131}I-TNT, including 97 patients with non-small cell lung (NSCL) carcinoma (77). Results demonstrated an overall response rate of 34.6% in the population studied and approximately 33% in the subset of patients with NSCL cancer. Complete responses, partial responses, no change in disease burden, and progressive disease were 3.7%, 30.8%, 55.1%, and 10.3% of the studied population, respectively. The most prominent toxicity was bone marrow suppression, which was noted to be minor and usually reversible. Obviously, additional trials are necessary to define the clinical role of this radioimmunoconjugate in patients with advanced lung disease.

Malignant Gliomas

Traditionally, gliomas have been treated with cytoreductive surgery, external-beam irradiation, and systemic chemotherapy. Despite the many modalities of treatment available, long-term results are disappointing due to tumor invasion into functional brain, chemoresistance, and, with respect to systemically delivered chemotherapy, the blood–brain barrier. As brain tumors rarely metastasize outside the craniospinal axis in the adult, locoregional RIT has been evaluated to treat glioblastoma multiforme (GBM) under the protocol of direct administration into surgically created resection cavities. This technique allows delivery of a highly localized radiation dose to residual tumor while minimizing exposure to normal brain. As previously described in the treatment of lung carcinoma, TNT (^{131}I-chTNT) has also been investigated in RIT applications for the treatment of GBM. A more specific target is tenascin-C (TN-C), an extracellular matrix glycoprotein expressed ubiquitously in high-grade gliomas, but absent in normal brain parenchyma. 81C6, a murine IgG_{2b} mAb, binds to this epitope within the alternatively spliced fibronectin type III region of TN-C, and intratumoral administration of ^{131}I-81C6 has shown promise in a phase I trial (78). In a more recent phase II study, the efficacy and toxicity of this ^{131}I-81C6 infused directly into the resection cavity was assessed in 33 patients with previously untreated malignant glioma (79). Median survival for all glioma patients and GBM patients was 86.7 weeks and 79.4 weeks, respectively. Even after accounting for established prognostic factors, these results exceed historic controls who were treated with conventional radiotherapy and chemotherapy. Reversible hematologic toxicity was observed in 27% of the population, symptomatic neurologic toxicity occurred in 15%, and a single patient required reoperation for radionecrosis. In another series of 43 patients with locally recurrent malignant brain tumors treated with 100 mCi of ^{131}I-m81C6 injected directly into a surgically created resection cavity, 63% of patients with GBM were alive at 1 year. Median overall survival for this group was 64 weeks (80). The results of this study showed a median survival that is greater than that of historical controls treated with surgery plus ^{125}I-brachytherapy. All these results serve to confirm the efficacy of ^{131}I-labeled 81C6 for patients with malignant gliomas and require a randomized phase III study for further evaluation.

Breast Cancer

Breast cancer RIT is being evaluated in multiple preclinical and clinical studies targeting MUC1, CEA, and L6. Monoclonal, humanized anti-MUC1 Abs, including BrE-3 and m170, have been studied in a number of different RIT settings. In a recent clinical trial, eight of 17 patients (47%) showed significant clinical response despite failing previous conventional therapies (81). The anti-MUC1 mAb, m170, radiolabeled with ^{90}Y has progressed to dosimetric studies with quantifiable tumor regression and partial responses (82). Synergistic effects in preclinical models with a combination of humanized ^{90}Y-labeled BrE-3 and capecitabine have been reported (83). While CEA was originally thought to be a specific colon cancer marker, it has been shown to be expressed in normal tissue and in multiple cancers, including breast carcinomas. NP-4, a murine anti-CEA antibody, labeled with ^{131}I, resulted in therapeutic responses in a phase I/II study (84). Modest antitumor activity was observed in 12 of 35 suitable patients treated with ^{131}I-NP-4, including one partial remission, four minor/mixed responses, and seven cases of stabilization of progressing disease. Finally, the L6 cell surface antigen is highly expressed in breast cancer and is related to a number of cell surface proteins implicated in cell growth. ^{90}Y-DOTA-peptide-ChL6 resulted in excellent tumor targeting and an effective therapeutic response in a number of different settings including when used alone (85); or when combined with an $\alpha_v\beta_3$-integrin inhibitor (86), paclitaxel (87), anti-EGFR mAb (88), or with a bcl-2 antisense oligonucleotide.

■ CONCLUSIONS

Radioimmunotherapy is becoming recognized as a feasible, safe, and efficacious treatment for NHL, and the FDA approval of Zevalin and Bexxar has fueled enthusiasm for the development of additional radiolabeled mAb therapeutics. However, actual clinical knowledge of the use of radiolabeled mAbs remains in its infancy, especially with respect to RIT's role for the treatment of solid tumors, in specific tumor settings, fractionated dosing, and integration within established chemotherapy regimens and external beam protocols. The successes of RIT in the field of the hematologic malignancies reflect the inherent accessibility and radiosensitivity of these cancers. Certainly, for solid tumors, the literature supports mAb-based therapies when applied in specific settings, such as the treatment of minimal residual micrometastatic disease and as an adjuvant component of a multimodality treatment regimen. Indeed, previous irrational investigations with poor targeting agents, suboptimal chelation chemistry, and poor radionuclide choice, in heavily pretreated or resistant or relapsed patients with gross, bulky disease have confounded results. However, this cumulative knowledge has aided the continuing efforts to refine and optimize all of the components of RIT and will improve efficacy and minimize toxicity. Presently, we stand to ultimately realize the full utility of radiolabeled mAbs in the field of oncology.

REFERENCES

1. Ehrlich P, et al. (1904) Ueber einige verwendungen der naphtochinosuflsaure. *Z Physiol Chem* 61:379–392.
2. Pressman D. Tissue localizing antibodies. *Ann NY Acad Sci* 1955;59(3):376–380.
3. Mach JP, Carrel S, Merenda C, et al. In vivo localization of radiolabeled antibodies to carcinoembryonic antigen in human colon carcinoma grafted into nude mice. *Nature* 1974;248(450):704–706.
4. Goldenberg DM, Preston DF, Primus FJ, Hansen HJ. Photoscan localization of GW-39 tumors in hamsters using radiolabeled anticarcinoembryonic antigen immunoglobulin G. *Cancer Res* 1974;34(1):1–9.
5. Schlom J. Monoclonal antibodies: They're more and less than you think. In: Broder S, ed. *Molecular Foundations of Oncology*. Williams and Wilkins: Baltimore, MD;1990:95–134.
6. Milenic DE. Radioimmunotherapy: Designer molecules to potentiate effective therapy. *Semin Radiat Oncol* 2000;10:139–155.
7. Baker M. Upping the ante on antibodies. *Nat Biotechnol* 2005;23(9):1065–1072.
8. Boswell CA, Brechbiel MW. Development of radioimmunotherapeutic and diagnostic antibodies: An inside-out view. *Nucl Med Biol* 2007;34(7):757–778.
9. Srivastava S, Dadachova E. Recent advances in radionuclide therapy. *Semin Nucl Med* 2001;31:330–341.
10. Trauth B, et al. Monoclonal antibody-mediated tumor regression by induction of apoptosis. *Science* 1989;245:301–305.
11. Baselga J, Mendelsohn J. Receptor blockade with monoclonal antibodies as anti-cancer therapy. *Pharmacol Ther* 1984;64:127–154.
12. Clynes RA, et al. Inhibitory Fc receptors modulate in vivo cytoxicity against tumor targets. *Nat Med* 2000;6:443–446.
13. Johnson P, Glennie M. The mechanisms of action of rituximab in the elimination of tumor cells. *Semin Oncol* 2003;30:3–8.
14. Cragg MS, et al. Signaling antibodies in cancer therapy. *Curr Opin Immunol* 1999;11:541–547.

15. Deans JP, et al. Association of tyrosine and serine kinases with the B cell surface antigen CD20. Induction via CD20 of tyrosine phosphorylation and activation of phospholipase C-gamma 1 and PLC phospholipase C-gamma 2. *J Immunol* 1993;151:4494–4504.
16. Maloney DG, et al. IDEC-C2B8 (Rituximab) anti-CD20 monoclonal antibody therapy in patients with relapsed low-grade non-Hodgkin's lymphoma. *Blood* 1998;90:2188–2195.
17. Sarup JC, et al. Characterization of an anti-p185HER2 monoclonal antibody that stimulates receptor function and inhibits tumor cell growth. *Growth Regul* 1991;1:72–82.
18. Uchiyama T, et al. A monoclonal antibody (anti-Tac) reactive with activated and functionally mature human T cells. II. Expression of Tac antigen on activated cytotoxic killer T cells, suppressor cells, and on one of two types of helper T cells. *J Immunol* 1981;126:1398–1340.
19. Goldenberg DM. Trastuzumab, a recombinant DNA-derived humanized monoclonal antibody, a novel agent for the treatment of metastatic breast cancer. *Clin Ther* 1999;21:309–318.
20. Waldmann TA. Daclizumab (anti-Tac, Zenapax) in the treatment of leukemia/lymphoma. *Oncogene* 2007;26:3699–3703.
21. Pietras RJ, et al. Monoclonal antibody to HER-2/neuroceptor modulates repair of radiation-induced DNA damage and enhances radiosensitivity of human breast cancer cells overexpressing this oncogene. *Cancer Res* 1999;59:1347–1355.
22. Hortobagyi GN, Perez EA. Integration of trastuzumab into adjuvant systemic therapy of breast cancer: Ongoing and planned clinical trials. *Semin Oncol* 2001;28:41–46.
23. DeNardo GL, Schlom J, Buchsbaum DJ, et al. Rationales, evidence, and design considerations for fractionated radioimmunotherapy. *Cancer* 2002;94(Suppl):1332–1348.
24. Kocher DC. Radioactive decay tables. Office of Scientific and Technical Information. Washington DC: U.S. Department of Energy:1981.
25. Milenic DE, et al. Antibody targeted radiation cancer therapy. *Nat Rev Drug Discov* 2004;6:488–499.
26. O'Donoghue JA, et al. Relationships between tumor size and curability for uniformly targeted therapy with beta-emitting radionuclides. *J Nucl Med* 1995;36:1902–1909.
27. Humm JL. Dosimetric aspects of radiolabeled antibodies for tumor therapy. *J Nucl Med* 1986;27:1490–1497.
28. Knox SJ, Meredith RF. Clinical radioimmunotherapy. *Semin Radiat Oncol* 2000;10:73–93.
29. Mulligan T, et al. Phase I study of intravenous Lu-labeled CC49 murine monoclonal antibody in patients with advanced adenocarcinoma. *Clin Cancer Res* 1995;1:1447–1454.
30. Alvarez RD, et al. Intraperitoneal radioimmunotherapy of ovarian cancer with 177Lu-CC49: A Phase I/II study. *Gynecol Oncol* 1997;65:94–101.
31. de Jong M, Breeman WA, Valkema R, et al. Combination radionuclide therapy using 177Lu- and 90Y-labeled somatostatin analogs. *J Nucl Med* 2005;46(Suppl 1):S13–S17.
32. Behr TM, et al. High-linear energy transfer (LET) α versus Low-LET β emitters in radioimmunotherapy of solid tumors: Therapeutic efficacy and dose-limiting toxicity of ^{213}Bi- versus ^{90}Y-labeled CO17-1A Fab' fragments in a human colonic cancer model. *Cancer Res* 1999;59:2635–2643.
33. Kurtzman SH, et al. ^{212}Bismuth linked to an antipancreatic carcinoma antibody: Model for alpha-particle-emitter radioimmunotherapy. *J Natl Cancer Inst* 1988;80:449–452.
34. Allen BJ, Raja C, Rizvi S, et al. Targeted alpha therapy for cancer. *Phys Med Biol* 2004;49:3703–3712.
35. McDevitt MR, et al. Radioimmunotherapy with alpha-emitting nuclides. *Eur J Nucl Med* 1988;25:1341–1351.

36. Hassfjell S, Brechbiel MW. The development of the α-particle emitting radionuclides ^{212}Bi and ^{213}Bi for therapeutic applications. *Chem Rev* 2001;101:2019–2036.
37. Allen BJ, Rizvi S, Li Y, et al. *In vitro* and pre-clinical targeted alpha therapy for melanoma, breast, prostate and colorectal cancers. *Crit Rev Oncol Hematol* 2001;39:139–146.
38. Milenic DE. Monoclonal antibody-based therapy strategies: Providing options for the cancer patient. *Curr Pharm Design* 2002;8:1749–1764.
39. Geerlings MW. Radionuclides for radioimmunotherapy: Criteria for selection. *Int J Biol Markers* 1993;8:180–186.
40. Bethge WA, et al. Selective T-cell ablation with bismuth-213 labeled anti-TCRαβ as nonmyeloablative conditioning for allogeneic canine marrow transplantation. *Blood* 2003;101:5068–5075.
41. Hartmann F, et al. Radioimmunotherapy of nude mice bearing a human IL2Rγ-expressing lymphoma utilizing the α-emitting radionuclide-conjugated monoclonal antibody ^{212}Bi-anti-Tac. *Cancer Res* 1994;54:4362–34370.
42. Kassis AI, et al. Kinetics of uptake, retention, and radiotoxicity of I-125 UDR in mammalian cells - implications of localized energy deposition by auger processes. *Radiat Res* 1987;109(1):78–89.
43. Kassis AI. The amazing world of auger electrons. *Int J Radiat Biol* 2004;80(11–12):789–803.
44. Goddu SM, et al. Multicellular Dosimetry for micrometastases: Dependence of self-dose versus cross-dose to cell nuclei on type and energy of radiation and subcellular distribution of radionuclides. *J Nucl Med* 1994;35(3):521–530.
45. Kassis AI, et al. Comparison of strand breaks in plasmid DNA after positional changes of auger electron-emitting iodine-125. *Radiat Res* 1999;151:167–176.
46. Makrigiorgos G, et al. Auger electron emitters: insights gained from in vitro experiments. *Radiat Environ Biophys* 1990;29:75–91.
47. Michel RB, et al. A comparison of radionuclides conjugated to antibodies for single-cell kill. *J Nucl Med* 2003;44:632–640.
48. Faraggi M, et al. The influence of tracer localization on the electron dose rate delivered to the cell nucleus. *J Nucl Med* 1994;35(1):113–119.
49. Behr TM, et al. Therapeutic Advantages of auger electron- over β-emitting radiometals or radioiodine when conjugated to internalizing antibodies. *Eur J Nucl Med* 2000;27(7):753–765.
50. Boswell CA, Brechbiel MW. Auger electrons: Lethal, low energy, and coming soon to a tumor cell nucleus near you. *J Nucl Med* 2005;46:1946–1947.
51. Ginj M, et al. Trifunctional somatostatin-based derivatives designed for targeted radiotherapy using auger electron emitters. *J Nucl Med* 2005;46:2097–2103.
52. Mattes MJ, et al. The advantage of residualizing radiolabels for targeting B-cell lymphomas with a radiolabeled anti-CD-22 monoclonal antibody. *Int J Cancer* 1997;71:429–435.
53. Milenic DE, et al. In vivo comparison of macrocyclic and acyclic ligands for radiolabeling of monoclonal antibodies with ^{177}Lu for radioimmunotherapeutic applications. *Nucl Med Biol* 2002;29:431–442.
54. Packard AB, et al. Metalloradiopharmaceuticals. In: Clarke MJ, Sadler PJ, eds. A Metallor adiopharmaceuticals II, Diagnosis and Therapy. NY, Springer-Verlag;1999:45–116.
55. Anderson KC, Bates MP, Slaughenhoupt BL, et al. Expression of human B cell-associated antigens on leukemias and lymphomas: A model of human B cell differentiation. *Blood* 1984;63:1424–1433.
56. Kamisnski M, Zelenetz AD, Press O, et al. Multicenter, phase III study of iodine-131 tositumab (anti-B1 antibody) for chemotherapy-refractory low-grade or transformed low-grade non-Hodgkin's lymphoma (Abstract 1296). *Blood* 1998;92:1296.

57. Witzig TE, Flinn IW, Gordon LI, et al. Treatment with ibritumomab tiuxetan radioimmunotherapy in patients with rituximab-refractory follicular non-Hodgkin's lymphoma. *J Clin Oncol* 2002;20:3262–3269.
58. Gordon LI, Molina A, Witzig T, et al. Durable responses after ibritumomab tiuxetan radioimmunotherapy for CD20+ B-cell lymphoma: Long-term follow-up of a phase 1/2 study. *Blood* 2004;103:4429–4431.
59. Witzig TE, Gordon LI, Cabanillas F, et al. Randomized controlled trial of yttrium-90-labeled ibritumomab tiuxetan radioimmunotherapy versus rituximab immunotherapy for patients with relapsed or refractory low-grade, follicular, or transformed B-cell non-Hodgkin's lymphoma. *J Clin Oncol* 2002;20:2453–2463.
60. Witzig TE, White CA, Wiseman GA, et al. Phase I/II trial of IDEC-Y2B8 radioimmunotherapy for treatment of relapsed or refractory CD20 (+) B-cell non-Hodgkin's lymphoma. *J Clin Oncol* 1999;17:3793–3803.
61. Knox SJ, Goris ML, Trisler K, et al. Yttrium-90-labeled anti-CD20 monoclonal antibody therapy of recurrent B-cell lymphoma. *Clin Cancer Res* 1996;2(3):457–470.
62. Wagner HN Jr., Wiseman GA, Marcus CS, et al. Administration guidelines for radioimmunotherapy of non-Hodgkin's lymphoma with (90) Y-labeled anti-CD20 monoclonal antibody. *J Nucl Med* 2002;43:267–272.
63. Du Y, Honeychurch J, Cragg MS, et al. Antibody- induced intracellular signaling works in combination with radiation to eradicate lymphoma in radioimmunotherapy. *Blood* 2004;103:1485–1494.
64. Press OW, Eary JF, Applebaum FR, et al. Phase II trial of 131-I-B1 (anti-CD20) antibody therapy with autologous stem cell transplantation for relapsed B cell lymphomas. *Lancet* 1995;346:336–340.
65. Press OW, Eary JF, Applebaum FR, et al. Radiolabeled- antibody therapy of B-cell lymphoma with autologous bone marrow support. *N Engl J Med* 1993;329:1219–1224.
66. Gopal AK, Gooley TA, Maloney DG, et al. High-dose radioimmunotherapy versus conventional high-dose therapy and autologous hematopoietic stem cell transplantation for relapsed follicular non-Hodgkin lymphoma: a multivariable cohort analysis. *Blood* 2003;102:2351–2357.
67. Wahl RL, Zasadny KR, Estes J, et al. Single center experience with iodine I131 tositumab radio-immunotherapy for previously untreated follicular lymphoma (FL) (Abstract 309). *J Nucl Med* 2000;41:78–79.
68. Kamisnski M, Estes J, Zasadny KR, et al. Radioimmunotherapy with iodine 131I tositumab for relapsed or refractory B-cell non-Hodgkin lymphoma: Updated results and long-term follow-up of the University of Michigan experience. *Blood* 2000;96:1259–1266.
69. Rana TM. Post Bexxar relapse in NHL responds to Zevalin and can be safely accomplished [Abstract]. *Proc Am Soc Clin Oncol* 2003;22:613.
70. Tsai DE, Maillard I, Schuster SJ, et al. Use of ibritumomab tiuxetan anti-CD20 radioimmunotherapy in a non-Hodgkin's lymphoma patient previously treated with a yttrium-90-labeled anti-CD22 monoclonal antibody. *Clin Lymphoma* 2003;4:56–59.
71. Ansell SM, Ristow KM, Haberman TM, et al. Subsequent chemotherapy regimens are well tolerated after radioimmunotherapy with yttrium-90 ibritumomab tiuxetan for non-Hodgkin's lymphoma. *J Clin Oncol* 2002;20:3885–3890.
72. Press OW, Unger JM, Braziel RM, et al. A phase II trial of CHOP chemotherapy followed by tositumab/iodine I 131 tositumab for previously untreated follicular non-Hodgkins lymphoma: Southwest Oncology Group Protocol S9911. *Blood* 2003;102:1606–1612.
73. Press OW, Eary JF, Gooley T, et al. A phase I/II trial of iodine-131 tositumab (anti-CD20), etoposide, cyclophosphamide, and autologous stem cell transplantation for relapsed B-cell lymphomas. *Blood* 2000;96:2934–2942.

74. Liersch T, Meller J, Kulle B, et al. Phase II trial of carcinoembryonic antigen radioimmunotherapy with 131I-labetuzumab after salvage resection of colorectal metastases in the liver: Five-year safety and efficacy results. *J Clin Oncol* 2005;23(27):6763–6770.
75. Juweid M, Sharkey RM, Behr T, et al. Radioimmunotherapy of medullary thyroid cancer with iodine-131-labeled anti-CEA antibodies. *J Nucl Med* 1996;37(6):905–911.
76. Chatal JF, Campion L, Kraeber-Bodere F, et al. Survival improvement in patients with medullary thyroid carcinoma who undergo pretargeted anti-carcinoembryonic-antigen radioimmunotherapy: A collaborative study with the French Endocrine Tumor Group. *J Clin Oncol* 2006;24(11):1705–1711.
77. Chen S, Yu L, Jiang C, et al. Pivotal study of iodine-131-labeled chimeric tumor necrosis treatment radioimmunotherapy in patients with advanced lung cancer. *J Clin Oncol* 2005;23(7):1538–1547.
78. Bigner DD, Brown M, Coleman RE, et al. Phase I studies of treatment of malignant gliomas and neoplastic meningitis with ^{131}I-radiolabeled monoclonal antibodies anti-tenascin 81C6 and anti-chondroitin proteoglycan Mel-14 F(ab')2 preliminary report. *J Neurooncol* 1995;24:109–122.
79. Reardon DA, Akabani G, Coleman RE, et al. Phase II trial of murine (131)I-labeled antitenascin monoclonal antibody 81C6 administered into surgically created resection cavities of patients with newly diagnosed malignant gliomas. *J Clin Oncol* 2002;20(5):1389–1397.
80. Reardon DA, Akabani G, Coleman RE, et al. Salvage radioimmunotherapy with murine iodine-131-labeled antitenascin monoclonal antibody 81C6 for patients with recurrent primary and metastatic malignant brain tumors: Phase II study results. *J Clin Oncol* 2006;24(1):115–122
81. DeNardo SJ, Richman CM, Goldstein DS, et al. Yttrium-90/Indium-111-DOTA-peptide-chimeric L6: Pharmacokinetics, dosimetry and initial results in patients with incurable breast cancer. *Anticancer Res* 1997;17:1735–1744.
82. Richman CM, DeNardo SJ, O'Donnell RT, et al. Combined modality radioimmunotherapy (RIT) in metastatic prostate and breast cancer using paclitaxel and a MUC-1 monoclonal antibody, m170, linked to ^{90}Y: A phase I trial. *J Clin Oncol* 2004;22(14S):2554.
83. Schrier DM, Stemmer SM, Johnson T, et al. High-dose ^{90}Y-Mx-diethylenetriaminepenta-acetic acid (DTPA)-BrE-3 and autologous hematopoietic stem cell support (AHSCS) for the treatment of advanced breast cancer: A phase I trial. *Cancer Res* 1995;55:S5921–S5924.
84. Behr TM, Sharkey RM, Juweid ME, et al. Phase I/II clinical radioimmunotherapy with an ^{131}I-labeled anti-carcinoembryonic antigen murine monoclonal antibody IgG. *J Nucl Med* 1997;38(6):858–870.
85. DeNardo GL, et al. Maximum tolerated dose of 67Cu-2IT-BAT-LYM-1 for fractionated radioimmunotherapy of non-Hodgkin's lymphoma: A pilot study. *Anticancer Res* 1998;18:2779–2788.
86. Burke PA, DeNardo SJ, Miers L, et al. Cilengitide targeting of alpha-v-beta-3 integrin receptor synergizes with radioimmunotherapy to increase efficacy and apoptosis in breast cancer xenografts. *Cancer Res* 2002;62:4263–4272.
87. DeNardo SJ, Kukis DL, Kroger LA, et al. Synergy of Taxol and radioimmunotherapy with ^{90}Y-labeled chimeric L6 antibody: Efficacy and toxicity in breast cancer xenografts. *Proc Natl Acad Sci USA* 1997;94:4000–4004.
88. Lee FT, Mountain AJ, Kelly MP, et al. Enhanced efficacy of radioimmunotherapy with ^{90}Y-CHX-A"-DTPA-hu3S193 by inhibition of epidermal growth factor receptor (EGFR) signaling with EGFR tyrosine kinase inhibitor AG1478. *Clin Cancer Res* 2005;11:S7080–S7086.

6 Targeted Therapies in Malignant Gliomas

SEAN GRIMM

The malignant gliomas [glioblastoma multiforme (GBM), anaplastic astrocytoma, anaplastic oligodendroglioma, and mixed oligoastrocytoma] are the most common primary brain tumors. With optimal treatment, median survival ranges from 14.6 months for GBM to 3–5 years for anaplastic oligodendroglioma (1–3). Radiotherapy is the most effective nonsurgical treatment (4). The small difference in sensitivity to radiotherapy between gliomas and normal glial tissue prohibits doses of external beam radiation large enough to cure. Combining cytotoxic chemotherapy with radiotherapy has improved outcome for several solid tumors, including GBM (2,5).

Although malignant gliomas display genetic heterogeneity, several key proliferation and survival signaling pathways have been identified (6). Recent work has focused on targeting these tumor-specific pathways in hopes of improving treatment efficacy and minimizing treatment toxicity. Because molecularly targeted agents have been mostly ineffective when used alone, combining them with radiotherapy is an appealing strategy (6).

■ VASCULAR ENDOTHELIAL GROWTH FACTOR PATHWAY INHIBITORS

Malignant gliomas are highly vascular tumors that depend on angiogenesis for growth and proliferation. Vascular endothelial growth factor (VEGF) pathway inhibitors were developed to inhibit tumor angiogenesis. Despite promising preclinical results, VEGF inhibitors failed to yield long-term survival benefits as single agents. Success has been achieved, however, by combining inhibitors of VEGF signaling with standard cytotoxic chemotherapy (7). Bevacizumab, an anti-VEGF antibody, has shown encouraging results when combined with irinotecan in a phase II trial for GBM (8,9). Based on a current hypothesis, VEGF inhibitors "normalize" abnormal tumor vasculature (10). Tumor blood vessels are structurally and functionally abnormal, contributing to a hostile microenvironment of low oxygen tension and high interstitial fluid pressure. This microenvironment promotes radioresistance and impairs delivery of chemotherapy (11). In animal models, VEGF inhibitors create a window of vascular "normalization" by passively pruning immature and leaky tumor vessels and actively remodeling the remaining vessels so that they resemble normal vasculature (12,13). Thus, by increasing tumor oxygenation, the response to radiation is enhanced.

Using magnetic resonance imaging techniques, Batchelor and colleagues demonstrated a "normalization window" for tumor vessels in recurrent GBM patients treated with daily cediranib (AZD2171), an oral tyrosine kinase (TK) inhibitor of VEGF receptors (VEGFRs) (14). The features of "vascular normalization" were maintained for at least 28 days, which suggests that combining radiotherapy or chemotherapy to cediranib during this window may prolong survival. An up-front phase II trial of combination cediranib, temozolomide, and radiotherapy is planned.

Mohile and colleagues performed a pilot study of bevacizumab and stereotactic intensity-modulated re-irradiation for recurrent high-grade gliomas (15). The authors demonstrated that the combination therapy was safe and well tolerated, with activity in recurrent glioma. An up-front phase II trial combining bevacizumab with temozolomide and radiotherapy followed by adjuvant bevacizumab and temozolomide is under way.

A phase I trial of the VEGFR TK inhibitor vatalanib, in combination with radiotherapy and temozolomide chemotherapy, has been reported, and a phase II portion is under way (16). A similar multicenter phase II trial with the combined VEGFR and epithelial growth factor receptor (EGFR) inhibitor vandetinib will soon begin accrual (17).

■ RAS SIGNALING

Radioresistance in gliomas may be mediated by radiation-resistant stem-like cells that repopulate the tumor after radiation via upregulation of the RAS pathway (18–20). Farnesyltransferase plays a critical role in the post-translational modification of RAS and other farnesyl protein transferases (21). Farnesyltransferase inhibitors have been shown to have radiosensitizing properties in preclinical models (20,22–24). The combination of radiotherapy and the farnesyltransferase inhibitors tipifarnib, perifosine, and lonafarnib are currently being studied in phase II clinical trials (17,25).

EPIDERMAL GROWTH FACTOR RECEPTOR

Epidermal growth factor receptor is a TK inhibitor involved in cellular proliferation. The EGFR gene is amplified in approximately 50% of GBMs and is overexpressed in malignant gliomas regardless of the amplification status (26). The most common mutated form in GBM is EGFRvIII, which is constitutively active in a ligand-independent manner because of a defect in the extracellular ligand-binding domain. EGFRvIII positivity is an independent, negative prognostic factor (27). The EGFR kinase inhibitors gefitinib and erlotinib have demonstrated minimal activity for patients with recurrent malignant gliomas. A Radiation Therapy Oncology Group (RTOG) phase I/II trial of 147 patients with newly diagnosed GBM investigated the combination of gefitinib and radiotherapy. The median survival was 11 months, which is comparable to historical controls receiving radiotherapy alone (28). Since the study did not restrict patients based on EGFR status, there may be a subset with overexpression of EGFR that would benefit from this combination therapy.

CONCLUSIONS

Most targeted agents of proliferation and survival pathways have failed to demonstrate survival benefit as single agents. Radiotherapy is the most effective nonsurgical treatment for malignant gliomas, and its combination with a targeted agent is an appealing strategy. Experience with this combination treatment is limited, but intense laboratory and clinical research is ongoing.

REFERENCES

1. Cairncross G, Berkey B, Shaw E, et al. Phase III trial of chemotherapy plus radiotherapy compared with radiotherapy alone for pure and mixed anaplastic oligodendroglioma: Intergroup Radiation Therapy Oncology Group Trial 9402. *J Clin Oncol* 2006;24(18):2707–2714.
2. Stupp R, Mason WP, van den Bent MJ, et al. Radiotherapy plus concomitant and adjuvant temozolomide for glioblastoma. *N Engl J Med* 2005;352(10):987–996.
3. van den Bent MJ, Chinot O, Boogerd W, et al. Second-line chemotherapy with temozolomide in recurrent oligodendroglioma after PCV (procarbazine, lomustine and vincristine) chemotherapy: EORTC Brain Tumor Group phase II study 26972. *Ann Oncol* 2003;14(4):599–602.
4. Walker MD, Alexander E Jr., Hunt WE, et al. Evaluation of BCNU and/or radiotherapy in the treatment of anaplastic gliomas. A cooperative clinical trial. *J Neurosurg* 1978;49(3):333–343.
5. Seiwert TY, Salama JK, Vokes EE. The concurrent chemoradiation paradigm—general principles. *Nat Clin Pract* 2007;4(2):86–100.
6. Sathornsumetee S, Reardon DA, Desjardins A, et al. Molecularly targeted therapy for malignant glioma. *Cancer* 2007;110(1):13–24.
7. Duda DG, Jain RK, Willett CG. Antiangiogenics: The potential role of integrating this novel treatment modality with chemoradiation for solid cancers. *J Clin Oncol* 2007;25(26):4033–4042.

8. Vredenburgh JJ, Desjardins A, Herndon JE 2nd, et al. Phase II trial of bevacizumab and irinotecan in recurrent malignant glioma. *Clin Cancer Res* 2007;13(4):1253–1259.
9. Vredenburgh JJ, Desjardins A, Herndon JE 2nd, et al. Bevacizumab plus irinotecan in recurrent glioblastoma multiforme. *J Clin Oncol* 2007;25(30):4722–4729.
10. Jain RK. Normalization of tumor vasculature: An emerging concept in antiangiogenic therapy. *Science* 2005;307(5706):58–62.
11. Jain RK. Normalizing tumor vasculature with anti-angiogenic therapy: A new paradigm for combination therapy. *Nat Med* 2001;7(9):987–989.
12. Lee CG, Heijn M, di Tomaso E, et al. Anti-vascular endothelial growth factor treatment augments tumor radiation response under normoxic or hypoxic conditions. *Cancer Res* 2000;60(19):5565–5570.
13. Winkler F, Kozin SV, Tong RT, et al. Kinetics of vascular normalization by VEGFR2 blockade governs brain tumor response to radiation: Role of oxygenation, angiopoietin-1, and matrix metalloproteinases. *Cancer Cell* 2004;6(6):553–563.
14. Batchelor TT, Sorensen AG, di Tomaso E, et al. AZD2171, a pan-VEGF receptor tyrosine kinase inhibitor, normalizes tumor vasculature and alleviates edema in glioblastoma patients. *Cancer Cell* 2007;11(1):83–95.
15. Mohile NA, Abrey LE, Lymberis SC, et al. A pilot study of bevacizumab and stereotactic intensity modulated re-irradiation for recurrent high grade gliomas. ASLO Meeting Abstracts 2007;25:202.
16. Brandes AA, Stupp R, Hau P, et al. EORTC Study 26041-22041: Phase I/II study on concomitant and adjuvant temozolomide (TMZ) and radiotherapy (RT) with or without PTK787/ZK222584 (PTK/ZK) in newly diagnosed glioblastoma: Results of a phase I trial. ASLO Meeting Abstracts 2007;25:2026.
17. Stupp R, Hegi ME, Gilbert MR, Chakravarti A. Chemoradiotherapy in malignant glioma: standard of care and future directions. *J Clin Oncol* 2007;25(26):4127–4136.
18. Bao S, Wu Q, McLendon RE, et al. Glioma stem cells promote radioresistance by preferential activation of the DNA damage response. *Nature* 2006;444(7120):756–760.
19. Caron RW, Yacoub A, Li M, et al. Activated forms of H-RAS and K-RAS differentially regulate membrane association of PI3K, PDK-1, and AKT and the effect of therapeutic kinase inhibitors on cell survival. *Mol Cancer Ther* 2005;4(2):257–270.
20. Wang CC, Liao YP, Mischel PS, et al. HDJ-2 as a target for radiosensitization of glioblastoma multiforme cells by the farnesyltransferase inhibitor R115777 and the role of the p53/p21 pathway. *Cancer Res* 2006;66(13):6756–6762.
21. Feldkamp MM, Lau N, Roncari L, Guha A. Isotype-specific Ras. GTP-levels predict the efficacy of farnesyl transferase inhibitors against human astrocytomas regardless of Ras mutational status. *Cancer Res* 2001;61(11):4425–4431.
22. Delmas C, Heliez C, Cohen-Jonathan E, et al. Farnesyltransferase inhibitor, R115777, reverses the resistance of human glioma cell lines to ionizing radiation. *Int J Cancer* 2002;100(1):43–48.
23. Ruiter GA, Verheij M, Zerp SF, van Blitterswijk WJ. Alkyl-lysophospholipids as anticancer agents and enhancers of radiation-induced apoptosis. *Int J Radiat Oncol Biol Phys* 2001;49(2):415–419.
24. Vink SR, Lagerwerf S, Mesman E, et al. Radiosensitization of squamous cell carcinoma by the alkylphospholipid perifosine in cell culture and xenografts. *Clin Cancer Res* 2006;12(5):1615–1622.
25. Reardon DA, Wen PY. Therapeutic advances in the treatment of glioblastoma: Rationale and potential role of targeted agents. *Oncologist* 2006;11(2):152–164.

26. Ekstrand AJ, James CD, Cavenee WK, et al. Genes for epidermal growth factor receptor, transforming growth factor alpha, and epidermal growth factor and their expression in human gliomas in vivo. *Cancer Res* 1991;51(8):2164–2172.
27. Pelloski CE, Ballman KV, Furth AF, et al. Epidermal growth factor receptor variant III status defines clinically distinct subtypes of glioblastoma. *J Clin Oncol* 2007;25(16):2288–2294.
28. Chakravarti A, Berkey B, Robins HI, et al. An update of phase II results from RTOG 0211: A phase I/II study of gefitinib with radiotherapy in newly diagnosed glioblastoma. ASLO Meeting Abstracts 2006;24:1527.

7 Targeted Therapies in Head and Neck Cancer

RANEE MEHRA
ROGER B. COHEN
PAUL M. HARARI

Squamous cell carcinoma of the head and neck (SCCHN) is diagnosed in over 500,000 patients worldwide each year. Despite advances in surgery, radiotherapy, and chemotherapy, SCCHN continues to be associated with high morbidity and mortality. In the United States, the estimated incidence will be 45,000 new cases in 2007 (1). Common risk factors include tobacco and alcohol use, with increasing evidence for human papilloma virus (HPV) in the pathogenesis of selected oral cavity and oropharynx squamous cell carcinomas, notably in patients who lack the usual risk factors (2).

Patients with stage I or II SCCHN are often cured with radiation therapy or surgery. More than half of patients present with locoregionally advanced disease, however, with a 5-year survival of less than 50% (3). Induction of DNA repair and survival pathways, accelerated repopulation, tumor hypoxia, and altered perfusion are known factors that can limit the effectiveness of radiation (4–6). The addition of chemotherapy as a radiosensitizing agent is one strategy for increasing treatment efficacy. Chemoradiotherapy is commonly given for locoregionally advanced disease, but survival gains are modest and such treatment is associated with significant short- and long-term side effects.

Promising new approaches in the treatment of SCCHN include emerging data supporting the use of taxane-based induction therapy, as well as the successful introduction of targeted biologic agents, with epidermal growth factor receptor (EGFR) inhibitors such as cetuximab in the lead (7–9). Despite these promising new therapies, many patients with locoregionally advanced SCCHN still die from their disease, so there remains an obvious need for novel therapies. This chapter reviews current data on the combination of targeted biologic agents with radiotherapy, with an emphasis on EGFR inhibitors and newer agents targeting angiogenesis and hypoxia.

CURRENT STATUS OF CHEMORADIOTHERAPY FOR SQUAMOUS CELL CARCINOMA OF THE HEAD AND NECK

Chemotherapy added to radiotherapy is indicated for medically fit patients with unresectable disease, or as adjuvant treatment for patients at a high risk of recurrence after primary tumor resection (10,11), with a number of randomized trials over the past 15 years providing support for the superiority of combined chemotherapy and radiotherapy compared to radiotherapy alone (12,13). A recent update of the meta-analysis of chemotherapy in head and neck cancer (MACH-NC) has confirmed an approximate 8% absolute benefit with combined therapy, noting that this advantage appears to benefit primarily patients younger than age 70 (14,15). In addition, the rate of laryngeal preservation in patients with advanced laryngeal cancer was higher in those who received the combination of cisplatin and radiotherapy, or cisplatin and fluorouracil induction therapy followed by radiotherapy compared to radiotherapy alone (3,16). High-dose cisplatin (100 mg/m^2 every 3 weeks) has emerged as one of the more common radiosensitizing agents used in the United States and Europe, but other agents, such as 5-fluorouracil, carboplatin, and taxanes, are also effective in combination with radiation (12,17). In addition, recent data support the administration of taxane-based induction chemotherapy followed by combined chemoradiotherapy for patients with locoregionally advanced SCCHN (7,18), with randomized comparisons of this approach versus concurrent chemoradiation in progress.

Combined chemotherapy and radiotherapy is quite toxic for most patients, with severe mucositis limiting their ability to take adequate nutrition by mouth. Indeed, it may not be possible because of unacceptable toxicity to further intensify combined modality regimens with additional cytotoxic agents in order to improve outcomes. The future of combined therapy therefore depends on the thoughtful, systematic integration of molecular targeted agents with radiotherapy and chemotherapy to improve the therapeutic index. The use of biologic agents in this setting has focused to date mainly on agents targeting the EGFR pathway.

EPIDERMAL GROWTH FACTOR INHIBITION IN SQUAMOUS CELL CANCER OF THE HEAD AND NECK

The EGFR is a transmembrane tyrosine kinase (TK) receptor with extracellular, transmembrane, and intracellular domains. The receptor was purified in 1980, and early investigations highlighted a role of EGFR in tumorigenesis, noting the antitumor effects of EGFR monoclonal antibodies in epithelial cancer cell lines (19,20). The EGFR is activated following ligand binding either by homodimerization with another EGFR, or via heterodimerization with another member of this type 1 receptor tyrosine kinase (RTK) family (21). Other receptors in this family include c-ErbB2 (HER-2/*neu*), c-ErbB3, and c-ErbB4, and associations between these receptors appear to play a role in SCCHN pathogenesis (22). EGFR stimulation results in activation of signal transduction pathways for phosphatidylinositol 3' kinase (PI3K)/AKT and RAS/RAF/mitogen-activated extracellular-regulated kinase (MEK)/mitogen-activate protein kinase (MAPK) (23). The EGFR may also translocate to the nucleus, where it can act as a transcription factor (24). In addition, a correlation exists between EGFR expression and that of signal transducers and activators of transcription 3 (STAT3), with these two molecules physically interacting to regulate gene transcription (25,26).

In addition to interacting with other members of the type 1 RTK family, TK receptors have been shown to interact with the vascular endothelial growth factor (VEGF) pathway that plays a critical role in angiogenesis. For instance, c-ErbB2 increases VEGF and hypoxia inducible factor (HIF) expression via activation of PI3K and mammalian target of rapamycin (mTOR) (27,28). EGFR (c-ErbB1) stimulation with the epidermal growth factor (EGF) also leads to increased VEGF release. The inhibition of EGFR suppresses this phenomenon (29).

The EGFR plays a critical role in SCCHN tumorigenesis. Elevated EGFR expression, as detected by immunohistochemistry, is associated with inferior survival and increased locoregional failure (30–32). In addition, EGFR expression predicts for response to radiotherapy, with increased expression correlating with radioresistance (33). One potential mechanism underlying this observation may be that high EGFR expression is related to failure of tumor cells to undergo radiation-induced apoptosis (34). EGFR status may be used in the future to guide selection of therapy as a predictive factor. For instance, continuous hyperfractionated accelerated radiotherapy has been shown to improve locoregional control in SCCHN patients with elevated EGFR levels in pretreatment tumor tissue, but not in those with low EGFR levels (6). The prognostic significance of EGFR expression for overall prognosis and radiosensitivity provides a strong rationale for targeting this receptor concurrently with radiation.

The role of EGFR inhibitors as radiosensitizers remains a very active area of research. Mechanisms for this advantageous interaction with radiation include EGFR effects on signal transduction cascades, cell cycle regulation, apoptosis, DNA repair, and angiogenesis. Radiation has been shown to stimulate EGFR autophosphorylation, which contributes to the phenomenon of accelerated repopulation (35). Treatment with EGF further augments cell survival during radiation (36). Increased EGFR expression correlates with radioresistance, as well as greater sensitivity to EGFR inhibition either with the monoclonal antibody cetuximab (C225) or small-molecule EGFR inhibitors (37–39). Numerous preclinical studies have confirmed that EGFR inhibition with a variety of agents sensitizes SCCHN cells to radiation and improves the response to treatment (36,40). For example, SCCs in tissue culture treated with cetuximab were found to be in G1 cell cycle arrest, with correspondingly fewer cells in the more radioresistant S phase (41–43). Similar observations have been made with SCC treated with the small-molecule inhibitors gefitinib or erlotinib in conjunction with radiation (44,45). All of the EGFR inhibitors result in decreased cell proliferation in tissue culture and xenograft models. These studies also showed that EGFR inhibition with radiation led to increased apoptosis (36,42,44,46). Blocking EGFR delays the repair of chemotherapy-induced DNA damage. This is felt to be via inhibition of MAPK, which is also activated by ionizing radiation and is implicated in the upregulation of DNA repair genes such as XRCC1 and ERCC1 (4,47). Treatment with cetuximab or gefitinib seems to affect these DNA repair mechanisms and could be another factor in their spectrum of activity (48,49). Finally, some data suggest that treatment with monoclonal antibody or small-molecule EGFR inhibitors in conjunction with radiation limits tumor neoangiogenesis (45,48).

THERAPEUTIC EPIDERMAL GROWTH FACTOR RECEPTOR INHIBITORS

Monoclonal Antibodies

Several EGFR-targeting antibodies are in varying stages of development (Table 7.1). Some differences among these agents may influence their activity. Each antibody consists of a domain that targets the EGFR epitope as well as an IgG (either IgG_1 or IgG_2) portion. Cetuximab is the most studied monoclonal antibody, and is a chimeric molecule that is 65% human and 35% murine. The mouse component may account for the low risk of infusional allergic reactions. Matuzumab (EMD72000) (50) and nimotuzumab (h-R3) (51) are humanized anti-EGFR antibodies (>95%), and panitumumab (ABX-EGF) is a fully human antibody. The risk of allergic reactions is lower with these latter agents. An interesting antibody, mAb 806, will only target tissue in which wild-type EGFR is overexpressed or tissues containing the mutant variant EGFRvIII. mAb 806 is also synergistic with the other anti-EGFR antibodies (52,53). The mAb 806 epitope is only exposed in a transitional form of the receptor between the inactive and the ligand-bound active states, which accounts for its unique properties (54).

Several mechanisms are involved in the anti-tumor activity of anti-EGFR monoclonal antibodies. One obvious mechanism is the interference by anti-

TABLE 7.1 Monoclonal antibodies that target EGFR

Antibody	Type	Phase of Development
Cetuximab (C225)	Chimeric	FDA approved: Locoregionally advanced SCCHN with radiation therapy and as monotherapy in platinum-refractory SCCHN (2006)
Panitumumab (ABX-EGF)	Fully human	III: Colon cancer II: SCCHN and various cancers
Matuzumab (EMD72000)	Humanized	II: Various cancers
Nimotuzumab (h-R3)	Humanized	I: SCCHN with radiation therapy
mAb 806	Humanized	I

body in the binding of natural ligands such as EGF and transforming growth factor (TGF-α) (55). Another established mechanism involves depletion of the receptors from the cell surface, which are then either recycled or degraded in lysosomes (56). Finally, cetuximab, matuzumab, and nimotuzumab are constructed on an IgG_1 framework that potentially allows these agents to mediate antibody-dependent cell-mediated cytotoxicity (ADCC) via natural killer (NK) cells and macrophages (57). Panitumumab is based on an IgG_2 framework and therefore will not mediate ADCC.

Cetuximab

The U.S. Food and Drug Administration (FDA) approved cetuximab in March 2006 for use in combination with radiation therapy in patients with locoregionally advanced SCCHN and as a single agent in the metastatic (incurable) setting (8,58). In the initial phase I trial with radiation therapy, patients with advanced SCCHN of the oropharynx, larynx, or hypopharynx received cetuximab at a loading dose of 100–500 mg/m^2 1 week before radiation therapy, followed by infusions of 100–250 mg/m^2 weekly during radiation therapy (59). Most patients received conventional once-a-day radiation therapy (2 Gy/day to a total dose of 70 Gy), and three patients received hyperfractionated radiation therapy (1.2 Gy/twice a day to a total dose of 76.8 Gy). The investigators determined that loading doses of cetuximab at 400–500 mg/m^2 followed by 250 mg/m^2 weekly could be administered safely with radiation therapy. At these cetuximab doses, a separate study showed high levels of EGFR binding in biopsies from SCCHN patients (60). Cetuximab plus radiation appeared to be an efficacious regimen, with 13 patients achieving a complete response and two showing a partial response. Common toxicities that were due to cetuximab included skin reactions in the radiation field (grade 3 in five patients) and infusion reactions (grade 4 in one patient).

The above study was followed by a phase III multicenter trial that randomized 424 patients between definitive radiation therapy alone and radiation therapy with cetuximab given as a 400-mg/m^2 loading dose followed by a 250-mg/m^2 weekly maintenance dose for eight planned doses (9). As in the phase I study, patients with tumors in the oropharynx (60%), larynx (25%), or hypopharynx (15%) were enrolled. When this study was designed and implemented, radiation therapy alone was considered by many experts to be a standard of care for definitive therapy of patients with locoregionally advanced SCCHN. Investigators in the phase III study could choose between once-daily fractionation, hyperfractionation (twice daily), or concomitant boost schedules but had to make this choice prior to randomization. Cetuximab in combination with radiation improved clinically relevant outcomes compared to radiation alone, with an increase in duration of locoregional control from 14.9 to 24.4 months ($p = 0.005$) and an improvement in median survival from 29.3 to 49 months ($p = 0.03$). The toxicity of radiation was not exacerbated by the addition of cetuximab. In particular, the rates of grade 3 and 4 mucositis were the same in both study arms. In an ad hoc subset analysis, patients with cancers in the oropharynx appeared to derive the greatest benefit, whereas there was little apparent benefit for patients with hypopharynx cancers. The results of this study are quite encouraging. This study did not include patients treated with chemoradiation, so we do not know at this time whether cetuximab plus radiation is equivalent to the concurrent chemoradiation that is presently a worldwide standard of care for medically fit patients who can tolerate platinum-based therapy.

Since cetuximab and platinum chemotherapy have nonoverlapping toxicity profiles, considerable interest exists in combining both agents with radiation in order to improve further locoregional control and overall survival. An exploratory phase II study enrolled 22 patients to receive cisplatin (100 mg/m^2 every 3 weeks) and cetuximab (400 mg/m^2 followed by 250 mg/m^2 weekly) in conjunction with concomitant boost radiotherapy (61). Long-term follow-up was encouraging, with 3-year overall survival and locoregional control of 76% and 71%, respectively. The study was terminated early as a result of two on-study deaths (1 pneumonia and 1 unknown), and other adverse events such as myocardial infarction, bacteremia, and atrial fibrillation; the relationship of these events to the therapy remains uncertain. Currently, a large randomized phase III effort is underway—RTOG 0522, a randomized phase III trial of concurrent accelerated radiation and cisplatin versus concurrent accelerated radiation, cisplatin, and cetuximab (C225) for stage III and IV head and neck carcinoma—that will further define the role and toxicities of cetuximab- and cisplatin-based chemoradiotherapy. Initial reports on a phase II trial of weekly cetuximab, carboplatin, and paclitaxel with daily radiation therapy provide further encouraging evidence that combining an EGFR inhibitor with chemoradiation is a worthy approach (62). These investigators reported that the first 18 patients in this study showed a 72% complete response rate. Toxicities included a grade 3 skin rash and a grade 3 radiation field skin desquamation.

Given the grave prognosis and multiple symptoms that require palliation in locally recurrent disease, the safety of reirradiation in this population is another active area of investigation. A recent abstract presented at the 2006 American Society of Clinical Oncology meeting reported on eight previously irradiated patients who received reirradiation (30 Gy, 2 Gy/day), carboplatin (AUC 6 every 3 weeks for three cycles), and cetuximab at standard doses (63). One patient died from pneumonia but the rest had a dramatic palliation of symptoms within 1 week of starting treatment, followed by an objective response in all patients (two complete responses). The overall time to progression of the seven patients who were followed ranged from 2–7+ months. All patients developed the characteristic rash, but did not appear to have excessive toxicities from the addition of cetuximab. Although the number of patients treated on this study is small, the early results support further investigation of this combination. Ongoing trials assessing cetuximab and radiation therapy are presented in Table 7.2.

Nimotuzumab and Other Anti-EGFR Monoclonal Antibodies

Nimotuzumab is a humanized monoclonal antibody that targets the EGFR. It has been studied in conjunction with radiation therapy in patients with locally advanced SCCHN, and has been well tolerated (51). Six weekly doses were administered ranging from 50 to 400 mg. In the initial analysis, patients who received the higher doses of 200 mg and 400 mg had a statistically significant improvement in median survival compared to those who received lower doses (44.3 months versus 8.6 months). Subsequently, the protocol was amended to enroll more patients at the higher dose levels, and the mean overall survival in this latter group is 22 months. Patients receiving nimotuzumab did not experience the skin toxicity that is typical for anti-EGFR agents, an observation that remains unexplained but may have to do with the affinity of this particular antibody for the EGFR in normal skin. Correlative studies for this trial included measures of tumor microvessel density (MVD), which decreased with treatment, suggesting decreased angiogenic activity. These data clearly support further evaluation of this agent with radiation, especially given the possibility of reduced skin toxicity.

Panitumumab, a fully human anti-EGFR monoclonal antibody, is another promising agent. In mouse SCCHN xenograft studies, the combination of panitumumab and radiation resulted in effective inhibition of tumor growth (64). Whether the lack of ADCC functionality in panitumumab (an IgG_2 antibody) will be important in the magnitude of response to this agent in patients with SCCHN is unknown at this time. Another emerging area of preclinical investi-

TABLE 7.2 Current or recent U.S. trials underway for SCCHN with radiation therapy and cetuximab

Trial	Phase	Stage	Schema	Projected Accrual	Sponsor
CDDP + RT vs. cisplatin/ RT/C225 (RTOG 0522)	III	III or IV	Randomized	720 patients	RTOG
C225/C/P/RT	II	Locally advanced	Single-arm, open-label	60	University of Maryland
D/C225/CDDP induction, then RT/C225/ cisplatin	II	Locally advanced	Single-arm, open-label	40	University of Pittsburgh
C225/CDDP/ RT→C225 *(ECOG 3303)	II	IV	Single-arm	69	ECOG
RT/C225/CDDP vs. RT/C225/D *(RTOG 0234) [163]	II	III or IV, treatment in adjuvant setting for high-risk disease	Randomized	238	RTOG
Induction → F/H/RT/C225 vs. CDDP/RT/ C225	II	Locally advanced, III/IV	Randomized	110	University of Chicago (EPIC)

C225, cetuximab; P, paclitaxel; RT, radiation; C, carboplatin; D, docetaxel; CDDP, cisplatin; * no longer recruiting. Available at www.clinicaltrials.gov. Accessed Jan. 3, 2008.

gation involves overcoming cetuximab resistance with second-generation antibodies such as pertuzumab (2C4), a monoclonal antibody that inhibits EGFR and HER-2 heterodimerization. It is hypothesized that the HER-2 pathway may play a role in the development of acquired resistance to EGFR inhibition. In vivo and in vitro studies indicate that cetuximab and pertuzumab do act synergistically to inhibit tumor growth in cetuximab-resistant SCC cell lines (65). At present, we do not have mature data regarding the use of these other antibodies either alone or with radiation in patients with SCCHN.

Small-Molecule Tyrosine Kinase Inhibitors

Tyrosine kinase inhibitors are oral agents that target EGFR. They are quinazoline-derived synthetic molecules that block the adenosine triphosphate (ATP) binding site of the intracellular TK domain of EGFR. Some of these agents are fairly specific for EGFR (gefitinib, erlotinib), whereas others have activity against other receptors as well, such as HER-2/*neu* (e.g., lapatinib) and the vascular endothelial growth factor receptor (VEGFR) (e.g., ZD6474/vandetanib). By inhibiting autophosphorylation of the receptor, downstream signal transduction cascades are inactivated. In general, TK inhibitors are well tolerated, with the exception of occasional dose-limiting gastrointestinal side effects such as nausea or diarrhea. The EGFR TK inhibitors all induce skin reactions. Key data from trials combining EGFR inhibitors with radiation therapy are summarized below, and ongoing studies are listed in Table 7.3.

Both erlotinib (66) and gefitinib (67,68) have modest activity as single agents in advanced SCCHN, affording a 4–10% objective response rate and a 40–50% rate of disease stabilization. Interestingly, there seems to be a dose response to treatment, with a 250-mg daily dose of gefitinib having less activity than a 500-mg dose. A phase I study was presented at the 2006 American Society of Clinical Oncology (ASCO) meeting that studied the safety of radiation therapy (70.2 Gy), and weekly docetaxel (15–20 mg/m^2) in conjunction with daily erlotinib (50–150 mg) (69). Erlotinib could be continued for up to 2 years following radiation therapy. Twenty-three patients with locally advanced disease of the oral cavity, pharynx, and larynx were enrolled. At the time of the ASCO presentation, the MTD had not been determined, with one dose-limiting toxicity observed at each of the three initial dose levels (two mucositis and

TABLE 7.3 Current U.S. trials for SCCHN with radiation therapy and EGFR small molecule inhibitors

Trial	Phase	Stage	Schema	Projected Accrual	Sponsor
G/ CDDP / radiation therapy	I/II	Locally advanced	Single-arm Open-label	29	Cornell
G/ CDDP / F/radiation therapy	I/II	Locally advanced	Single-arm Open-label	60	Case Comprehensive Cancer Center
CDDP/radiation therapy +/- E	II	III/IV	Randomized Open-label	204	Seattle Cancer Care Alliance
E + RT or E/CDDP/RT	I	II-IV	Open-label, dose escalation (E)	24–48	Johns Hopkins
E/D/RT	I	III, IV, M0	Open-label, nonrandomized	24	MD Anderson
L/CDDP/RT→ L vs. CDDP/RT	II	III, IVA, IVB	Randomized, double-blind	100	GlaxoSmithKline

G, gefitinib; F, fluorouracil; E, erlotinib; L, lapatinib.
Available at www.clinicaltrials.gov. Accessed Jan. 3, 2008.

one death). Fifteen complete responses were observed and three patients who had a planned neck dissection all had a pathologic complete response. This regimen seems to be active, but further safety data have yet to mature. A phase I/II study was also presented at ASCO 2006 that assessed the tolerability of erlotinib with cisplatin and radiation therapy in patients with locally advanced SCCHN (70). Cisplatin and radiation therapy were given at standard doses, and erlotinib was escalated from 50 mg to 150 mg in three dose levels, with establishment of oral 150 mg daily as the recommended phase II dose. Tumor tissue was sampled after treatment and 11 patients (84.6%) had a pathologic complete response. Grade 3 or 4 toxicities that were relevant to erlotinib included dermatitis, skin rash, and cutaneous infections.

Although the role of induction therapy has yet to be fully defined in SCCHN, trials are underway adding gefitinib to induction and concurrent chemoradiation regimens. One trial treated 45 patients with locally advanced disease with carboplatin, docetaxel, fluorouracil, and gefitinib at a dose of 250 mg, followed by radiation therapy, docetaxel, and gefitinib (71). Eleven complete responses (32%) and 18 partial responses (53%) were achieved. Gefitinib did not substantially increase the toxicity of this regimen. Another trial of carboplatin and paclitaxel induction therapy incorporated gefitinib in the subsequent concurrent chemoradiation treatment (72). The combined modality treatment consisted of gefitinib 250 mg, fluorouracil, hydroxyurea, and twice-daily radiation, followed by maintenance gefitinib. Treatment resulted in an 88% complete response rate. Although these results are encouraging and provide strong support for the continued study of both erlotinib and gefitinib with radiation therapy, it is not known how these treatments will compare to the present standard of concurrent cisplatin-based chemoradiation for locally advanced disease.

Lapatinib is an oral quinazoline that targets EGFR and HER-2/*neu*, and has recently been approved by the FDA for the treatment of patients with metastatic breast cancer who have received trastuzumab (73). It is an attractive agent for development in SCCHN because of its ability to inhibit two key receptors that are known to heterodimerize. As well, preclinical data suggest that alterations in HER2 signaling may contribute to responsiveness to gefitinib (74). Common toxicities attributable to lapatinib include diarrhea and rash (75). As a single agent in advanced SCCHN, the activity of lapatinib was limited, with the best response being stable disease in a minority of patients (75). A phase I study of escalating doses of lapatinib with cisplatin and radiation therapy at standard doses has been conducted (77). At the recommended phase II dose of lapatinib, 1500 mg daily, treatment was well tolerated. Observed toxicities were those typically seen with cisplatin and radiation therapy, including grade 1/2 nausea, vomiting, and tinnitus. Efficacy data are immature. Dual EGFR receptor targeting in conjunction with radiation therapy is an interesting approach, but one that remains investigational.

Toxicities Associated with Epidermal Growth Factor inhibition and Radiation Therapy

Because of the nonoverlapping toxicity profiles of EGFR inhibitors and cytotoxic agents, safety evaluations of combination regimens have consistently supported the administration of chemotherapy, biologic agents, and radiation therapy at full therapeutic doses. In addition, the pivotal trial of cetuximab and radiation therapy was notable for documenting no significant differences in the rate, intensity, or duration of mucositis, xerostomia, pain, or dysphagia in patients in the two treatment arms (9,78). Thus, there is considerable excitement about the potential to improve efficacy with agents such as cetuximab without adding significantly to the toxicity of an already very intense treatment program. One unique risk posed by the chimeric monoclonal antibodies, but not the humanized antibodies or the small-molecule inhibitors, is hypersensitivity infusion reactions that on occasion may be severe, life-threatening, and dose-limiting. Most EGFR inhibitors cause a characteristic skin toxicity, and this may be exacerbated in the radiation therapy field. The EGFR is expressed at the basal layer of the epidermis, and therefore it is not surprising that the skin expresses this mechanism-based toxicity (79). In the study by Bonner and colleagues, eight of nine patients who discontinued cetuximab did so because of the characteristic rash. Treatment recommendations for management of the rash remain anecdotal, and this is an active area of investigation. Early trials with nimotuzumab are exceptional, with the data so far showing that this anti-EGFR agent does not cause rash, but this observation also requires confirmation and further study.

More mature data from the registration study for cetuximab with radiation therapy in SCCHN suggest that the overall incidence of late radiation toxicities was greater with cetuximab and radiation therapy compared with radiation therapy alone (80). This includes the following sites: salivary glands (65%/56%), larynx (52%/36%), subcutaneous tissue (49%/45%), mucous membranes (48%/39%), esophagus (44%/35%), skin (42%/33%), brain (11%/9%), lung (11%/8%), spinal cord (4%/3%), and bone (4%/5%) in the cetuximab-radiation therapy versus radiation therapy alone arms, respectively. The incidence of grade 3 or 4 late radiation toxicities, however, was similar between the two groups. This area obviously needs to be followed further prospectively, especially with regard to studies that combine cetuximab, radiation therapy, and cytotoxic therapy.

Another potential toxicity of anti-EGFR agents is the development of oral dysesthesias, characterized by pain with a "burning" quality. This was reported in a pilot study of gefitinib, paclitaxel, and radiation therapy in patients with locally advanced SCCHN (81). Seven of nine patients treated on this protocol developed this type of oral neuropathic pain; all seven of these patients had received 50–70 Gy of radiation to the oral tongue. This phenomenon should be monitored further in future studies, as it is not clear at this time to what degree this toxicity is due to radiation, gefitinib, or paclitaxel, especially as the latter is a known neurotoxic agent.

Despite the typical skin toxicities caused by EGFR inhibitors, the risk of poor wound healing appears to be low. In an analysis of a subset of patients who were treated with radiation therapy plus cetuximab or radiation therapy alone and subsequently underwent neck dissection, no significant difference in time to healing or complication rates was noted between the two groups of patients (82).

Relevant Biomarkers for the Epidermal Growth Factor Receptor

The EGFR is present, if not overexpressed, on the majority of SCCHN cells. It remains to be determined if the population of patients who will benefit from anti-EGFR treatment can be characterized further. Some preclinical data suggest that high levels of EGFR expression may contribute to increased radiosensitization by erlotinib (83). A subset analysis of the outcomes of patients treated with cetuximab in the setting of advanced SCCHN, however, suggests that patients with low to moderate levels of EGFR expression, in fact, had the best response to cetuximab (8). This latter observation may be due to the fact that patients with high EGFR–expressing tumors have a worse prognosis at baseline regardless of the therapeutic intervention (32) but could also reflect a dose response (pharmacodynamic) effect if tumors with higher EGFR levels require greater doses of antibody to achieve a clinical benefit. Presently, no standard assay is available for EGFR immunohistochemical (IHC) analysis of patient samples. Given that EGFR expression by IHC is not a reliable, validated predictor of clinical benefit for SCCHN, this type of analysis should not be used to guide clinical practice at this time.

Unlike data obtained in patients with non-small cell lung cancer (NSCLC) who were treated with EGFR small-molecule inhibitors (84,85), little evidence suggests that the presence of somatic activating EGFR mutations is clinically relevant in SCCHN (74,86). The majority of mutations described in lung cancer patients are in exons 19 or 21, and are more prevalent in female nonsmokers with adenocarcinoma. Similar EGFR mutations have been detected in a very small number of patients in limited series of SCCHN tissue samples. In one of these, two patients out of 24 were found to have activating mutations in exons 19 and 20 (87). An analysis of Korean SCCHN patients also detected in-frame mutations in exon 19 in three of 41 patients with SCCHN (88). In contrast with the NSCLC mutations that are far more common in nonsmokers, all three of these Korean patients were smokers with laryngeal cancer. Whether these mutations in SCCHN confer responsiveness to anti-EGFR therapy is unknown.

Recent data by Chung have shown that high gene copy numbers of EGFR detected by fluorescence in situ hybridization (FISH) are present in 63% of

41 SCCHN samples that were analyzed (89). FISH-positive tumors were associated with a trend toward a worse recurrence-free survival. Further data will be needed to know whether EGFR copy number will predict therapeutic response in SCCHN. As radiation therapy itself has been shown to activate EGFR autophosphorylation (35), increased EGFR levels or copy number may not be required to achieve a clinical benefit from the use of EGFR inhibitors in conjunction with radiation therapy. Again, this is a complex topic that warrants continued investigation.

VASCULAR ENDOTHELIAL GROWTH RECEPTOR INHIBITORS AND RADIATION

Brief Review of Vascular Biology in Cancer

The generation of new vasculature from existing vessels has long been thought to play a role in tumor pathogenesis (90,91). Tumor growth beyond a certain size depends on the development of new blood vessels at the growing edge, a process that is stimulated by angiopoietins, including VEGF (92). Vascular endothelial growth factor and its associated receptors, VEGFR-1 and VEGFR-2, play a prominent role in normal and pathologic angiogenesis (93). In addition to increasing the supply of nutrients, angiogenesis results in the proliferation of endothelial cells that in turn produce paracrine growth factors that can further stimulate tumor growth (94). Evidence to support targeting of angiogenesis for cancer therapy is illustrated best by preclinical experiments in which xenografts were treated with a monoclonal antibody against VEGFR (95). Treatment resulted in a decrease in tumor size and tumor blood vessel density. Antibody treatment had no effects on the growth of tumor cell lines in vitro, suggesting that its activity was not directly against tumor cells.

Antiangiogenic agents are thought to inhibit tumor growth via several mechanisms: (a) blocking the formation of new blood vessels needed to sustain growth; (b) blocking tumor metastasis, as shown in xenograft studies in which antiangiogenesis therapy reduced the number of metastatic foci (96); (c) enhancing drug delivery to tumors by normalizing tumor blood flow and reducing tumor interstitial pressure (97); (d) promoting endothelial cell apoptosis after radiation (98); and, (e) inhibiting the paracrine production of growth factors by tumor-associated endothelial cells.

Preclinical Data on Antiangiogenesis Therapy and Radiation

One obvious concern about interference with tumor vasculature is that this might adversely limit the effects of radiation by inducing tumor hypoxia. The production of VEGF as well as upregulation of VEGFR both increase under hypoxic conditions (99,100). The available data suggest, however, that induction of tumor hypoxia by antiangiogenic agents does not occur, with preclinical studies showing that radiation effects are, in fact, enhanced by treatment with antiangiogenesis agents such as TNP-470 (101). One explanation for this observation may be that antiangiogenesis therapy blocks new vessel formation, but does not affect existing vasculature, thereby preserving tumor oxygen delivery. In fact, antiangiogenesis therapy seems to reduce the extent of dysfunctional tumor vessels, with the result that tumor oxygenation may be transiently improved in the same way that chemotherapy drug delivery may be promoted (102). Xenograft studies have confirmed that treatment with the antiangiogenesis agents TNP-470 and minocycline reduces tumor hypoxia (103). Antiangiogenic agents also must be distinguished from true antivascular agents. The latter are designed to destroy existing blood vessels in a tumor and may well cause tumor hypoxia.

A wide spectrum of antiangiogenic drugs work in concert with radiation therapy in various animal models. Thus, O'Reilly and colleagues have shown that mice bearing A431 xenografts treated with radiation in combination with endostatin had an improved tumor response compared with radiation or endostatin alone or given sequentially (104). AZD2171 is a small-molecule inhibitor that targets all three VEGFRs. In model systems, radiation and AZD2171 resulted in a decrease of radiation-induced VEGFR-2 phosphorylation, decreased tumor proliferation, and increased apoptosis (105). ZD6474 (vandetinib) is a dual inhibitor of EGFR and VEGFR-2 (106). In combination with radiation in mouse orthotopic lung cancer models, optimal antitumor effects were seen with sequential treatment, whereas concurrent treatment with ZD6474 and radiation was less effective (107). These data suggest that concurrent antiangiogenesis therapy with ZD6474 may reduce tumor perfusion, thereby antagonizing the effects of radiation. On the other hand, angiostatin enhanced the benefits of radiotherapy in lung cancer xenografts when given concurrently, but not after radiation therapy (108). These somewhat divergent observations underscore the need for careful preclinical work to determine the optimal schedules of radiation and antiangiogenesis therapy, as well as the mechanistic basis for these interactions. In this regard, neoadjuvant treatment prior to surgical tumor resection could provide useful data regarding the effects of this type of treatment on tumor vasculature. In one such clinical study, neoadjuvant chemoradiation plus a single dose of bevacizumab was administered to patients with rectal cancer. Treatment resulted in a decrease in tumor perfusion, vascular volume, microvascular density, and interstitial fluid pressure (109). This approach could be pursued with relative ease in patients with head and neck cancer, and might provide an elegant approach to learn more about the biologic effects of antiangiogenesis treatment to improve the design of future clinical trials.

Resistance to Radiation Therapy

The production of VEGF, and that of other vascular growth factors such as basic fibroblast growth factor (bFGF), may be a contributing factor for resistance to radiation therapy. Radiation induces VEGF expression in vitro (110). Treatment with VEGF neutralizing antibodies together with radiation in xenograft models increased the antitumor effects of radiation, likely by countering this resistance mechanism (110). The appearance of recurrent tumors shortly after completion of radiation in model systems may be related to a burst of angiogenesis that occurs within 20 days after radiation (111). Increased tumor angiogenesis may also be one of the key mechanisms for tumor escape from EGFR inhibition. Inhibition of EGFR normally suppresses VEGF production and angiogenesis (29,112). However, in A431 squamous cell carcinoma cell lines with an acquired resistance to EGFR inhibition, increased levels of VEGF expression have been detected (112). Since inhibiting EGFR does not completely block VEGF because of redundancy from other pathways, angiogenesis is still active in the presence of anti-EGFR therapy. Preclinical studies have indicated that total blockade of VEGF is required for the maximum effect on tumor growth (113). Therefore, dual inhibition of both EGFR and VEGF is a rational approach to optimize blockade of two critical pathways in cancer proliferation and limit resistance to therapy. In this regard, treatment with the dual VEGFR-EGFR inhibitor ZD6474 has been shown to overcome EGFR resistance in mouse xenograft models (114). In addition, phase I/II clinical data by Vokes and colleagues, combining erlotinib and bevacizumab in the treatment of SCCHN patients with recurrent or metastatic disease, provide further indication for a benefit of these therapies based on an objective and encouraging response rate of 14.6% (115).

Vascular Endothelial Growth Factor Expression in Squamous Cell Carcinoma of the Head and Neck

A full description of the role of angiogenic factors such as VEGF in SCCHN biology is still emerging and much of the evidence is indirect. SCCHN cell lines have been shown to produce VEGF and fibroblast growth factor (FGF). Both proteins are able to activate human umbilical vein endothelial cells (HUVECs) (116). A meta-analysis has indicated that VEGF+ tumors (by IHC) are associated with decreased overall survival (117). In one series, positive VEGF expression was detected in 55% of tumor specimens. Although increased VEGF did not correlate with tumor stage or grade, it was associated with increased microvascular density and p53 mutations, which would be regarded as adverse features (118). Squamous cell carcinomas of the head and neck are known to be characterized by hypoxia (119,120), and hypoxia is associated with radiation resistance (121). Tumor hypoxia results via the hypoxia inducible factor (HIF)-1α pathway in the increased production of angiogenic factors, such as VEGF (122). A correlation exists between HIF-1α and VEGF expression in lower lip and laryngeal cancers, although this association was not noted in oral cavity tumors (123). These observations provide some of the emerging rationale for angiogenic targeting in the treatment of SCCHN.

Current Antiangiogenesis Agents in Clinical Development in Squamous Cell Carcinoma of the Head and Neck

Bevacizumab, a monoclonal antibody against VEGF, initially received FDA approval for the treatment of advanced colon cancer (124). It has since been studied in a multitude of malignancies, showing clinical benefits in lung and breast cancer (125,126). In SCCHN, trials combining bevacizumab 10 mg/kg every 2 weeks with radiation therapy are currently in progress (Table 7.4). A phase I trial of bevacizumab, fluorouracil, hydroxyurea, and concurrent radiation therapy (B-FHX) for high-risk locally advanced SCCHN was presented at the 2006 ASCO meeting (127). This was found to be a tolerable regimen, with the occurrence of the typical bevacizumab-associated toxicities. One and 2-year survivals were 52% and 26%, respectively, providing support to study

TABLE 7.4 Current U.S. trials for SCCHN with radiation therapy and antiangiogenesis agents

Trial	Phase	Stage	Schema	Projected Accrual	Sponsor
B/E/CDDP/RT	II	Locally advanced	Open-label	30	Duke
Neoadjuvant C/P/F/BV—then RT/P/B/E	II	Locally advanced	Single-arm Open-label	61	Sarah Cannon
CDDP/BV/IMRT	II	III/IV	Single-arm Open-label	42	Memorial Sloan Kettering
BV/D/RT	II	III/IV	Single-arm Open-label	30	Case
RT + BV-FHX vs. RT + FHX	II	II, III	Randomized	30	University of Chicago
Z/CDDP/RT	I	III, IV	Single-arm Open-label		AstraZeneca
Z/RT or Z/CDDP/RT	I	III, IV	Nonrandomized, Open-label	48	M.D. Anderson

BV, bevacizumab; H, hydroxyurea; Z, ZD6474.
Available at www.clinicaltrials.gov. Accessed Jan. 3, 2008.

this approach further in the phase II setting. In another study, bevacizumab at a dose of 5 mg/kg every 2 weeks was administered in combination with weekly docetaxel and standard fractionation radiation therapy as first-line treatment for locally advanced SCCHN (128). Bevacizumab could then continue for up to a year after the initial treatment or until progression. Of the nine patients who were treated, all five who underwent a planned neck dissection had a complete response. No expected or severe toxicities, including bleeding or delayed wound-healing, were noted. A third trial studying the addition of bevacizumab to cisplatin and radiotherapy is treating patients with locally advanced disease with one dose of neoadjuvant bevacizumab, followed by a dose escalation of bevacizumab with standard doses of cisplatin and radiation therapy (129). Correlative studies, including functional imaging, are planned after the neoadjuvant bevacizumab, as well as during and after chemoradiotherapy.

ZD6474 (vandetinib), a dual VEGFR-2 and EGFR inhibitor, has preclinical activity when combined with radiation therapy. It has been tested as a single agent in the phase I setting, with dose-limiting toxicities of diarrhea, hypertension, and rash (130). The recommended phase II dose is 300 mg/day. An effort is presently underway to evaluate cisplatin and radiation therapy with or without ZD6474. Sorafenib is an oral inhibitor of Raf kinase and VEGFR-2, among others, and there is evidence that it blocks neovascularization. In a phase II study of this agent in metastatic SCCHN, antitumor activity was minimal (131). Correlative studies, however, indicated that sorafenib results in inhibition of protein kinase-like endoplasmic reticulum kinase (pERK) levels, decreased proliferation, and an increase in markers of apoptosis. Thus, this agent seems to target some of the relevant signaling pathways in SCCHN, supporting further development of sorafenib in combination with other agents and radiation. A phase II trial combining sorafenib with radiotherapy and chemotherapy in SCCHN is underway at the Princess Margaret Hospital in Canada. A summary of antiangiogenesis agents in clinical development in SCCHN is provided in Table 7.4.

Toxicities Associated with Antiangiogenic Therapy

In the pivotal phase III study of bevacizumab in patients with metastatic colon cancer, toxicities included hypertension, proteinuria, and gastrointestinal perforations (124). Other mechanism-based toxicities included increased risk of bleeding, poor wound healing, and a small risk of arterial thromboembolism. Each of these is a concern in the SCCHN population (132). The current label for bevacizumab warns against the treatment of patients with brain metastases or its use immediately before or after planned surgical procedures. Also, the pivotal study of bevacizumab in NSCLC specifically excluded patients with squamous cell histology because they were felt to be at an excess risk for potentially fatal bleeding events (125,133). It is not known if bevacizumab is associated with an excess risk of bleeding in all squamous cell tumors, or whether this toxicity reflects more the biology and growth patterns of lung cancers (with a tendency to present centrally in close proximity to major vessels along with tracheobronchial invasion). In the phase I/II trial of erlotinib and bevacizumab in SCCHN patients, two grade 3/4 bleeding events occurred at the tumor site, and one fatal grade 5 event, suggesting that this could be a toxicity that occurs more frequently in tumors with squamous histology (115). In future studies of patients with SCCHN, the bleeding risk will need to be monitored vigilantly, although these patients should not be excluded from these trials a priori.

TISSUE HYPOXIA AND RADIATION

Tumor hypoxia in SCCHN is associated with resistance to radiotherapy, increased metastatic potential, and a poor prognosis (121,134). This is in part due to increased angiogenesis, reduced apoptosis, and hypoxia-induced expression of EGFR (135). Proteins that are associated with the presence of hypoxic cells include carbonic anhydrase 9 (CA-9, a marker of HIF-1α activity) in tissue and osteopontin levels in plasma (136). Elevated serum osteopontin levels correlate with tissue hypoxia in SCCHN and, in one study, patients with higher osteopontin levels had a decreased 1-year survival, compared with those with lower levels (137). In an analysis of the U.K. CHART trial, which did not detect a benefit for continuous hyperfractionated accelerated radiotherapy, resistance to radiotherapy was associated with increased CA-9 and HIF-2 expression, indicating activation of these hypoxia pathways (138). These markers also correlated with decreased survival and inferior locoregional control.

Another gene of interest in SCCHN is LOX (lysyl oxidase), which shows increased expression in tissue microarrays of hypoxic tumor cells (139). Lysyl oxidase plays a role in cell migration and the invasive potential of metastasizing tumors (140). Increased expression of LOX is induced by HIF-1, and SCCHN tumors that express LOX had a worse prognosis, with reduced metastasis-free survival in retrospective analyses (140). Other proteins with increased expression in hypoxic tissue include galectin-1 (141), IKKβ (142), and XBP-1 (143). Each of these could serve as a potential future therapeutic target and/or biomarker for patient selection or measurement of effect.

Functional Imaging of Hypoxia

Tissue hypoxia cannot easily be measured using noninvasive techniques. Hypoxia can be measured directly in SCCHN tumors with a polarographic electrode (121). Developing simple and reproducible biomarkers to serve as surrogate measures for hypoxia could help guide patient selection for clinical trials of hypoxia-targeting agents and strategies. In this regard, functional imaging of hypoxia is an emerging technique for noninvasive patient assessment. Positron emission tomography (PET) imaging with [18F]-misonidazole (FMISO) (144) can detect hypoxia in SCCHN tumors and assess if there is a clinically relevant reduction of hypoxia after treatment (145).

Hypoxia Targeting in the Clinic

Anemia and Erythropoietin

As anemia reduces tissue oxygenation and results in increased tissue hypoxia, it was hypothesized several years ago that raising hemoglobin levels with erythropoietin might improve outcomes in SCCHN patients undergoing potentially curative therapy with radiation. A large randomized phase III study compared the outcomes of patients with carcinoma of the oral cavity, oropharynx, or larynx who received radiation therapy with curative intent and were randomized to placebo or epoietin-β (146). Surprisingly, epoietin-β did correct anemia but did not improve locoregional control or survival. In fact, patients who received erythropoietin actually did worse than the control group. A second recently reported trial evaluating darbepoetin with radiation therapy yielded very similar results (147). Together, these data have led to global concerns about the use of erythropoiesis-stimulating agents, especially in potentially curable SCCHN populations receiving radiation therapy. The reasons for these unexpected results are not known, although one analysis of the patients in the Henke and colleagues trial indicated that those patients with tumors that expressed the erythropoietin receptor on the cell surface had a reduced progression-free survival if they received epoietin-β (148). This observation suggests that the erythropoietin receptor may be protective to cancer cells by stimulating angiogenesis and tumor survival, via STAT5 signaling (149). These data also remind us of the importance of randomized clinical trials to validate therapeutic hypotheses, including interference with angiogenesis, in which the regulatory pathways are highly complex and difficult to model completely in preclinical studies.

Studies of Hypoxia-Targeting Drugs with Radiation

Tirapazamine is a hypoxic cell cytotoxin that targets cells in hypoxic conditions and triggers apoptosis. Tirapazamine also has antiangiogenic activity (150). Preclinical data support the combination of tirapazamine, which also causes DNA damage in tumor cells, with cisplatin and radiation therapy (151,152). The results of the initial clinical trials are encouraging. In a phase II trial, 39 patients with stage III or IV SCCHN were treated with conventional fractionation radiation therapy (70 Gy in 7 weeks) along with tirapazamine (153). This regimen was well-tolerated, with the more common toxicities being nausea and muscle cramps. Preliminary data suggested efficacy with a 1-year locoregional control rate of 64%. Rischin and colleagues performed a phase I study of tirapazamine with radiation therapy and cisplatin, with dose-limiting toxicities of febrile neutropenia (154). A follow-up phase II trial from the Trans Tasman Radiation Oncology Group (TROG 98.02) randomized patients between the recommended tirapazamine schedule determined from the phase I study and a standard chemoradiotherapy regimen of cisplatin, 5-fluorouracil (5FU) and radiation therapy. Although the study was not designed for statistical comparisons between the two arms, the group treated with tirapazamine had a better 3-year failure-free survival of 55%, versus 44% in the group that received chemotherapy only (155). FMISO was assayed in the TROG 98.02 study as well; patients with tumors showing increased hypoxia by FMISO experienced a greater risk of locoregional failure if they did not receive tirapazamine (156). The investigators hypothesized that detecting hypoxia by FMISO could indicate which patients would respond best to hypoxia-targeted therapy. A phase III study (HeadSTART), comparing standard dosing of cisplatin and radiation therapy to tirapazamine, cisplatin and radiation therapy, has completed accrual with results expected in the near future. Another phase III trial (TRACE) evaluating the same regimen was stopped early due to excessive deaths in the tirapazamine arm. In HeadSTART, no differences in toxicities were detected between the two arms. Le and colleagues performed a randomized phase II study of induction cisplatin, 5FU with or without tirapazamine followed by cisplatin, and 5FU and radiation therapy with or without tirapazamine. No significant improvement in outcome was noted in the patients treated with tirapazamine, and there was an increase in hematologic toxicity (157). This was a small study, however, with only 62 patients treated.

Another hypoxic radiosensitizer of interest is nimorazole. In phase I studies, this agent was well tolerated without significant toxicity, including neurotoxicity (158). This agent was studied by the Danish Head and Neck Cancer Study Group in a randomized, double–blind phase III study of radiation therapy (62-68 Gy) with and without nimorazole (DAHANCA 5-85) (159). The addition of nimorazole to radiation therapy for the treatment of supraglottic and pharyngeal tumors resulted in improved locoregional control and a trend toward a survival benefit. Further studies with this agent are ongoing. Higher osteopontin levels were associated with a worse prognosis and predicted for increased sensitivity to nimorazole treatment. Thus, osteopontin is a promising biomarker for future trials in this area (160).

A novel approach to improve tissue oxygenation in patients undergoing radiation for SCCHN was evaluated in the Accelerated Radiotherapy with Carbogen and Nicotinamide (ARCON) study (161). In this trial, 215 patients with SCCHN were treated with accelerated radiation with carbogen inhalation and nicotinamide infusions. Nicotinamide required a dose adjustment during the study because of severe nausea and vomiting, and mucositis was a common toxicity as well. The 3-year local control rates were encouraging at 80% for laryngeal tumors, but only 29% for oral cavity tumors. This approach is being tested in Europe in a phase III trial for the treatment of laryngeal cancer.

FUTURE DIRECTIONS

There is great optimism and enthusiasm for molecular targeted therapies in oncology and their potential to provide meaningful benefits to cancer patients. Whereas trials involving the presently available prototypical molecular targeted agents have been very encouraging (162), there remains much to learn regarding the optimal strategies for incorporation of these therapies. Future areas of research should attempt to answer the following questions, among others:

- Define those anatomic tumor settings in which monoclonal antibodies and/or small-molecule inhibitors provide optimal efficacy when combined with radiation therapy.
- Identify preferred sequencing regimens for molecular targeted agents with chemotherapy and/or radiation therapy. The sequences may vary depending on the specific molecular agents involved and the underlying mechanisms of action.
- Examine logical combinations of molecular targeted agents. Is it preferable, for example, to accomplish multitarget approaches with drugs that possess multiple functionalities or with distinct drugs?
- Optimize efficacy/toxicity ratios: In patients with favorable prognostic features, will integration or substitution of targeted agents allow for decrease in the intensity of chemoradiotherapy? For instance, could targeted therapies be used alone with radiation therapy instead of conventional chemotherapy, thereby avoiding the known toxicities of cytotoxic chemotherapy?
- Acquire further data regarding the acute and chronic toxicities of antiangiogenesis therapy in SCCHN patients, with a particular emphasis on bleeding risk, impaired wound-healing, and any late radiation effects.
- Identify and validate biomarkers that could guide patient selection and treatment choices to enrich the design of future clinical trials.

■ REFERENCES

1. Jemal A, Siegel R., et al., Cancer statistics, 2007. *CA Cancer J Clin* 2007; 57(1):43-66.
2. Herrero R, Castellsague X, et al. Human papillomavirus and oral cancer: The International Agency for Research on Cancer multicenter study. *J Natl Cancer Inst* 2003;95(23):1772–1783.
3. Forastiere AA, Weber RS, et al. Long-term results of Intergroup RTOG 91-11: A phase III trial to preserve the larynx—Induction cisplatin/5-FU and radiation therapy versus concurrent cisplatin and radiation therapy versus radiation therapy. Paper presented at American Society of Clinical Oncology (ASCO) annual meeting, Atlanta GA, 2006.
4. Yacoub A, McKinstry R, et al. Epidermal growth factor and ionizing radiation up-regulate the DNA repair genes XRCC1 and ERCC1 in DU145 and LNCaP prostate carcinoma through MAPK signaling. *Radiat Res* 2003;159(4):439–452.
5. Bentzen SM. Repopulation in radiation oncology: Perspectives of clinical research. *Int J Radiat Biol* 2003;79(7):581–585.
6. Bentzen SM, Atasoy BM, et al. Epidermal growth factor receptor expression in pretreatment biopsies from head and neck squamous cell carcinoma as a predictive factor for a benefit from accelerated radiation therapy in a randomized controlled trial. *J Clin Oncol* 2005;23(24):5560–5567.
7. Posner MR, Le Lann L, et al. TAX 324: A phase III trial at TPF vs. PF induction chemotherapy followed chemoradiotherapy in locally advanced SCCHN. Paper presented at American Society of Clinical Oncology (ASCO) annual meeting, Atlanta GA, 2006.
8. Burtness B, Goldwasser MA, et al. Phase III randomized trial of cisplatin plus placebo compared with cisplatin plus cetuximab in metastatic/recurrent head and neck cancer: An Eastern Cooperative Oncology Group study. *J Clin Oncol* 2005;23(34):8646–8654.
9. Bonner JA, Harari PM, et al. Radiotherapy plus cetuximab for squamous-cell carcinoma of the head and neck. *N Engl J Med* 2006;354(6):567–578.
10. Bernier J, Domenge C, et al. Postoperative irradiation with or without concomitant chemotherapy for locally advanced head and neck cancer. *N Engl J Med* 2004;350(19):1945–1952.
11. Cooper JS, Pajak TF, et al. Postoperative concurrent radiotherapy and chemotherapy for high-risk squamous-cell carcinoma of the head and neck. *N Engl J Med* 2004;350(19):1937–1944.
12. Calais G, Alfonsi M, et al. Randomized trial of radiation therapy versus concomitant chemotherapy and radiation therapy for advanced-stage oropharynx carcinoma. *J Natl Cancer Inst* 1999;91(24):2081–2086.
13. Adelstein DJ, Li Y, et al. An intergroup phase III comparison of standard radiation therapy and two schedules of concurrent chemoradiotherapy in patients with unresectable squamous cell head and neck cancer. *J Clin Oncol* 2003;21(1):92–98.
14. Pignon JP, Bourhis J, et al. Chemotherapy added to locoregional treatment for head and neck squamous-cell carcinoma: three meta-analyses of updated individual data. MACH-NC Collaborative Group. Meta-Analysis of Chemotherapy on Head and Neck Cancer. *Lancet* 2000;355(9208):949–955.
15. Bourhis J, Pignon JP, et al. Update of MACH-NC (Meta-Analysis of Chemotherapy in Head & Neck Cancer) database focused on concomitant chemoradiotherapy. Paper presented at American Society of Clinical Oncology (ASCO) annual meeting, 2004.
16. Forastiere AA, Goepfert H, et al. Concurrent chemotherapy and radiotherapy for organ preservation in advanced laryngeal cancer. *N Engl J Med* 2003;349(22):2091–2098.

17. Brizel DM, Albers ME, et al. Hyperfractionated irradiation with or without concurrent chemotherapy for locally advanced head and neck cancer. *N Engl J Med* 1998;338(25):1798–1804.
18. Calais G, Alfonsi M, et al. Randomized phase III trial comparing induction chemotherapy using cisplatin (P) fluorouracil (F) with or without docetaxel (T) for organ preservation in hypopharynx and larynx cancer. Preliminary results of GORTEC 2000-01. Paper presented at American Society of Clinical Oncology (ASCO) annual meeting, Atlanta GA, 2006.
19. Cohen S, Carpenter G, King L Jr. Epidermal growth factor-receptor-protein kinase interactions. Co-purification of receptor and epidermal growth factor-enhanced phosphorylation activity. *J Biol Chem* 1980;255(10):4834–4842.
20. Masui H, Kawamoto T, et al. Growth inhibition of human tumor cells in athymic mice by anti-epidermal growth factor receptor monoclonal antibodies. *Cancer Res* 1984;44(3):1002–1007.
21. Prigent SA, Lemoine NR. The type 1 (EGFR-related) family of growth factor receptors and their ligands. *Prog Growth Factor Res* 1992;4(1):1–24.
22. O-charoenrat P, Rhys-Evans PH, Modjtahedi H, Eccles SA. The role of C-ErbB receptors and ligands in head and neck squamous cell carcinoma. *Oral Oncol* 2002;38(7):627–640.
23. Hambek M, Baghi M, et al. Iressa (ZD 1839) inhibits phosphorylation of three different downstream signal transducers in head and neck cancer (SCCHN). *Anticancer Res* 2005;25(3B):1871–1875.
24. Schlessinger J, Lemmon MA. Nuclear signaling by receptor tyrosine kinases: The first robin of spring. *Cell* 2006;127(1):45–48.
25. Haura EB, Zheng Z, et al. Activated epidermal growth factor receptor-Stat-3 signaling promotes tumor survival in vivo in non-small cell lung cancer. *Clin Cancer Res* 2005;11(23):8288–8294.
26. Lo HW, Hsu SC, et al. Nuclear interaction of EGFR and STAT3 in the activation of the iNOS/NO pathway. *Cancer Cell* 2005;7(6):575–589.
27. Klos KS, Wyszomierski SL, et al. ErbB2 increases vascular endothelial growth factor protein synthesis via activation of mammalian target of rapamycin/p70S6K leading to increased angiogenesis and spontaneous metastasis of human breast cancer cells. *Cancer Res* 2006;66(4):2028–2037.
28. Li YM, Zhou BP, et al. A hypoxia-independent hypoxia-inducible factor-1 activation pathway induced by phosphatidylinositol-3 kinase/Akt in HER2 overexpressing cells. *Cancer Res* 2005;65(8):3257–3263.
29. Sini P, Wyder L, et al. The antitumor and antiangiogenic activity of vascular endothelial growth factor receptor inhibition is potentiated by ErbB1 blockade. *Clin Cancer Res* 2005;11(12):4521–4532.
30. Rubin Grandis J, Melhem MF, et al. Levels of TGF-alpha and EGFR protein in head and neck squamous cell carcinoma and patient survival. *J Natl Cancer Inst* 1998;90(11):824–832.
31. Dassonville O, Formento JL, et al. Expression of epidermal growth factor receptor and survival in upper aerodigestive tract cancer. *J Clin Oncol* 1993;11(10):1873–1878.
32. Ang KK, Berkey BA, et al. Impact of epidermal growth factor receptor expression on survival and pattern of relapse in patients with advanced head and neck carcinoma. *Cancer Res* 2002;62(24):7350–7356.
33. Sheridan MT, O'Dwyer T, et al. Potential indicators of radiosensitivity in squamous cell carcinoma of the head and neck. *Radiat Oncol Investig* 1997;5(4):180–186.

34. Akimoto T, Hunter NR, et al. Inverse relationship between epidermal growth factor receptor expression and radiocurability of murine carcinomas. *Clin Cancer Res* 1999;5(10): 2884–2890.
35. Schmidt-Ullrich RK, Mikkelsen RB, et al. Radiation-induced proliferation of the human A431 squamous carcinoma cells is dependent on EGFR tyrosine phosphorylation. *Oncogene* 1997;15(10):1191–1197.
36. Balaban N, Moni J, et al. The effect of ionizing radiation on signal transduction: Antibodies to EGF receptor sensitize A431 cells to radiation. *Biochim Biophys Acta* 1996;1314(1–2):147–156.
37. Milas L, Fan Z, et al. Epidermal growth factor receptor and tumor response to radiation: In vivo preclinical studies. *Int J Radiat Oncol Biol Phys* 2004;58(3):966–971.
38. Bonner JA, Buchsbaum DJ, et al. Anti-EGFR-mediated radiosensitization as a result of augmented EGFR expression. *Int J Radiat Oncol Biol Phys* 2004;59(Suppl 2):2–10.
39. Shintani S, Kiyota A, et al. Enhancement of radiosensitivity in head and neck cancer cells by ZD1839 ("Iressa"), a selective epidermal growth factor receptor tyrosine kinase inhibitor. *Am J Clin Oncol* 2003;26(5):E150–E156.
40. Milas L, Mason K, et al. In vivo enhancement of tumor radioresponse by C225 antiepidermal growth factor receptor antibody. *Clin Cancer Res* 2000;6(2):701–708.
41. Harari PM, Huang SM. Head and neck cancer as a clinical model for molecular targeting of therapy: Combining EGFR blockade with radiation. *Int J Radiat Oncol Biol Phys* 2001;49(2):427–433.
42. Huang SM, Bock JM, Harari PM. Epidermal growth factor receptor blockade with C225 modulates proliferation, apoptosis, and radiosensitivity in squamous cell carcinomas of the head and neck. *Cancer Res* 1999;59(8):1935–1940.
43. Kiyota A, Shintani S, et al. Anti-epidermal growth factor receptor monoclonal antibody 225 upregulates p27(KIP1) and p15(INK4B) and induces G1 arrest in oral squamous carcinoma cell lines. *Oncology* 2002;63(1):92–98.
44. Chinnaiyan P, Huang S, et al. Mechanisms of enhanced radiation response following epidermal growth factor receptor signaling inhibition by erlotinib (Tarceva). *Cancer Res* 2005;65(8):3328–3335.
45. Huang SM, Li J, et al. Modulation of radiation response and tumor-induced angiogenesis after epidermal growth factor receptor inhibition by ZD1839 (Iressa). *Cancer Res* 2002;62(15):4300–4306.
46. Bonner JA, Raisch KP, et al. Enhanced apoptosis with combination C225/radiation treatment serves as the impetus for clinical investigation in head and neck cancers. *J Clin Oncol* 2000;18(Suppl 21):S47–S53.
47. Friedmann B, Caplin M, et al. Modulation of DNA repair in vitro after treatment with chemotherapeutic agents by the epidermal growth factor receptor inhibitor gefitinib (ZD1839). *Clin Cancer Res* 2004;10(19):6476–6486.
48. Huang SM, Harari PM. Modulation of radiation response after epidermal growth factor receptor blockade in squamous cell carcinomas: Inhibition of damage repair, cell cycle kinetics, and tumor angiogenesis. *Clin Cancer Res* 2000;6(6):2166–2174.
49. Friedmann BJ, Caplin M, et al. Interaction of the epidermal growth factor receptor and the DNA-dependent protein kinase pathway following gefitinib treatment. *Mol Cancer Ther* 2006;5(2):209–218.
50. Vanhoefer U, Tewes M, et al. Phase I study of the humanized antiepidermal growth factor receptor monoclonal antibody EMD72000 in patients with advanced solid tumors that express the epidermal growth factor receptor. *J Clin Oncol* 2004;22(1):175–184.

51. Crombet T, Osorio M, et al. Use of the humanized anti-epidermal growth factor receptor monoclonal antibody h-R3 in combination with radiotherapy in the treatment of locally advanced head and neck cancer patients. *J Clin Oncol* 2004;22(9):1646–1654.
52. Jungbluth AA, Stockert E, et al. A monoclonal antibody recognizing human cancers with amplification/overexpression of the human epidermal growth factor receptor. *Proc Natl Acad Sci USA* 2003;100(2):639–644.
53. Perera RM, Narita Y, et al. Treatment of human tumor xenografts with monoclonal antibody 806 in combination with a prototypical epidermal growth factor receptor-specific antibody generates enhanced antitumor activity. *Clin Cancer Res* 2005;11(17):6390–6399.
54. Johns TG, Adams TE, et al. Identification of the epitope for the epidermal growth factor receptor-specific monoclonal antibody 806 reveals that it preferentially recognizes an untethered form of the receptor. *J Biol Chem* 2004;279(29):30375–30384.
55. Li S, Schmitz KR, et al. Structural basis for inhibition of the epidermal growth factor receptor by cetuximab. *Cancer Cell* 2005;7(4):301–311.
56. Sigismund S, Woelk T, et al. Clathrin-independent endocytosis of ubiquitinated cargos. *Proc Natl Acad Sci USA* 2005;102(8):2760–2765.
57. Cartron G, Dacheux L, et al. Therapeutic activity of humanized anti-CD20 monoclonal antibody and polymorphism in IgG Fc receptor FcgammaRIIIa gene. *Blood* 2002;99(3):754–758.
58. Vermorken, JB, et al., Open-label, uncontrolled, multicenter phase II study to evaluate the efficacy and toxicity of cetuximab as a single agent in patients with recurrent and/or metastatic squamous cell carcinoma of the head and neck who failed to respond to platinum-based therapy. *J Clin Oncol* 2007;25(16):2171-2177.
59. Robert F, Ezekiel MP, et al. Phase I study of anti—epidermal growth factor receptor antibody cetuximab in combination with radiation therapy in patients with advanced head and neck cancer. *J Clin Oncol* 2001;9(13):3234–3243.
60. Shin DM, Donato NJ, et al. Epidermal growth factor receptor-targeted therapy with C225 and cisplatin in patients with head and neck cancer. *Clin Cancer Res* 2001;7(5):1204–1213.
61. Pfister DG, Su YB, et al. Concurrent cetuximab, cisplatin, and concomitant boost radiotherapy for locoregionally advanced, squamous cell head and neck cancer: A pilot phase II study of a new combined-modality paradigm. *J Clin Oncol* 2006;24(7):1072–1078.
62. Suntharalingam M, Taylor R, Wolf J, et al. Initial report of phase II trial of weekly cetuximab, CBDCA, paclitaxel and daily RT in patients with locally advanced SCCHN. In: *Multidisciplinary Head and Neck Cancer Symposium*. Rancho Mirage, CA: 2007.
63. Numico G, Colantonio I, Heouaine A, et al. Compassionate treatment (CTr) with re-irradiation, Carboplatin (Cb) and Cetuximab (C) in very advanced head and neck cancer (HNC). Paper presented at American Society of Clinical Oncology (ASCO) annual meeting, Atlanta GA, 2006.
64. Cannon MJ, Armstrong E, Huang E, et al. Panitumumab, a fully human anti-EGFR monoclonal antibody, augments radiation response in xenograft modles of squamous cell carcinoma of the head and neck (SCCHN). In: *Multidisciplinary Head and Neck Cancer Symposium*. Rancho Mirage, CA: 2007.
65. Kruser TJ, Wheeler DL, Huang S, et al. Dual agent targeting of EGFR and ErbB2 with cetuximab and 2C4: A strategy to pvercome acquired resistance. In: *Multidiscliplinary Head and Neck Cancer Symposium*. Rancho Mirage, CA: 2007.
66. Soulieres D, Senzer NN, et al. Multicenter phase II study of erlotinib, an oral epidermal growth factor receptor tyrosine kinase inhibitor, in patients with recurrent or metastatic squamous cell cancer of the head and neck. *J Clin Oncol* 2004;22(1):77–85.

67. Cohen EE, Kane MA, et al. Phase II trial of gefitinib 250 mg daily in patients with recurrent and/or metastatic squamous cell carcinoma of the head and neck. *Clin Cancer Res* 2005;11(23):8418–8424.
68. Cohen EE, Rosen F, et al. Phase II trial of ZD1839 in recurrent or metastatic squamous cell carcinoma of the head and neck. *J Clin Oncol* 2003;21(10):1980–1987.
69. Savvides P, Agarwala SS, Greskovich J, et al. Phase I study of the EGFR tyrosine kinase inhibitor erlotinib in combination with docetaxel and radiation in locally advanced squamous cell cancer of the head and neck (SCCHN). Paper presented at American Society of Clinical Oncology (ASCO) annual meeting, Atlanta GA, 2006.
70. Herchenhorn D, Dias FL, Ferreira CG, et al. Phase I/II study of erlotinib combined with cisplatin and radiotherapy for locally advanced squamous cell carcinoma of the head and neck (SCCHN). Paper presented at American Society of Clinical Oncology (ASCO) annual meeting, Atlanta GA, 2006.
71. Doss HH, Greco FA, Meluch AA, et al. Induction chemotherapy + gefitinib followed by concurrent chemotherapy/radiation therapy/gefitinib for patients (pts) with locally advanced squamous carcinoma of the head and neck: A phase I/II trial of the Minnie Pearl Cancer Research Network. Paper presented at American Society of Clinical Oncology (ASCO) annual meeting, Atlanta, GA, 2006.
72. Cohen EE, Haraf DJ, Stenson KM, et al. Integration of gefitinib (G), into a concurrent chemoradiation (CRT) regimen followed by G adjuvant therapy in patients with locally advanced head and neck cancer (HNC): A Phase II Trial. Paper presented at the American Society of Clinical Oncology (ASCO) annual meeting, Orlando, FL, 2005.
73. Geyer CE, Forster J, et al. Lapatinib plus capecitabine for HER2-positive advanced breast cancer. *N Engl J Med* 2006;355(26):2733–2743.
74. Cohen EE, Lingen MW, et al. Response of some head and neck cancers to epidermal growth factor receptor tyrosine kinase inhibitors may be linked to mutation of ERBB2 rather than EGFR. *Clin Cancer Res* 2005;11(22):8105–8108.
75. Burris HA 3rd, Hurwitz HI, et al. Phase I safety, pharmacokinetics, and clinical activity study of lapatinib (GW572016), a reversible dual inhibitor of epidermal growth factor receptor tyrosine kinases, in heavily pretreated patients with metastatic carcinomas. *J Clin Oncol* 2005;23(23):5305–5313.
76. Abidoye OO, Cohen EE, Wong SJ. A phase II study of lapatinib (GW572016) in recurrent/metastatic (R/M) squamous cell carcinoma of the head and neck (SCCHN). Paper presented at American Society of Clinical Oncology (ASCO) annual meeting, Atlanta GA, 2006.
77. Harrington K, Bourhis J, Nutting CM, et al. A phase I, open-label study of lapatinib plus chemoradiation in patients with locally advanced squamous cell carcinoma of the head and neck (SCCHN). Paper presented at American Society of Clinical Oncology (ASCO) annual meeting, Atlanta GA, 2006.
78. Bonner JA, Harari PM, Giralt J, et al. Duration of mucositis and dysphagia following radiotherapy (+ cetuximab) for locoregionally advanced head and neck cancer. In: *Multidisciplinary Head and Neck Cancer Symposium*. Rancho Mirage, CA: 2007.
79. Yano S, Kondo K, et al. Distribution and function of EGFR in human tissue and the effect of EGFR tyrosine kinase inhibition. *Anticancer Res* 2003;23(5A):3639–3650.
80. Erbitux package insert, ImClone Systems, Incorporated.
81. Sharp HJ, VanWaes C, et al. A high incidence of oral dysesthesias unrelated to mucositis in a pilot trial of Gefitinib, Paclitaxel and concurrent external beam radiation in patients with locally advanced Squamous Cell Carcinoma of the Head and Neck (SCCHN). Paper presented at American Society of Therapeutic Radiology and Oncology annual meeting, Phildelphia PA, 2006.

82. Harari PM, Durland WF, Chinnaiyan P, et al. Impact of the EGFR inhibitor C225 on wound healing in advanced head & neck cancer patients undergoing neck dissection Paper presented at American Society of Clinical Oncology (ASCO) annual meeting, Chicago IL, 2003.
83. Kim JC, Ali MA, et al. Correlation of HER1/EGFR expression and degree of radiosensitizing effect of the HER1/EGFR-tyrosine kinase inhibitor erlotinib. *Indian J Biochem Biophys* 2005;42(6):358–365.
84. Lynch TJ, Bell DW, et al. Activating mutations in the epidermal growth factor receptor underlying responsiveness of non-small-cell lung cancer to gefitinib. *N Engl J Med* 2004;350(21):2129–2139.
85. Pao W, Miller V, et al. EGF receptor gene mutations are common in lung cancers from "never smokers" and are associated with sensitivity of tumors to gefitinib and erlotinib. *Proc Natl Acad Sci USA* 2004;101(36):13306–13311.
86. Loeffler-Ragg J, Witsch-Baumgartner M, et al. Low incidence of mutations in EGFR kinase domain in Caucasian patients with head and neck squamous cell carcinoma. *Eur J Cancer* 2006;42(1):109–111.
87. Willmore-Payne C, Holden JA, Layfield LJ. Detection of EGFR- and HER2-activating mutations in squamous cell carcinoma involving the head and neck. *Mod Pathol* 2006;19(5):634–640.
88. Lee JW, Soung YH, et al. Somatic mutations of EGFR gene in squamous cell carcinoma of the head and neck. *Clin Cancer Res* 2005;11(8):2879–2882.
89. Chung, CH, Ely K, et al. Increased epidermal growth factor receptor gene copy number is associated with poor prognosis in head and neck squamous cell carcinomas. *J Clin Oncol* 2006;24(25):4170-4176.
90. Folkman J. Tumor angiogenesis: Therapeutic implications. *N Engl J Med* 1971;285(21): 1182–1186.
91. Griffioen AW, Molema G. Angiogenesis: Potentials for pharmacologic intervention in the treatment of cancer, cardiovascular diseases, and chronic inflammation. *Pharmacol Rev* 2000;52(2):237–268.
92. Holash J, Maisonpierre PC, et al. Vessel cooption, regression, and growth in tumors mediated by angiopoietins and VEGF. *Science* 1999;284(5422):1994–1998.
93. Ferrara N, Gerber HP, LeCouter J. The biology of VEGF and its receptors. *Nat Med* 2003;9(6):669–676.
94. Folkman J. Tumor angiogenesis and tissue factor. *Nat Med* 1996;2(2):167–168.
95. Kim KJ, Li B, et al. Inhibition of vascular endothelial growth factor-induced angiogenesis suppresses tumour growth in vivo. *Nature* 1993;362(6423):841–844.
96. Yamaoka M, Yamamoto T, et al. Inhibition of tumor growth and metastasis of rodent tumors by the angiogenesis inhibitor O-(chloroacetyl-carbamoyl)fumagillol (TNP-470; AGM-1470). *Cancer Res* 1993;53(18):4262–4267.
97. Jain RK, Tong RT, Munn LL. Effect of vascular normalization by antiangiogenic therapy on interstitial hypertension, peritumor edema, and lymphatic metastasis: Insights from a mathematical model. *Cancer Res* 2007;67(6):2729–2735.
98. Garcia-Barros M, Paris F, et al. Tumor response to radiotherapy regulated by endothelial cell apoptosis. *Science* 2003;300(5622):1155–1159.
99. Forsythe JA, Jiang BH, et al. Activation of vascular endothelial growth factor gene transcription by hypoxia-inducible factor 1. *Mol Cell Biol* 1996;16(9):4604–4613.
100. Brown LF, Detmar M, et al. Vascular permeability factor/vascular endothelial growth factor: A multifunctional angiogenic cytokine. *EXS* 1997;79:233–269.
101. Teicher BA, Dupuis NP, et al. Increased efficacy of chemo- and radio-therapy by a hemoglobin solution in the 9L gliosarcoma. *In Vivo* 1995;9(1):11–18.

102. Jain RK. Normalization of tumor vasculature: An emerging concept in antiangiogenic therapy. *Science* 2005;307(5706):58–62.
103. Teicher BA, Holden SA, et al. Influence of an anti-angiogenic treatment on 9L gliosarcoma: Oxygenation and response to cytotoxic therapy. *Int J Cancer* 1995;61(5):732–737.
104. Itasaka S, Komaki R, et al. Endostatin improves radioresponse and blocks tumor revascularization after radiation therapy for A431 xenografts in mice. *Int J Radiat Oncol Biol Phys* 2007;67(3):870–878.
105. Cao C, Albert JM, et al. Vascular endothelial growth factor tyrosine kinase inhibitor AZD2171 and fractionated radiotherapy in mouse models of lung cancer. *Cancer Res* 2006;66(23):11409–11415.
106. Wu W, Onn A, et al. Targeted therapy of orthotopic human lung cancer by combined vascular endothelial growth factor and epidermal growth factor receptor signaling blockade. *Mol Cancer Ther* 2007;6(2):471–483.
107. Williams KJ, Telfer BA, et al. ZD6474, a potent inhibitor of vascular endothelial growth factor signaling, combined with radiotherapy: Schedule-dependent enhancement of antitumor activity. *Clin Cancer Res* 2004;10(24):8587–8593.
108. Gorski DH, Mauceri HJ, et al. Potentiation of the antitumor effect of ionizing radiation by brief concomitant exposures to angiostatin. *Cancer Res* 1998;58(24):5686–5689.
109. Willett CG, Boucher Y, et al. Direct evidence that the VEGF-specific antibody bevacizumab has antivascular effects in human rectal cancer. *Nat Med* 2004;10(2):145–147.
110. Gorski DH, Beckett MA, et al. Blockage of the vascular endothelial growth factor stress response increases the antitumor effects of ionizing radiation. *Cancer Res* 1999;59(14):3374–3378.
111. Hast J, Schiffer IB, et al. Angiogenesis and fibroblast proliferation precede formation of recurrent tumors after radiation therapy in nude mice. *Anticancer Res* 2002;22(2A):677–688.
112. Viloria-Petit A, Crombet T, et al. Acquired resistance to the antitumor effect of epidermal growth factor receptor-blocking antibodies in vivo: A role for altered tumor angiogenesis. *Cancer Res* 2001;61(13):5090–5101.
113. Gerber HP, Kowalski J, et al. Complete inhibition of rhabdomyosarcoma xenograft growth and neovascularization requires blockade of both tumor and host vascular endothelial growth factor. *Cancer Res* 2000;60(22):6253–6258.
114. Ciardiello F, Bianco R, et al. Antitumor activity of ZD6474, a vascular endothelial growth factor receptor tyrosine kinase inhibitor, in human cancer cells with acquired resistance to antiepidermal growth factor receptor therapy. *Clin Cancer Res* 2004;10(2):784–793.
115. Vokes EE, Cohen EE, Mauer AM, et al. A phase I study of erlotinib and bevacizumab for recurrent or metastatic squamous cell carcinoma of the head and neck (HNC). Paper presented at American Society of Clinical Oncology (ASCO) annual meeting, Orlando FL, 2005.
116. Shemirani B, Crowe DL. Head and neck squamous cell carcinoma lines produce biologically active angiogenic factors. *Oral Oncol* 2000;36(1):61–66.
117. Kyzas PA, Cunha IW, Ioannidis JP. Prognostic significance of vascular endothelial growth factor immunohistochemical expression in head and neck squamous cell carcinoma: A meta-analysis. *Clin Cancer Res* 2005;11(4):1434–1440.
118. Riedel F, Gotte K, et al. Vascular endothelial growth factor expression correlates with p53 mutation and angiogenesis in squamous cell carcinoma of the head and neck. *Acta Otolaryngol* 2000;120(1):105–111.
119. Adam MF, Gabalski EC, et al. Tissue oxygen distribution in head and neck cancer patients. *Head Neck* 1999;21(2):146–153.

120. Lartigau E, Le Ridant AM, et al. Oxygenation of head and neck tumors. *Cancer* 1993; 71(7):2319–2325.
121. Nordsmark M, Bentzen SM, et al. Prognostic value of tumor oxygenation in 397 head and neck tumors after primary radiation therapy. An international multi-center study. *Radiother Oncol* 2005;77(1):18–24.
122. Tsuzuki Y, Fukumura D, et al. Vascular endothelial growth factor (VEGF) modulation by targeting hypoxia-inducible factor-1alpha–> hypoxia response element–> VEGF cascade differentially regulates vascular response and growth rate in tumors. *Cancer Res* 2000;60(22):6248–6252.
123. Kyzas PA, Stefanou D, et al. Hypoxia-induced tumor angiogenic pathway in head and neck cancer: An in vivo study. *Cancer Lett* 2005;225(2):297–304.
124. Hurwitz H, Fehrenbacher L, et al. Bevacizumab plus irinotecan, fluorouracil, and leucovorin for metastatic colorectal cancer. *N Engl J Med* 2004;350(23):2335–2342.
125. Sandler A, Gray R, et al. Paclitaxel-carboplatin alone or with bevacizumab for non-small-cell lung cancer. *N Engl J Med* 2006;355(24):2542–2550.
126. Miller KD. E2100: A phase III trial of paclitaxel versus paclitaxel/bevacizumab for metastatic breast cancer. *Clin Breast Cancer* 2003;3(6):421–422.
127. Seiwert TY, Haraf DJ, Cohen EE, et al. A phase I study of bevacizumab (B) with fluorouracil (F) and hydroxyurea (H) with concomitant radiotherapy (X) (B-FHX) for poor prognosis head and neck cancer (HNC. Paper presented at American Society of Clinical Oncology (ASCO) annual meeting, Atlanta GA, 2006.
128. Savvides P, Greskovich J, Bokar J, et al. Phase II study of bevacizumab in combination with docetaxel and radiation in locally advanced squamous cell cancer of the head and neck (SCCHN). In: *Multidisciplinary Head and Neck Cancer Symposium*. Rancho Mirage, CA: 2007.
129. Khuntia D, Jeraj R, Kruser TJ, et al. Phase I trial of neoadjuvant bevacizumab followed by concurrent radiation, cisplatin and bevacizumab for locoregionally advanced squamous cell carcinoma of the head and neck. In: *Multidisciplinary Head and Neck Cancer Symposium*. Ranch Mirage, CA: 2007.
130. Holden SN, Eckhardt SG, et al. Clinical evaluation of ZD6474, an orally active inhibitor of VEGF and EGF receptor signaling, in patients with solid, malignant tumors. *Ann Oncol* 2005;16(8):1391–1397.
131. Elser C, Siu L, Winquist E, et al. Phase II trial of sorafenib in patients with recurrent or metastatic squamous cell carcinoma of the head and neck (SCCHN) or nasopharyngeal carcinoma (NPC): Final Results. EORTC Conference, Prague, 2006.
132. Gray R, Giantonio BJ, O'Dwyer PJ, et al. The safety of adding angiogenesis inhibition into treatment for colorectal, breast, and lung cancer: The Eastern Cooperative Oncology Group's (ECOG) experience with bevacizumab (anti-VEGF). Paper presented at American Society of Clinical Oncology (ASCO) annual meeting, Chicago IL, 2003.
133. Johnson DH, Fehrenbacher L, et al. Randomized phase II trial comparing bevacizumab plus carboplatin and paclitaxel with carboplatin and paclitaxel alone in previously untreated locally advanced or metastatic non-small-cell lung cancer. *J Clin Oncol* 2004;22(11):2184–2191.
134. Le QT, Denko NC, Giaccia AJ. Hypoxic gene expression and metastasis. *Cancer Metastasis Rev* 2004;23(3–4):293–310.
135. Laderoute KR, Grant TD, et al. Enhanced epidermal growth factor receptor synthesis in human squamous carcinoma cells exposed to low levels of oxygen. *Int J Cancer* 1992;52(3):428–432.
136. Le QT, Chen E, et al. An evaluation of tumor oxygenation and gene expression in patients with early stage non-small cell lung cancers. *Clin Cancer Res* 2006;12(5):1507–1514.

137. Le QT, Sutphin PD, et al. Identification of osteopontin as a prognostic plasma marker for head and neck squamous cell carcinomas. *Clin Cancer Res* 2003;9(1):59–67.
138. Koukourakis MI, Bentzen SM, et al. Endogenous markers of two separate hypoxia response pathways (hypoxia inducible factor 2 alpha and carbonic anhydrase 9) are associated with radiotherapy failure in head and neck cancer patients recruited in the CHART randomized trial. *J Clin Oncol* 2006;24(5):727–735.
139. Denko NC, Fontana LA, et al. Investigating hypoxic tumor physiology through gene expression patterns. *Oncogene* 2003;22(37):5907–5914.
140. Erler JT, Bennewith KL, et al. Lysyl oxidase is essential for hypoxia-induced metastasis. *Nature* 2006;440(7088):1222–1226.
141. Le QT, Shi G, et al. Galectin-1: a link between tumor hypoxia and tumor immune privilege. *J Clin Oncol* 2005;23(35):8932–8941.
142. Chen Y, Shi G, et al. Identification of hypoxia-regulated proteins in head and neck cancer by proteomic and tissue array profiling. *Cancer Res* 2004;64(20):7302–7310.
143. Romero-Ramirez L, Cao H, et al. XBP1 is essential for survival under hypoxic conditions and is required for tumor growth. *Cancer Res* 2004;64(17):5943–5947.
144. Koh WJ, Bergman KS, et al. Evaluation of oxygenation status during fractionated radiotherapy in human nonsmall cell lung cancers using [F-18]fluoromisonidazole positron emission tomography. *Int J Radiat Oncol Biol Phys* 1995;33(2):391–398.
145. Hicks RJ, Rischin D, et al. Utility of FMISO PET in advanced head and neck cancer treated with chemoradiation incorporating a hypoxia-targeting chemotherapy agent. *Eur J Nucl Med Mol Imaging* 2005;32(12):1384–1391.
146. Henke M, Laszig R, et al. Erythropoietin to treat head and neck cancer patients with anaemia undergoing radiotherapy: Randomised, double-blind, placebo-controlled trial. *Lancet* 2003;362(9392):1255–1260.
147. Overgaard J. Interim analysis of DAHANCA 10. Available at: http://frejacms.au.dk/dahanca/get_media_file.php?mediaid=125. Accessed January 5, 2008.
148. Henke M, Mattern D, et al. Do erythropoietin receptors on cancer cells explain unexpected clinical findings? *J Clin Oncol* 2006;24(29):4708–4713.
149. Yasuda Y, Fujita Y, et al. Erythropoietin regulates tumour growth of human malignancies. *Carcinogenesis* 2003;24(6):1021–1029.
150. Nagasawa H, Mikamo N, et al. Antiangiogenic hypoxic cytotoxin TX-402 inhibits hypoxia-inducible factor 1 signaling pathway. *Anticancer Res* 2003;23(6a):4427–4434.
151. Dorie MJ, Kovacs MS, et al. DNA damage measured by the comet assay in head and neck cancer patients treated with tirapazamine. *Neoplasia* 1999;1(5):461–467.
152. Denny WA, Wilson WR. Tirapazamine: A bioreductive anticancer drug that exploits tumour hypoxia. *Expert Opin Investig Drugs* 2000;9(12):2889–2901.
153. Lee DJ, Trotti A, et al. Concurrent tirapazamine and radiotherapy for advanced head and neck carcinomas: A Phase II study. *Int J Radiat Oncol Biol Phys* 1998;42(4):811–815.
154. Rischin D, Peters L, et al. Phase I trial of concurrent tirapazamine, cisplatin, and radiotherapy in patients with advanced head and neck cancer. *J Clin Oncol* 2001;19(2):535–542.
155. Rischin D, Peters L, et al. Tirapazamine, Cisplatin, and Radiation versus Fluorouracil, Cisplatin, and Radiation in patients with locally advanced head and neck cancer: A randomized phase II trial of the Trans-Tasman Radiation Oncology Group (TROG 98.02). *J Clin Oncol* 2005;23(1):79–87.
156. Rischin D, Hicks RJ, et al. Prognostic significance of [18F]-misonidazole positron emission tomography-detected tumor hypoxia in patients with advanced head and neck cancer randomly assigned to chemoradiation with or without tirapazamine: A substudy of Trans-Tasman Radiation Oncology Group Study 98.02. *J Clin Oncol* 2006;24(13):2098–2104.

157. Le QT, Taira A, et al. Mature results from a randomized Phase II trial of cisplatin plus 5-fluorouracil and radiotherapy with or without tirapazamine in patients with resectable Stage IV head and neck squamous cell carcinomas. *Cancer* 2006;106(9):1940–1949.
158. Timothy AR, Overgaard J, Overgaard M. A phase I clinical study of Nimorazole as a hypoxic radiosensitizer. *Int J Radiat Oncol Biol Phys* 1984;10(9):1765–1768.
159. Overgaard J, Hansen HS, et al. A randomized double-blind phase III study of nimorazole as a hypoxic radiosensitizer of primary radiotherapy in supraglottic larynx and pharynx carcinoma. Results of the Danish Head and Neck Cancer Study (DAHANCA) Protocol 5-85. *Radiother Oncol* 1998;46(2):135–146.
160. Overgaard J, Eriksen JG, et al. Plasma osteopontin, hypoxia, and response to the hypoxia sensitiser nimorazole in radiotherapy of head and neck cancer: Results from the DAHANCA 5 randomised double-blind placebo-controlled trial. *Lancet Oncol* 2005;6(10):757–764.
161. Kaanders JH, Pop LA, et al. ARCON: experience in 215 patients with advanced head-and-neck cancer. *Int J Radiat Oncol Biol Phys* 2002;52(3):769–778.
162. Clinical trials listing is available at: www.clinicaltrials.gov. Accessed on January 5, 2008.

8 Targeted Therapies in Lung Cancer

GREGORY M.M. VIDETIC

The treatment of lung cancer remains one of the most challenging areas in oncology practice, and much is needed to improve the survival and quality of life for patients suffering from this disease. Lung cancer is the leading cause of cancer deaths in the United States, with an estimated 160,390 Americans dying of the malignancy in 2007 (1). The 5-year survival rate remains below 20% (1), despite increased sophistication in surgical practice, radiation technology, and the introduction, during the 1990s, of new combinations of chemotherapy. Even as new data reveal improved neoadjuvant and adjuvant strategies for early-stage non-small cell lung (NSCL) cancer patients (2,3), and some progress in the treatment of locally advanced and advanced disease (4,5) such improvements have also come with the risk of increased toxicity, especially when the intensification of radiation delivery was involved, although radiotherapy techniques have improved with the advent of three-dimensional treatment planning, and the availability, although limited use, of thiol-based radioprotectants (6).

Clinical research of new treatment strategies is therefore warranted. Advances in the knowledge of tumor biology and the mechanisms of oncogenesis have led to the discovery and study of a whole range of potential molecular targets for NSCL cancer treatment, thus creating the field of so-called biologic or "targeted therapies." Targeted therapies are designed to interfere with specific aberrant biologic pathways involved in tumorigenesis. A large amount of preclinical in vivo and in vitro data has been gathered on the antitumor properties of a number of new biologic agents, both as single agents and combined with other conventional treatment modalities, such as chemotherapy and radiotherapy. Maione and colleagues have provided a comprehensive review on combining targeted therapies and drugs with multiple targets in the treatment of NSCL cancer (7). With respect to chemotherapy, they noted that the first generation of clinical trials of targeted agents in NSCL cancer treatment concluded that only a few of these new agents offered any substantial impact on the natural history of the disease, with negative results from studies more commonly reported than positive outcomes. And yet some clinically meaningful advances have been reported. In chemotherapy-refractory advanced NSCL cancer patients, erlotinib (Tarceva), an epidermal growth factor receptor tyrosine kinase inhibitor (EGFR-TKI), may extend survival, improve tumor control and help in symptom palliation for a subset of patients otherwise eligible only for supportive care (8). In chemotherapy-naive advanced NSCL cancer patients (with nonsquamous histology), an anti–vascular endothelial growth factor (anti-VEGF) monoclonal antibody bevacizumab (Avastin) produced better survival when given with chemotherapy than seen with chemotherapy alone (9).

Given that the emphasis in the majority of clinical publications is on the relationship between chemotherapy and targeted therapies, the goal of the present review is to provide an overview of the targeted therapies from a specific radiotherapy perspective and to understand the rationale, biology, and preclinical and clinical data that support the potential benefits to employing such agents in combination with radiation treatment for lung cancer, with a particular focus on NSCL cancer.

RATIONALE FOR COMBINING DRUGS WITH RADIOTHERAPY

Wilson and colleagues recently provided a comprehensive review on the biologic basis for combining drugs with radiation (10). In brief, radiation therapy has been a mainstay of lung cancer treatment for over a century (11), whereas chemotherapy's role has evolved over the last 40 years (12). Interactions between radiation and chemotherapy were described soon after they were employed in patient treatments (13), but without the precise mechanisms underlying the enhancement of radiation therapy by chemotherapy being fully understood. Nevertheless, combined modality chemotherapy and radiation therapy became the standard of care for the majority of patients with solid tumors, including lung cancer, based on demonstrated improvements in locoregional disease control and survival.

The classic framework defining the possible basis for interactions between combined radiation and chemotherapy was defined by Steel (13). The Steel paradigm involved the concepts of spatial cooperation, toxicity independence, normal tissue protection, and varying degrees of additivity resulting in enhanced tumor response. Interactions were defined as supra-additive, synergistic, or radiosensitizing when the effect of combined therapy was greater than the sum of the respective single responses. On the other hand, if the drug caused selective protection of normal tissues, when used with radiation therapy, then the decrease in radiation toxicity along with a preserved antitumor effect was an indicator of infra-additive or radioprotecting effects. It was proposed that any radiosensitization or radioprotection had to involve some form of molecular interaction between the drug and radiation. In this classic model, radiation and drug interactions are felt to be diverse but nonspecific and involve direct damage to DNA, interference with DNA repair processes, cell-cycle disruptions, inhibition of proliferation, and enhancement of apoptosis.

The emergence of novel agents with mechanisms that do not necessarily involve direct cytotoxicity has meant that the conceptual framework for understanding drug–radiation interactions proposed by Steel may no longer be optimal (10). The new molecular agents may sensitize through classic pathways but also may function through inhibition of tumor vasculature and angiogenesis, modification of hypoxia, and interference with signal transduction pathways that sensitize cells to radiation therapy (10). Thus, Bentzen and colleagues proposed a revised paradigm for describing such interactions: in addition to the classical rationales of spatial cooperation and radiosensitization, they have added the concepts of biologic cooperation, kinetic cooperation, and normal-tissue protection as new rationales for combining drugs with radiation. Biologic cooperation refers to strategies in which the drug and the radiation have different biologic targets. Kinetic cooperation refers to a broad class of strategies modulating the cell-cycle/proliferative response to fractionated radiotherapy (10). Specific drug schedules to be used with radiation therapy would ideally attempt to exploit more than one of the proposed mechanisms.

EPIDERMAL GROWTH FACTOR RECEPTOR AS A TARGET IN LUNG CANCER TREATMENT

Rationale

Advances in the understanding of tumor biology have led to the identification of the epidermal growth factor receptor (EGFR) (Fig. 8.1) (14–16) as a key molecular pathway that drives tumor growth. The EGFR is a transmembrane glycoprotein belonging to the human EGFR family, made up of an extracellular ligand-binding domain, a transmembrane region, and a cytoplasmic domain that contains a tyrosine kinase (TK) region (14). Tyrosine kinases are ubiquitously expressed proteins that are implicated in many intracellular signaling pathways, including both normal and aberrant cell growth (17). Both epidermal growth factor (EGF) and transforming growth factor (TGF)-α bind to the EGFR to trigger its biologic and mitogenic effects. Ligand binding to the EGFR induces receptor dimerization and activation of the TK activity of the receptor

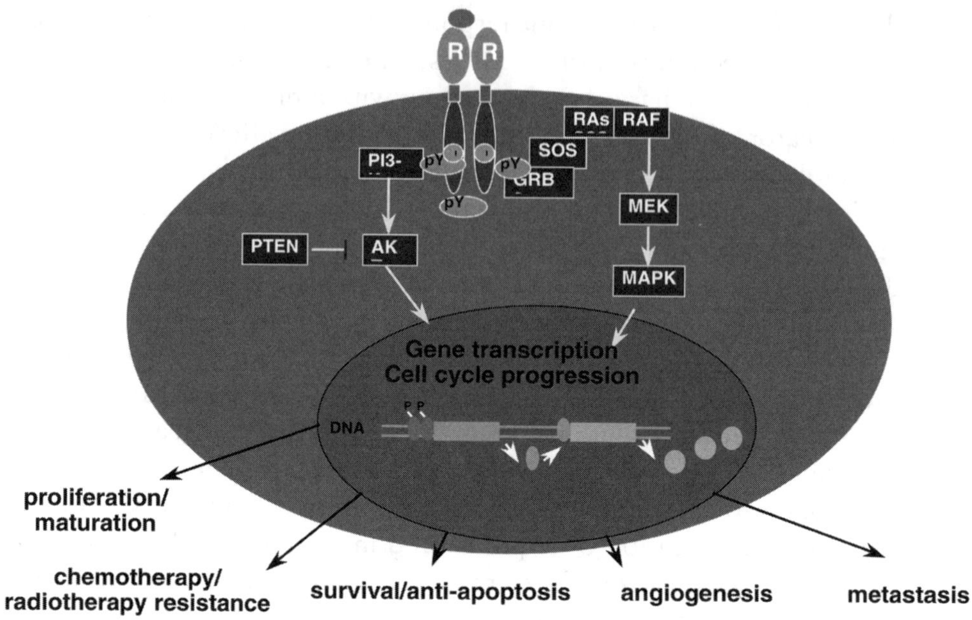

FIGURE 8.1 Epidermal growth factor receptor (EGFR) signal transduction in tumor cells. R, EGFR receptor; PTEN, PTEN tumor suppressor gene product; AKT, antiapoptotic downstream cellular kinase; P13K, phosphatidylinositol 3' kinase; GRB2, growth factor receptor bound protein-2; SOS, son of sevenless; RAS/RAT/MEK, RAS- associated pathway; MAPK, mitogen-activated protein kinase.

(Fig. 8.1). This then leads to receptor autophosphorylation, initiating signal transduction pathways that result in cell proliferation, inhibition of apoptosis, and angiogenesis (15,16). Dysregulation of these pathways can result in oncogenesis and malignant progression.

Substantial evidence suggests a direct link between EGFR and human cancers (15), and abnormal TK activity is in fact characteristic of malignant cells. Non-small cell lung cancer has increased or altered expression of EGFR-TK or its ligands (18). Overexpression of EGFR is reported to occur in 40–80% of NSCL cancer cases (16) and is most commonly reported in squamous cell (84%), followed by large-cell (68%) and adenocarcinoma (65%) (17,19). Several studies (14,15,17) have indicated that the level of EGFR expression correlates with poor disease prognosis and reduced survival.

The idea of treating NSCL cancer by inhibiting EGFR signaling is inherently different from the effect expected from conventional chemotherapy since the agents that target the EGFR are expected to act selectively on malignant cells because of the limited role of the EGFR in normal nonembryonic tissue (7). As summarized by Kim and Choy (20) (Fig. 8.2), there would theoretically be four main strategies for interfering with EGFR function: (a) monoclonal antibodies to the extracellular domain of the receptors, (b) small molecules that

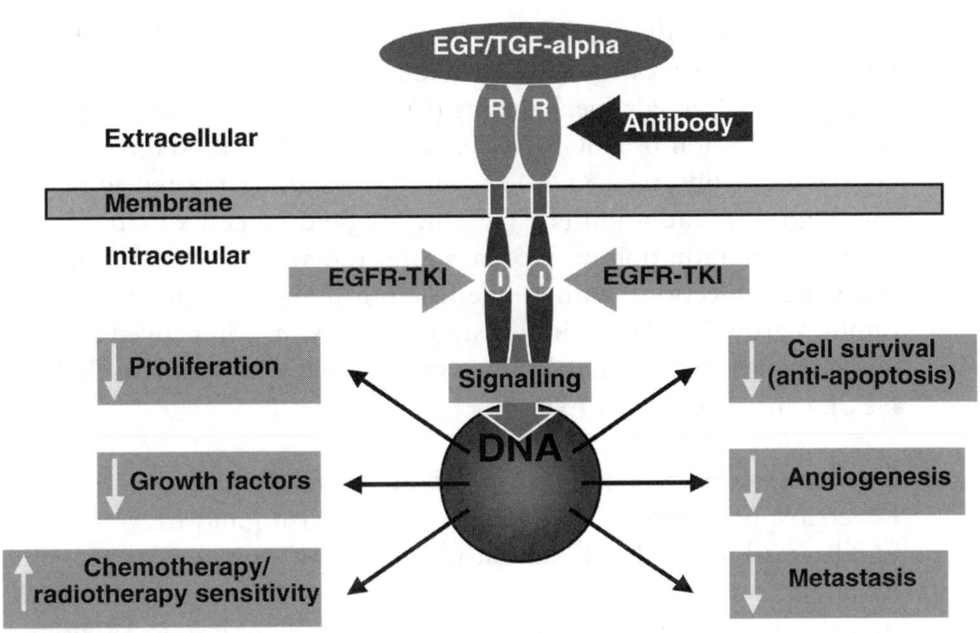

FIGURE 8.2 Mode of action of epidermal growth factor receptor (EGFR) inhibitors. EGF, epidermal growth factor; TGF, transforming growth factor; EGFR-TKI, epidermal growth factor receptor-tyrosine kinase inhibitor, R, epidermal growth factor receptor.

inhibit receptor autophosphorylation by inhibiting adenosine triphosphate (ATP) binding, (c) antisense oligonucleotides, and (d) toxins attached to EGFR ligands/antibodies. The specific rationale for investigation of EGFR inhibitors as radiation sensitizers in cancer therapy is based on the following observations: (a) there exists a positive correlation between EGFR expression and cellular resistance to radiation in many cell types (21–25), (b) radioresistance appears to correlate positively with the degree of EGFR overexpression (23), (c) cell survival and repopulation during a course of radiotherapy are influenced by activation of EGFR/TGF-α that is induced after exposure to radiation (26), and (d) inhibition of EGFR signaling–enhanced radiation sensitivity (27,28).

Preclinical Studies

Anti-EGFR Antibodies and Radiotherapy

Raben and colleagues have recently published a comprehensive review of preclinical studies relevant to targeted therapies and radiotherapy for NSCL cancer (6). Preclinical studies using mouse anti-EGFR monoclonal antibodies showed tumor growth inhibition alone and in combination with chemotherapy or radiation (29,30). These experimental data led to the development of cetuximab, a human–mouse chimeric mAb with high binding affinity to the extracellular domain of the human EGFR, and which reduces human antimouse antibody reactions. Cetuximab prevents EGFR–EGFR or EGFR–HER-2/*neu* dimerization (6). Through downstream mechanisms, cetuximab perturbs DNA repair mechanisms (6). Cetuximab monotherapy also causes growth inhibition in NSCL cancer cell lines (31). Marked tumor growth delay has been observed in A431 tumor xenografts treated with single fraction high-dose radiation (18 Gy) and single-dose cetuximab administered 6 hours before radiation or 3–6 days after radiation (32). Combining multiple cetuximab injections with single-fraction high-dose radiation also delayed tumor regrowth (32). In similar studies, cetuximab improved both radiation- and chemotherapy-induced tumor growth delay in a human EGFR+ (H226) NSCL cancer xenograft (31).

Small-molecule Tyrosine Kinase Inhibitors and Radiotherapy

Reversible (gefitinib, ZD6464, erlotinib, PKI-166) and irreversible (CI-1033) EGFR small-molecule TK inhibitors have shown preclinical antitumor activity alone or with radiation and chemotherapy. Gefitinib blocks EGFR signal transduction pathways by interfering with the cytoplasmic TK domain of the EGFR (6). Its activity has been demonstrated in a wide variety of human cancer models (6).

In vivo, oral gefitinib inhibits the growth of well-established NSCL cancer tumor xenografts alone or in combination with chemotherapy (33). Growth inhibition by up to one-half has been observed in NSCL cancer xenografts, with very low levels of EGFR expression treated with gefitinib alone (33). The in vitro growth inhibitory effects of gefitinib in combination with radiation in human cell lines have been described. Clonogenic assays have demonstrated that treatment of human squamous cell carcinomas (SCCs) with gefitinib reduced cell survival after exposure to ionizing radiation (6,28). In vivo, oral gefitinib (0.5 mg/day for 2.5 weeks) in combination with radiation (single fraction of 3 Gy given twice weekly for 7 weeks) resulted in significant tumor regression and growth delay in mice bearing human SCC xenografts compared with either agent alone (34). Concurrent administration of gefitinib and fractionated radiation in nude mice bearing GEO xenografts revealed a synergistic effect, with a significant survival benefit noted in combination-treated animals in contrast to untreated animals or animals treated with gefitinib or radiation alone (6). Raben and colleagues have demonstrated a cooperative effect between fractionated radiation and gefitinib in an NSCL cancer tumor xenograft with high EGFR expression, and triplet therapy with the addition of cisplatin appeared to further enhance tumor growth inhibition (6). Erlotinib appears similar to gefitinib in preclinical studies with respect to its enhancement of radiation cytotoxicity in NSCL cancer models (6).

Clinical Studies

Anti-EGFR Antibodies and Radiotherapy

In the clinical setting, phase I studies of cetuximab and in combination with cisplatin have been reported. Baselga and colleagues (35) have reported a summary of three initial studies, which included a single-dose trial of cetuximab (CP02-9401), a weekly multiple-dose trial (once weekly for 4 weeks) (CP02-9502), or a weekly dose in combination with cisplatin (CP02-9503). In CP02-9503, patients were required to have head-and-neck cancer (n = 16) or NSCL cancer (n = 6). A total of 52 patients were treated in these three studies. Overall, cetuximab was well tolerated with five episodes of grade 3 or higher toxicity occurring with 317 doses of cetuximab. There was also no relationship of toxicity to the dose level or number of cycles administered, with the possible exception of the acneiform rashes that occurred. The most frequent adverse reactions included fever and chills, asthenia, transaminase elevations, nausea, and skin toxicities [flushing (four cases), seborrheic dermatitis (one case), and acneiform rash (six cases)]. Overall, in these studies, the maximum tolerated dose was not reached.

A phase II study of cetuximab in combination with docetaxel in chemotherapy-refractory patients with advanced NSCL cancer was reported by Kim and colleagues (36). Cetuximab was administered intravenously as 400 mg/m^2 during the first week, followed by 250 mg/m^2 intravenous weekly. Docetaxel was administered intravenously at 75 mg/m^2 every 3 weeks. Preliminary results showed that after two cycles of therapy, four patients had a partial response and six had stable disease. Toxicities included acneiform rash (grade 2/3) in five patients and febrile neutropenia in two patients (grade 2/3).

To date, the only phase III study involving only cetuximab and radiotherapy in combination has been in the setting of head and neck malignancies and was published by Bonner and colleagues in the *New England Journal of Medicine* (37). Patients with locoregionally advanced head and neck cancer were randomly assigned to treatment with high-dose radiotherapy alone (213 patients) or high-dose radiotherapy plus weekly cetuximab (211 patients) at an initial dose of 400 mg/m^2, followed by 250 mg/m^2 weekly for the duration of radiotherapy. The primary end-point was the duration of control of locoregional disease. The results showed a significant improvement in the median duration of locoregional control, 24.4 months among patients treated with cetuximab plus radiotherapy compared to 14.9 months among those given radiotherapy alone (p = 0.005). With a median follow-up of 54.0 months, the median duration of overall survival was 49.0 months among patients treated with combined therapy and 29.3 months among those treated with radiotherapy alone (p = 0.03). Radiotherapy plus cetuximab appeared therefore to significantly prolong progression-free survival and reduce mortality, without added toxicity. These novel findings are the first to suggest a direct clinical benefit to the combination of targeted therapies and radiotherapy in the nonmetastatic setting. The Radiation Therapy Oncology Group (RTOG) has recently completed a phase II study of cetuximab in combination with chemoradiation in patients with stage IIIA/B NSCL cancer. Toxicity data have been reported and show tolerability of this combination (38).

Small-molecule Tyrosine Kinase Inhibitors and Radiotherapy

Gefitinib

Gefitinib has been tested clinically in a number of phase I studies, with variable doses of drug ranging from 50 to 1,000 mg/day. Two-hundred fifty-two patients, 100 of whom had advanced NSCL cancer, in four trials received at least one dose of the drug (39–42). Adverse reactions included dose-related skin changes (mainly rash, most often involving the head, neck, and upper trunk), nausea, vomiting, diarrhea, and rare transaminase elevations. Based on safety and antitumor activity data, doses tested in phase II trials have been 250 mg/day and 500 mg/day and were judged to have antitumor activity.

Two important randomized phase II studies of gefitinib, the Iressa Dose Evaluation in Advanced Lung Cancer (IDEAL 1 and IDEAL 2) studies, involved advanced NSCL cancer patients only (43,44). In IDEAL 1208 patients (from Europe, Australia, South Africa, and Japan) with locally advanced/metastatic NSCL cancer were randomized to receive either 250 mg or 500 mg of gefitinib daily (43). Entry criteria included one to two prior chemotherapy regimens, one of which contained a platinum-based agent. Adverse reactions were generally mild. Response rates were 18.4% versus 19%, and overall survival was 7.6 versus 8.1 months for the 250- and 500-mg doses, respectively. In IDEAL 2 (44), 216 patients (from the United States) were randomized to receive either 250 mg or 500 mg of gefitinib daily. Entry criteria for IDEAL 2 included two or more prior chemotherapy regimens, including a platinum-based regimen and docetaxel administered concurrently or as separate regimens. Response rates for the 250-mg and 500-mg arms were 11.8% and 8.8%, respectively. Median survival was 6.1 months and 6 months for the 250-mg and 500-mg arms, respectively. The toxicity profile was similar to IDEAL 1. Both studies indicated that 250 mg is a well-tolerated dose, with evidence of clinically significant antitumor activity in patients who had failed one or two previous chemotherapy regimens. Many patients in both IDEAL 1 and IDEAL 2 reported significant improvement in disease-related symptoms and quality of life (40.3% and 43.1% for IDEAL 1 and IDEAL 2, respectively) (45).

Three phase III studies using gefitinib in advanced NSCL cancer have been conducted. The Iressa NSCL Cancer Trial Assessing Combination Treatment (INTACT) 1 (46) and 2 (47) were three-arm studies testing: (a) chemotherapy plus 250 mg/day gefitinib, (b) chemotherapy plus 500 mg/day gefitinib, and (c) chemotherapy plus placebo, all of which were to be followed by continuation of gefitinib or placebo until disease progression. The chemotherapy regimen was gemcitabine and cisplatin in INTACT 1, and paclitaxel and carboplatin in INTACT 2. More than 1000 patients were treated in each of these studies. The primary end-point for both trials was survival. Median survival was 9.92 months for the placebo arm and 9.82 months for the 250-mg arm and the 500-mg arm. Therefore, it was concluded that gefitinib showed no added benefit in survival for these patients who were being treated with a standard chemotherapy regimen.

The Iressa Survival Evaluation in Lung Cancer (ISEL) trial (48) was a double-blind, placebo-controlled, parallel-group, multicenter, phase III survival study that randomly assigned 1692 patients with previously treated, locally advanced or metastatic NSCL cancer in a 2:1 ratio to receive gefitinib 250 mg/day or placebo, plus best supportive care. Gefitinib was associated with a trend to improvement in survival in the overall ($p = 0.087$) but failed to reach statistical significance. Preplanned subset analyses showed marked heterogeneity in survival between patient groups; those who never smoked, patients of Asian origin, and females achieved a significant survival improvement with gefitinib versus placebo.

A number of ongoing and completed but not yet fully published trials have looked at the addition of gefitinib to combinations of chemotherapy and radiation therapy in the treatment of locally advanced lung cancer. For example, Southwest Oncology Group (SWOG)-0023 was a phase III, multi-institution, randomized double-blind study designed to assess whether maintenance therapy with gefitinib compared with placebo after induction cisplatin/etoposide/radiation therapy, plus consolidation docetaxel improves overall survival and progression-free survival in patients with unresectable stage III NSCL cancer. It was closed early due to results from the ISEL trial (48), described above, suggesting no survival benefit to gefitinib. Toxicity data have been reported for SWOG 0023 with respect to radiation pneumonitis rates, but preliminary survival data suggest no advantage to the addition of the drug (49). A multi-institution phase II trial has been conducted by the University of Colorado and Memorial Sloan-Kettering Cancer Center as a nonrandomized trial designed to study the safety and tolerability (in particular the treatment-related mortality, esophagitis, and pneumonitis) of preoperative gefitinib in combination with chemoradiation therapy in patients with stage IIIA NSCL cancer (cited in 20). Objectives are to determine the impact of concurrent preoperative gefitinib with cisplatin/etoposide and radiation therapy on the rates of operability and resectability, to evaluate the radiographic and pathologic response rate of preoperative ZD1839 with cisplatin/etoposide and radiation therapy, and to perform molecular correlation studies. Final results are pending.

Erlotinib

In phase I studies, erlotinib has found to be a safe and well-tolerated oral drug without severe toxicity. In this study, Hidalgo and colleagues treated 40 patients with erlotinib who had advanced solid malignancies refractory to conventional therapy, four of whom had NSCL cancer. Diarrhea and skin rash were the primary toxicities and precluded treatment with doses greater than 150 mg/day. Among patients with advanced, platinum-refractory NSCL cancer, 14.3% had an objective responses, and 28.6% had stable disease (50).

Three phase II trials with erlotinib have been conducted in patients with advanced refractory malignancies, including SCC of the head and neck, ovarian carcinoma, and NSCL cancer (51–53). Patients in each of these studies received 150 mg/day of the drug. One study enrolled 56 patients (all evaluable) with progressive, recurrent NSCL cancer previously treated with a platinum-based chemotherapy regimen (53). Eight patients (14.3%) achieved any response whereas 16 patients (28.6%) had stable disease lasting 12 weeks, and 28 patients (57.1%) had documented progression of their underlying malignancy. A relationship between response and the degree of EGFR overexpression was not established.

In a recent phase III study, a survival benefit of erlotinib compared with best supportive care was reported in previously treated NSCL cancer patients (8). Patients with stage IIIB or IV NSCL cancer were randomly assigned in a 2:1 ratio to receive oral erlotinib, at a dose of 150 mg daily, or placebo. The response rate was 8.9% in the erlotinib group and less than 1% in the placebo group. Progression-free survival was 2.2 months and 1.8 months, respectively. In contrast to trials with gefitinib (ISEL, 48), this study comparing erlotinib with best supportive care did show improved survival for erlotinib-treated patients. After the publication of these trials, clinicians favored the use of erlotinib over gefitinib. However, a trial directly comparing the two drugs was never started.

A subsequent series of phase III trials [TALENT (54) and TRIBUTE (55)] in NSCL cancer patients and involving erlotinib have been reported; there was no additional benefit of erlotinib in combination with chemotherapy, compared to chemotherapy alone. This has mimicked the experience noted in similarly designed trials with gefitinib. To date, no published trials deal exclusively with clinical testing of radiation therapy and TK inhibitors alone.

ANTIANGIOGENESIS AND TUMOR VASCULATURE TARGETING AGENTS IN LUNG CANCER TREATMENT

Rationale

Angiogenesis, or the development of new blood vessels, is integral to a number of physiologic but also pathophysiologic processes (56). Under physiologic conditions stimulating new vessel formation, angiogenesis is tightly controlled. However, during tumorigenesis, the process is sustained and requires ongoing production of stimulators by tumor and stromal cells over and above inhibitors. In a comprehensive review by O'Reilley (56), malignant angiogenesis is summarized as being notable for: (a) new vessels being markedly disorganized and lacking pericytes and other support cells, (b) impaired flow, (c) plasma proteins that act as neostroma, and (d) increased vascular permeability. In addition to their normal expected physiologic functions, proliferating endothelial cells also produce multiple growth factors that can promote tumor cell growth, invasion, and survival (57). In the end, neoangiogenesis may support malignancy directly through perfusion effects and indirectly via paracrine effects.

Vascular endothelial growth factor (VEGF) is the prime stimulus of angiogenic signaling (58). Upon VEGF binding, intrinsic receptors (VEGFRs) initiate a cascade of intracellular signaling pathways to trigger new vessel formation via gene-expression products that promote proliferation, migration, and survival (58). Of further interest, new tumor vasculature may arise from other mechanisms, including circulating endothelial progenitor cells (58). The abnormal pathways stimulating neovasculature formation are then reflected in the grossly abnormal vessel architecture seen in tumors. Immaturity and tortuosity is characteristic of cancer-associated vessels, as are leakiness and vacillating perfusion pressures (58). The latter can lead to transient hypoxia, which in turn can activate proangiogenic transcript factors. Such activation then leads to increased VEGF levels and other stimulating proteins, creating a circuitous cascade furthering growth and invasion (58).

Radiation therapy may also have a systemic and/or local effect on angiogenesis. Increased expression of proangiogenic factors such as VEGF has been observed after irradiation (59). For example, animals with recurrences at a primary site after being treated by radiotherapy had a higher likelihood of metastatic disease (60). It has been shown that the formation of recurrent tumors after radiotherapy is preceded by angiogenesis, most of which occurs within 20 days of irradiation (61), and that radiation therapy to a primary tumor can decrease the mobilization of angiogenesis inhibitors such as angiostatin (62). Administration of an angiogenesis inhibitor can also prevent accelerated metastatic growth in the lungs of mice after radiation treatment of a primary Lewis lung carcinoma (62). However, the effects of irradiation may seem paradoxical, with impairment of angiogenesis also possible. For example, irradiation of a primary tumor in rodents was associated with an inhibition of angiogenesis at a distant site (63), while plasma levels of endostatin, a proangiogenic peptide, in the irradiated mice were twice those found in the nonirradiated mice. These data suggest that irradiation may exert both pro- or antiangiogenic effects.

Preclinical Studies of Antiangiogenic Agents and Radiotherapy

It had long been assumed that an angiogenesis inhibitor would impair the effect of ionizing radiation by inducing tumor hypoxia (58). However, in a now-classic experiment, Teicher and colleagues (64) observed that antiangiogenic therapy given in combination with the angiogenesis inhibitors TNP-470 and minocycline, a weak inhibitor of metalloproteinase activity, improved tumor oxygenation and the antitumor effect of radiation therapy. In the first study of a specific inhibitor of angiogenesis combined with radiation therapy, Mauceri and colleagues (65) showed a synergistic effect when angiostatin and ionizing radiation were combined. The studies were designed using low doses of each modality and established murine lung carcinomas or human glioblastomas, SCCs, or prostate carcinomas. Other agents with antiangiogenic activity have been tested in combination with concurrent radiation therapy in preclinical models. These include celecoxib, a selective inhibitor of the cyclooxygenase-2 enzyme; cetuximab, an antibody directed against EGFR; platelet-derived growth factor (PDGFR); and sunitinib, a small-molecule inhibitor of VEGFR-2, PDGF, and c-kit, which has demonstrated enhanced radiation-induced tumor vascular destruction and control when combined with fractionated radiotherapy in murine tumor models (58). It would appear then that agents targeting EGFR, PDGFR, and other receptor TKs offer the potential for both indirect and direct effects on both the tumor and endothelial cell compartments and enhance the effects of radiotherapy.

Increased tumor responses to radiation therapy have been shown when it is combined with anti-VEGF agents (59), even for tumors that were markedly hypoxic (66,67) with an increase in tumor growth delay and an augmentation of tumor curability in the combined modality groups. Kozin and coworkers (68) treated mice with human small-cell lung cancer with fractionated radiation therapy combined with antibodies directed against VEGFR-2 and found that the dose of radiation was diminished 1.3-fold to achieve 50% control. The antiangiogenic agent semaxinib, a small-molecule antagonist of VEGFR signaling, had an additive effect when combined with radiation therapy in a glioblastoma tumor line, and permanent vascular changes were seen with combined treatment, resulting in complete remission (69).

A number of preclinical models have examined the pharmacologic and pharmacodynamic activities of the anti-VEGF humanized, monoclonal antibody, bevacizumab (70). In a review by Gerber and Ferrara (71), bevacizumab has been noted to inhibit tumor growth in a wide range of tumor lines. Several studies also observed significant inhibition of tumor metastases. Various studies examined the feasibility of combining anti-VEGF therapy with cytotoxic or biologic agents. Combining bevacizumab with doxorubicin, topotecan, paclitaxel, docetaxel, or radiotherapy resulted in additive or synergistic tumor growth inhibition. Changes in vascular functions were frequently reported, including decreased vessel diameter, density, and permeability in response to treatment. Combination treatment with radiation increased tumor oxygenation and tumor growth inhibition.

Some studies suggest that the timing of radiation therapy and drug administration may be of critical importance. Semaxinib increased the antitumor effects of fractionated radiation in SCC xenografts, regardless of whether it was administered before or after radiotherapy (72). In contrast, when PTK787, a small-molecule inhibitor of VEGFR-2, was administered before, concurrent with, or after fractionated irradiation, only adjuvant application retarded regrowth of human SCC xenografts, and long-term inhibition of angiogenesis after radiotherapy significantly reduced the growth rate of local recurrences but did not improve local tumor control (73). Clearly, there is potential for combining antiangiogenic agents with radiation in the clinical setting, but further preclinical study will better define the possible interactions of these agents in the clinical setting.

Clinical Studies of Antiangiogenic Agents and Radiotherapy

A number of antiangiogenesis agents are under clinical study (Fig. 8.3) and these can be categorized into the following categories: (a) direct endothelial cell inhibitors, inhibiting proliferation or migration without affecting other cell types; (b) VEGF and VEGFR inhibitors, either blocking the growth factor directly or indirectly, inhibiting the receptor, or interfering with its downstream signaling; and (c) agents with multiple overlapping effects. We review those agents with current trial-based relevance for clinical radiation.

Bevacizumab

Initial clinical studies involved phase I trials that established the safety and tolerability of bevacizumab in the advanced disease setting for a number of solid tumors including colorectal, kidney, pancreatic, breast, and lung tumors (74).

Bevacizumab has been studied in NSCL cancer in the randomized phase II setting. In a key study of 99 patients treated with carboplatin/paclitaxel with or without bevacizumab, those receiving the experimental drug had improved response and progression-free survival rates (75). However, an increased risk of fatal hemoptysis was noted, in particular for patients with central tumors, in close proximity to major vessels and/or with squamous histology.

In a subsequent landmark phase III trial, the Eastern Cooperative Oncology Group (ECOG) conducted a randomized study in which 878 patients with recurrent or advanced NSCL cancer (stage IIIB or IV) were assigned to chemotherapy with paclitaxel and carboplatin alone, or paclitaxel and carboplatin plus bevacizumab (76). Patients with squamous-cell tumors and clinically sig-

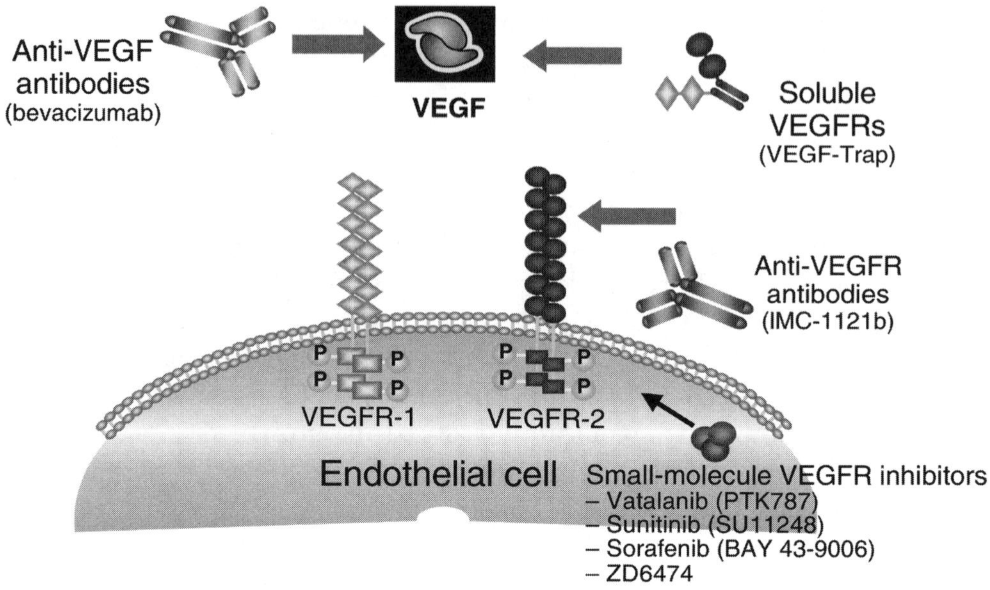

FIGURE 8.3 Agents targeting the vascular endothelial growth factor (VEGF) pathway. VEGF, vascular endothelial growth factor; VEGFR, VEGF receptor.

nificant hemoptysis were specifically excluded. The median survival was 12.3 months in the group assigned to chemotherapy plus bevacizumab, as compared with 10.3 months in the chemotherapy-alone group ($p = 0.003$). Rates of clinically significant bleeding were 4.4% and 0.7%, respectively ($P < 0.001$). There were 15 treatment-related deaths in the chemotherapy-plus-bevacizumab group, including five from pulmonary hemorrhage.

Because of the association with potentially fatal hemoptysis in central lung tumors, there have been concerns about the use of radiotherapy concurrently with bevacizumab for such tumors (77). However, a recent report suggests that this association may not be significant (78). Nonetheless, current trials in which the drug is being tested in locally advanced lung cancer have been mindful of this concern in the designs of their studies, for example, in SWOG 30533, a pilot study of cisplatin/etoposide/radiation therapy/docetaxel and three cohorts of bevacizumab in stage III NSCL cancer.

Other Vascular-Targeting Agents

Combretastatin A4-phosphate is a small-molecule vascular-targeting agent (VTA) that acts as a microtubule destabilizing agent (58). A phase Ib study combining the drug with radiation therapy in patients with locally advanced NSCL cancer or prostate carcinoma demonstrated no significant increase in radiation-related toxicity at early follow-up, and no untoward vascular events were noted (79).

Agents That Target Multiple Sites

Antiangiogenic/anti-EGFR Therapies and Radiotherapy: Preclinical Studies

A variety of small-molecule agents that target multiple receptors are currently under investigation. ZD6474 is a VEGFR-TK inhibitor that has dual anti-EGFR and anti-VEGFR properties. When a variety of EGFR-positive human epithelial cancer cell lines, including lung, were treated with ZD6474, reduced colony formation in soft agar assays was seen and a dose-dependent potentiation of the effect was noted with either paclitaxel or docetaxel. A marked reduction in angiogenesis has also been seen in ZD6474-treated GEO xenografts (80,81).

Another strategy directed at multiple targets can include anti-EGFR treatments with concurrent administration of anti-VEGFR agents. This strategy is based on the rationale that cancer cells may override EGFR blockade by upregulating signaling through angiogenic pathways. This hypothesis is supported in part from preclinical investigations, such as one that showed increased VEGF production in A431 human cancer variants derived from recurrent tumor xenograft models resistant to anti-EGFR antibodies (81). In another example, combining an EGFR-TK inhibitor with a VEGFR-TK inhibitor produced synergism in mice containing human small-cell lung cancer xenografts, reducing by 50% the daily dosage requirement of each compound required for growth inhibition (82).

MISCELLANEOUS BIOLOGIC THERAPIES WITH RADIOTHERAPY IN LUNG CANCER TREATMENT

Clinical Studies

Celecoxib

Overexpression of cyclo-oxygenase (COX)-2 is frequently present in lung cancer and may play a significant role in carcinogenesis, invasion, and metastasis. It has been associated with shortened survival in patients with resected early-stage adenocarcinoma of the lung (83). COX-2 inhibition decreases tumor cell proliferation in vivo and has been shown to enhance tumor radiosensitivity. Additionally, COX-2 inhibition may protect normal pulmonary tissue from radiation fibrosis. Clinical studies are under way to assess the potential benefits and risks of COX-2 inhibition in the treatment of lung cancer. A recently completed RTOG study (0213) using celecoxib and concurrent radiation therapy (doses of either 45 Gy/15 fractions or 66 Gy/33 fractions) for NSCL cancer in poor-risk patients with medically inoperable nonmetastatic disease (83). Celecoxib was used concurrently with radiation therapy and then as maintenance. Results remain to be reported. A similar study from Liao and colleagues at the M.D. Anderson Cancer Center has been published (84). This phase I clinical trial of thoracic radiotherapy and concurrent celecoxib for patients with unfavorable performance status in inoperable/unresectable NSCL cancer involved celecoxib being administered on a daily basis 5 days before and throughout the course of radiotherapy. Celecoxib doses were escalated from 200, 400, 600, to 800 mg/day, given in two equally divided doses. Two to eight patients of each cohort were assigned to each dose level of celecoxib. These results showed that celecoxib could be safely administered concurrently with thoracic radiotherapy when given up to the highest U.S. Food and Drug Administration (FDA)-approved dose of 800 mg/day. A maximal tolerated dose was not reached in this study. The treatment resulted in actuarial local progression-free survival of 66.0% at 1 year and 42.2% at 2 years.

Proteosome Inhibitors

The ubiquitin/proteasome pathway plays an essential role in the degradation of most short- and long-lived intracellular proteins in eukaryotic cells, and therefore in regulating the cell cycle, neoplastic growth, and metastasis. Bortezomib is a selective 26S proteasome inhibitor that has been approved for the treatment of multiple myeloma (85). Edelman has reviewed the potential role of bortezomib in NSCL cancer (85). Bortezomib has demonstrated in vitro chemotherapy- and radiotherapy-sensitizing properties as well as single-agent activity in lung cancer. To date, no studies are under way of bortezomib as a single-agent radiation therapy sensitizer alone or as part of a combination regimen for lung cancer. However, Van Waes and colleagues have reported on bortezomib concurrent with radiation therapy in patients with recurrent or metastatic head and neck SCCs who had previous chemotherapy or radiation therapy; they noted responses with the drug, although it was felt to be too toxic (86).

■ SMALL-CELL LUNG CANCER

Small-cell lung (SCL) cancer remains as much a therapeutic challenge as NSCL cancer. For reasons not yet fully understood, the incidence of the disease in the West has decreased over the past 20 years and is now close to 15% of diagnosed lung cancers (1). Survival rates, as with NSCL cancer, also remain modest, with optimal median survivals not greater than 24 months in limited disease (87). In the setting of targeted therapy development and trials, the infrequency of this disease presentation has not made it an optimal setting for the testing of new therapies; however, there are clinical reports detailing new approaches to SCL cancer treatment with a perspective relevant to radiation therapy.

The Minnie Pearl Cancer Research Network conducted a multicenter phase II trial to assess the tolerability and response rate of concurrent radiotherapy and carboplatin plus irinotecan followed by bevacizumab in 41 patients with limited stage (LS) SCL cancer (88). Patients were restaged after the fourth cycle, and those without progression or undue toxicity received bevacizumab 10 mg/kg intravenously every 14 days for ten doses. Complete and partial responses were observed in 12 (32%) and 18 patients (49%), respectively. Overall survival from this trial has not yet been reported.

Vaccines have been evaluated in pilot studies for the prevention of relapse in SCL cancer, namely the BEC2 (mitumomab) anti-idiotypic mouse monoclonal antibody combined with Bacillus Calmette-Guérin (BCG) (89). A phase III trial called Survival in an International Phase III Prospective Randomized Limited Disease Small Cell Lung Cancer Vaccination Study with BEC2 and BCG (SILVA) enrolled 515 LS-SCLC patients with response after chemoradiation to an observation arm or a vaccine. Unfortunately, no difference was seen between the observation and vaccine arms in terms of median survival (16.3 compared with 14.3 months, respectively) or progression-free survival (6.6 compared with 5.7 months) (90).

The Cancer and Leukemia Group B (CALGB) performed a phase III trial of tamoxifen with cisplatin/etoposide and radiation, based on data that suggested tamoxifen enhanced the effectiveness of cisplatin-based chemotherapy regimens. The trial enrolled 307 patients and randomized them to standard chemotherapy with or without high-dose tamoxifen. There was no significant difference in response rates or overall survival (20.6 months compared with 18.4 months) (91).

The SWOG 0004 studied the use of a bioreductive agent, tirapazamine, in conjunction with chemoradiation consisting of etoposide, cisplatin, and radiation (92). The preliminary phase I data suggested that survival was favorable but the addition of tirapazamine increased the incidence of vomiting, neutropenia, and febrile neutropenia.

■ FUTURE DIRECTIONS

Preclinical studies remain a pressing requirement in determining the effectiveness of the new targeted or biologic agents in combination with radiation therapy. In that regard, numerous examples of innovative research are currently addressing this question. For example, Garkavij and colleagues have explored combined external radiation therapy and radioimmunotargeting to enhance tumor radiation without affecting morbidity using antibody-guided targeting of NSCL cancer using ^{111}In-labeled human milk-fat globule (HMFG1) F(ab')2 fragments (93). Anscher and colleagues used thalidomide to determine if it might protect normal tissues in patients when used in combination with vinorelbine plus thoracic radiotherapy (94). Unfortunately, they found increased toxicity with this combination. Adusumilli and colleagues have found that radiation therapy potentiates effective oncolytic viral therapy in the treatment of lung cancer (95). The rationale for their study was that replication-competent oncolytic herpes simplex viruses with deletion of the γ(1)34.5 gene preferentially replicate in and kill malignant cells. The γ(1)34.5 gene codes for ICP 34.5, a protein that enhances viral replication and is homologous to growth arrest and DNA damage protein 34 (GADD34), a radiation-inducible DNA repair gene. The authors showed that radiation therapy could potentiate efficacy of oncolytic viral therapy by upregulating GADD34 and promoting viral replication. Cerna and colleagues have looked at histone deacetylation as a target for radiosensitization (96). Histone acetylation plays a role in regulating chromatin structure and gene expression—two parameters that may influence radioresponse. A structurally diverse set of histone deacetylase (HDAC) inhibitors has been shown to enhance the in vitro radiosensitivity of human tumor cell lines generated from a spectrum of solid tumors (96).

The current era of clinical research in lung cancer is active and rapidly evolving, as witnessed by the number of clinical trials listed on the National Cancer Institute's website, at least a dozen of which are testing currently developed and newer targeted therapies along with radiotherapy and/or chemotherapy. Not only efficacy, but safety must be established for any and all these agents, especially in the context of multimodal therapy that will continue to remain the standard of care for lung cancer. Radiation oncologists will therefore need to be leaders in elucidating the potential benefits and interactions between all forms of radiation therapy delivery as the diversity of drugs increases.

REFERENCES

1. Jemal A, Siegel R, Ward E, et al. Cancer statistics, 2007. *CA Cancer J* Clin 2007;57:43–66.
2. Depierre A, Milleron B, Moro-Sibilot D, et al. Preoperative chemotherapy followed by surgery compared with primary surgery in resectable stage I (except T1N0), II, and IIIa non-small-cell lung cancer. *J Clin Oncol* 2002;20:247–253.
3. Hotta K, Matsuo K, Ueoka H, et al. Role of adjuvant chemotherapy in patients with resected non-small-cell lung cancer: Reappraisal with a meta-analysis of randomized controlled trials. *J Clin Oncol* 2004;22:3860–3867.
4. Curran WJ, Scott CB, Langer CJ, et al. Long-term benefit is observed in a phase III comparison of sequential vs concurrent chemo-radiation for patients with unresected stage III NSCLC: ROT 9410. *Proc Am Soc Clin Oncol* 2003;22:621.
5. Hotta K, Matsuo K, Ueoka H, et al. Addition of platinum compounds to a new agent in patients with advanced non-small-cell lung cancer: A literature based meta-analysis of randomised trials. *Ann Oncol* 2004;15:1782–1789.
6. Raben D, Helfrich B, Bunn PA Jr. Targeted therapies for non-small-cell lung cancer: Biology, rationale, and preclinical results from a radiation oncology perspective. Int J Radiat Oncol Biol Phys 2004;59(Suppl 2):27–38.
7. Maione P, Gridelli C, Troiani T, Ciardiello F. Combining targeted therapies and drugs with multiple targets in the treatment of NSCLC. *Oncologist* 2006;11:274–284.

8. Shepherd FA, Rodrigues Pereira J, Ciuleanu T, et al. Erlotinib in previously treated non-small-cell lung cancer. *N Engl J Med* 2005;353:123–132.
9. Vokes E, Herbst R, Sandler A. Angiogenesis inhibition in the treatment of lung cancer. *Clin Adv Hematol Oncol* 2006;4(11 Suppl 23):1–12.
10. Wilson GD, Bentzen SM, Harari PM. Biologic basis for combining drugs with radiation. *Semin Radiat Oncol* 2006;16:2–9.
11. Bernier J, Hall EJ, Giaccia A. Radiation oncology: A century of achievements. *Nat Rev Cancer* 2004;4:737–747.
12. Bengtson EM, Rigas JR. A brief historical review of the development of chemotherapy for the treatment of advanced non-small cell lung cancer: why we should look beyond platinum. *Semin Oncol* 1999;26(5 Suppl 16):1–6.
13. Steel GG. Terminology in the description of drug-radiation interactions. *Int J Radiat Oncol Biol Phys* 1979;5:1145–1150.
14. Arteaga C. Targeting HER1/EGFR: A molecular approach to cancer therapy. *Semin Oncol* 2003;30(3 Suppl 7):3–14.
15. Raymond E, Faivre S, Armand JP. Epidermal growth factor receptor tyrosine kinase as a target for anticancer therapy. *Drugs* 2000;60 (Suppl 1):15–23.
16. Salomon DS, Brandt R, Ciardiello F, Normanno N. Epidermal growth factor-related peptides and their receptors in human malignancies. *Crit Rev Oncol Hematol* 1995;19:183–232.
17. Veale D, Kerr N, Gibson GJ, et al. The relationship of quantitative epidermal growth factor receptor expression in non-small cell lung cancer to long term survival. *Br J Cancer* 1993;68:162–165.
18. Silvestri GA, Rivera MP. Targeted therapy for the treatment of advanced non-small cell lung cancer: A review of the epidermal growth factor receptor antagonists. *Chest* 2005;128:3975–3984.
19. Cerny T, Barnes DM, Hasleton P, et al. Expression of epidermal growth factor receptor (EGF-R) in human lung tumours. *Br J Cancer* 1986;54:265–269.
20. Kim DW, Choy H. Potential role for epidermal growth factor receptor inhibitors in combined-modality therapy for non-small-cell lung cancer. *Int J Radiat Oncol Biol Phys* 2004;59(Suppl 2):11–20.
21. Contessa JN, Reardon DB, Todd D, et al. The inducible expression of dominant-negative epidermal growth factor receptor-CD533 results in radiosensitization of human mammary carcinoma cells. *Clin Cancer Res* 1999;5:405–411.
22. Sheridan MT, O'Dwyer T, Seymour CB, Mothersill CE. Potential indicators of radiosensitivity in squamous cell carcinoma of the head and neck. *Radiat Oncol Investig* 1997;5:180–186.
23. Akimoto T, Hunter NR, Buchmiller L, et al. Inverse relationship between epidermal growth factor receptor expression and radiocurability of murine carcinomas. *Clin Cancer Res* 1999;5:2884–2890.
24. Bowers G, Reardon D, Hewitt T, et al. The relative role of ErbB1-4 receptor tyrosine kinases in radiation signal transduction responses of human carcinoma cells. *Oncogene* 2001;20:1388–1397.
25. Bonner JA, De Los Santos J, Waksal HW, et al. Epidermal growth factor receptor as a therapeutic target in head and neck cancer. *Semin Radiat Oncol* 2002;12(3 Suppl 2):11–20.
26. Schmidt-Ullrich RK, Mikkelsen RB, Dent P, et al. Radiation-induced proliferation of the human A431 squamous carcinoma cells is dependent on EGFR tyrosine phosphorylation. *Oncogene* 1997;15:1191–1197.
27. Harari PM, Huang SM. Modulation of molecular targets to enhance radiation. *Clin Cancer Res* 2000;6:323–325.

28. Huang SM, Li J, Armstrong EA, Harari PM. Modulation of radiation response and tumor-induced angiogenesis after epidermal growth factor receptor inhibition by ZD1839 (Iressa). *Cancer Res* 2002;62:4300–4306.
29. Beerli RR, Hynes NE. Epidermal growth factor-related peptides activate distinct subsets of ErbB receptors and differ in their biological activities. *J Biol Chem* 1996;271:6071–6076.
30. Riese DJ 2nd, Bermingham Y, van Raaij TM, et al. Betacellulin activates the epidermal growth factor receptor and erbB-4, and induces cellular response patterns distinct from those stimulated by epidermal growth factor or neuregulin-beta. *Oncogene* 1996;12:345–353.
31. Raben D, Helfrich B, Chan DC, et al. The effects of cetuximab alone and in combination with radiation and/or chemotherapy in lung cancer. *Clin Cancer Res* 2005;11:795–805.
32. Milas L, Mason K, Hunter N, et al. In vivo enhancement of tumor radioresponse by C225 antiepidermal growth factor receptor antibody. *Clin Cancer Res* 2000;6:701–708.
33. Sirotnak FM, Zakowski MF, Miller VA, et al. Efficacy of cytotoxic agents against human tumor xenografts is markedly enhanced by coadministration of ZD1839 (Iressa), an inhibitor of EGFR tyrosine kinase. *Clin Cancer Res* 2000;6:4885–4892.
34. Moasser MM, Basso A, Averbuch SD, Rosen N. The tyrosine kinase inhibitor ZD1839 ("Iressa") inhibits HER2-driven signaling and suppresses the growth of HER2-overexpressing tumor cells. *Cancer Res* 2001;61:7184–7188.
35. Baselga J, Pfister D, Cooper MR, et al. Phase I studies of anti-epidermal growth factor receptor chimeric antibody C225 alone and in combination with cisplatin. *J Clin Oncol* 2000;18:904–914.
36. Kim ES, Mauer AM, Fosella FV et al. A phase II study of Erbitux (IMC-C225), an epidermal growth factor receptor (EGFR) blocking antibody, in combination with docetaxel in chemotherapy refractory/resistant patients with advanced non-small cell lung cancer (NSCLC). *Proc Am Soc Clin Oncol* 2002;21:A293.
37. Bonner JA, Harari PM, Giralt J, et al. Radiotherapy plus cetuximab for squamous-cell carcinoma of the head and neck. *N Engl J Med* 2006;354:567–578.
38. Robert F, Blumenschein G, Herbst RS, et al. Phase I/IIa study of cetuximab with gemcitabine plus carboplatin in patients with chemotherapy-naive advanced non-small-cell lung cancer. *J Clin Oncol* 2005;23:9089–9096.
39. Baselga J, Rischin D, Ranson M, et al. Phase I safety, pharmacokinetic, and pharmacodynamic trial of ZD1839, a selective oral epidermal growth factor receptor tyrosine kinase inhibitor, in patients with five selected solid tumor types. *J Clin Oncol* 2002;20:4292–4302.
40. Ferry D, Hammond L, Ranson M, et al. Intermittent oral ZD1839 (Iressa), a novel epidermal growth factor receptor tyrosine kinase inhibitor (EGFR-TKI) shows evidence of good tolerability and activity: Final results from a phase I study. *Proc Am Soc Clin Oncol* 2000;19:A3.
41. Goss G, Lorimer I, Miller W, et al. Phase I, dose escalation, pharmacokinetics (PK) and pharmacodynamic (PD) study of ZD1839: NCIC CTG IND.122. *Clin Cancer Res* 2000;6: Abstract, 382.
42. Kusaba H, Tamura T, Nakagawa K, et al. A phase I intermittent dose-escalation trial of ZD1839 (Iressa) in Japanese patients with solid malignant tumours. *Clin Cancer Res* 2000;6:Abstract, 381.
43. Fukuoka M, Yano S, Giaccone G, et al. Multi-institutional randomized phase II trial of gefitinib for previously treated patients with advanced non-small-cell lung cancer. *J Clin Oncol* 2003;21:2237–2246.
44. Kris MG, Natale RB, Herbst RS, et al. Efficacy of gefitinib, an inhibitor of the epidermal growth factor receptor tyrosine kinase, in symptomatic patients with non-small cell lung cancer: A randomized trial. *JAMA* 2003;290:2149–2158.

45. Cella D, Herbst RS, Lynch TJ, et al. Clinically meaningful improvement in symptoms and quality of life for patients with non-small-cell lung cancer receiving gefitinib in a randomized controlled trial. *J Clin Oncol* 2005;23:2946–2954.
46. Giaccone G, Herbst RS, Manegold C, et al. Gefitinib in combination with gemcitabine and cisplatin in advanced non-small-cell lung cancer: A phase III trial–INTACT 1. *J Clin Oncol* 2004;22:777–784.
47. Herbst RS, Giaccone G, Schiller JH, et al. Gefitinib in combination with paclitaxel and carboplatin in advanced non-small-cell lung cancer: A phase III trial–INTACT 2. *J Clin Oncol* 2004;22:785–794.
48. Thatcher N, Chang A, Parikh P, et al. Gefitinib plus best supportive care in previously treated patients with refractory advanced non-small-cell lung cancer: Results from a randomised, placebo-controlled, multicentre study (Iressa Survival Evaluation in Lung Cancer). *Lancet* 2005;366:1527–1537.
49. Kelly K, Gaspar LE, Chansky K, et al. Low incidence of pneumonitis on SWOG 0023: A preliminary analysis of an ongoing phase III trial of concurrent chemoradiotherapy followed by consolidation docetaxel and gefitinib/placebo maintenance in patients with inoperable stage III non-small cell lung cancer. *Proc Am Soc Clin Oncol* 2005;23:S634.
50. Hidalgo M, Siu LL, Nemunaitis J, et al. Phase I and pharmacologic study of OSI-774, an epidermal growth factor receptor tyrosine kinase inhibitor, in patients with advanced solid malignancies. *J Clin Oncol* 2001;19:3267–3279.
51. Senzer NN, Soulieres D, Siu L, et al. Phase 2 evaluation of OSI-774, a potent oral antagonist of the EGFR-TK in patients with advanced squamous cell carcinoma of the head and neck. *Proc Am Soc Clin Oncol* 2001;20:A2.
52. Finkler N, Gordon A, Crozier M, et al. Phase 2 evaluation of OSI-774, a potent oral antagonist of the EGFR-TK in patients with advanced ovarian carcinoma. *Proc Am Soc Clin Oncol* 2001;20:A209.
53. Perez-Soler R, Chachoua A, Huberman M, et al. A phase II trial of the epidermal growth factor receptor (EGFR) tyrosine kinase inhibitor OSI-774, following platinum-based chemotherapy, in patients (pts) with advanced, EGFR-expressing, non-small cell lung cancer (NSCLC). *Proc Am Soc Clin Oncol* 2001;20:A310.
54. Gatzemeier U, Pluzanska A, Szczesna A, et al. Results of a phase III trial of erlotinib (OSI-774) combined with cisplatin and gemcitabine (GC) chemotherapy in advanced non-small cell lung cancer (NSCLC). *J Clin Oncol* 2007;25(12):1545–1552.
55. Herbst RS, Prager D, Hermann R, et al. TRIBUTE: A phase III trial of erlotinib HCl (OSI-774) combined with carboplatin and paclitaxel (CP) chemotherapy in advanced non-small cell lung cancer (NSCLC). *J Clin Oncol* 2005; 23(25):5892–5899.
56. O'Reilly MS. Radiation combined with antiangiogenic and antivascular agents. *Semin Radiat Oncol* 2006;16:45–50.
57. Rak J, Filmus J, Kerbel RS. Reciprocal paracrine interactions between tumour cells and endothelial cells: The "angiogenesis progression" hypothesis. *Eur J Cancer* 1996;32A:2438–2450.
58. Raben D, Ryan A. Vascular-targeting agents and radiation therapy in lung cancer: Where do we stand in 2005? *Clin Lung Cancer* 2005;7:175–179.
59. Gorski DH, Beckett MA, Jaskowiak NT, et al. Blockage of the vascular endothelial growth factor stress response increases the antitumor effects of ionizing radiation. *Cancer Res* 1999;59:3374–3378.
60. Suit HD, Sedlacek RS, Gillette EL. Examination for a correlation between probabilities of development of distant metastasis and of local recurrence. *Radiology* 1970;95:189–194.

61. Hast J, Schiffer IB, Neugebauer B, et al. Angiogenesis and fibroblast proliferation precede formation of recurrent tumors after radiation therapy in nude mice. *Anticancer Res* 2002;22:677–688.
62. Camphausen K, Moses MA, Beecken WD, et al. Radiation therapy to a primary tumor accelerates metastatic growth in mice. *Cancer Res* 2001;61:2207–2211.
63. Hartford AC, Gohongi T, Fukumura D, Jain RK. Irradiation of a primary tumor, unlike surgical removal, enhances angiogenesis suppression at a distal site: potential role of host-tumor interaction. *Cancer Res* 2000;60:2128–2131.
64. Teicher BA, Dupuis NP, Robinson MF, et al. Antiangiogenic treatment (TNP-470/minocycline) increases tissue levels of anticancer drugs in mice bearing Lewis lung carcinoma. *Oncol Res* 1995;7:237–243.
65. Mauceri HJ, Hanna NN, Beckett MA, et al. Combined effects of angiostatin and ionizing radiation in antitumour therapy. *Nature* 1998;394:287–291.
66. Lee CG, Heijn M, di Tomaso E, et al. Anti-Vascular endothelial growth factor treatment augments tumor radiation response under normoxic or hypoxic conditions. *Cancer Res* 2000;60:5565–5570.
67. Hess C, Vuong V, Hegyi I, et al. Effect of VEGF receptor inhibitor PTK787/ZK222584 [correction of ZK222548] combined with ionizing radiation on endothelial cells and tumour growth. *Br J Cancer* 2001;85:2010–2016.
68. Kozin SV, Boucher Y, Hicklin DJ, et al. Vascular endothelial growth factor receptor-2-blocking antibody potentiates radiation-induced long-term control of human tumor xenografts. *Cancer Res* 2001;61:39–44.
69. Schuuring J, Bussink J, Bernsen HJ, et al. Irradiation combined with SU5416: Microvascular changes and growth delay in a human xenograft glioblastoma tumor line. *Int J Radiat Oncol Biol Phys* 2005;61:529–534.
70. Jain RK. Normalizing tumor vasculature with anti-angiogenic therapy: A new paradigm for combination therapy. *Nat Med* 2001;7:987–989.
71. Gerber HP, Ferrara N. Pharmacology and pharmacodynamics of bevacizumab as monotherapy or in combination with cytotoxic therapy in preclinical studies. *Cancer Res* 2005;65:671–680.
72. Ning S, Laird D, Cherrington JM, Knox SJ. The antiangiogenic agents SU5416 and SU6668 increase the antitumor effects of fractionated irradiation. *Radiat Res* 2002;157:45–51.
73. Zips D, Hessel F, Krause M, et al. Impact of adjuvant inhibition of vascular endothelial growth factor receptor tyrosine kinases on tumor growth delay and local tumor control after fractionated irradiation in human squamous cell carcinomas in nude mice. *Int J Radiat Oncol Biol Phys* 2005;61:908–914.
74. Verhoef C, de Wilt JH, Verheul HM. Angiogenesis inhibitors: Perspectives for medical, surgical and radiation oncology. *Curr Pharm Des* 2006;12:2623–2630.
75. Herbst RS, Johnson DH, Mininberg E, et al. Phase I/II trial evaluating the anti-vascular endothelial growth factor monoclonal antibody bevacizumab in combination with the HER-1/epidermal growth factor receptor tyrosine kinase inhibitor erlotinib for patients with recurrent non-small-cell lung cancer. *J Clin Oncol* 2005;23:2544–2555.
76. Sandler A, Gray R, Perry MC, et al. Paclitaxel-carboplatin alone or with bevacizumab for non-small-cell lung cancer. *N Engl J Med* 2006;355:2542–2550.
77. Hennequin C. Targeted therapies and radiotherapy in lung cancer. *Cancer Radiother* 2007;11(1–2):77–83. Epub 2006 Oct. 27.
78. Sandler AB, Johnson DH, Brahmer J, et al. Retrospective study of clinical and radiographic risk factors associated with early onset, severe pulmonary hemorrhage in bevacizumab-

treated patients with advanced non-small cell lung cancer (NSCLC). *Proc Am Soc Clin Oncol* 2006;24:381.

79. Ng QS, Carnell D, Milner J, et al. Phase Ib trial of Combretastatin A4 Phosphate (CA4P) in combination with radiotherapy (RT): Initial clinical results. *J Clin Oncol* 2005;23(16 suppl):221s.
80. Ciardiello F, Caputo R, Damiano V, et al. Antitumor effects of ZD6474, a small molecule vascular endothelial growth factor receptor tyrosine kinase inhibitor, with additional activity against epidermal growth factor receptor tyrosine kinase. *Clin Cancer Res* 2003;9:1546–1556.
81. Viloria-Petit A, Crombet T, Jothy S, et al. Acquired resistance to the antitumor effect of epidermal growth factor receptor-blocking antibodies in vivo: A role for altered tumor angiogenesis. *Cancer Res* 2001;61:5090–5101.
82. Bianco C, Bianco R, Tortora G, et al. Antitumor activity of combined treatment of human cancer cells with ionizing radiation and anti-epidermal growth factor receptor monoclonal antibody C225 plus type I protein kinase A antisense oligonucleotide. *Clin Cancer Res* 2000;6:4343–4350.
83. Gore E. Celecoxib and radiation therapy in non-small-cell lung cancer. *Oncology (Williston Park)* 2004;18(14 Suppl 14):10–14.
84. Liao Z, Komaki R, Milas L, et al. A phase I clinical trial of thoracic radiotherapy and concurrent celecoxib for patients with unfavorable performance status inoperable/unresectable non-small cell lung cancer. *Clin Cancer Res* 2005;11:3342–3348.
85. Edelman MJ. The potential role of bortezomib in combination with chemotherapy and radiation in non-small-cell lung cancer. *Clin Lung Cancer* 2005;7(Suppl 2):S64–S66.
86. Van Waes C, Chang AA, Lebowitz PF, et al. Inhibition of nuclear factor-kappaB and target genes during combined therapy with proteasome inhibitor bortezomib and reirradiation in patients with recurrent head-and-neck squamous cell carcinoma. *Int J Radiat Oncol Biol Phys* 2005;63:1400–1412.
87. Turrisi AT 3rd. Limited-disease small-cell lung cancer research: Sense and nonsense. *Int J Radiat Oncol Biol Phys* 2004;59:925–927.
88. Patton JF, Spigel DR, Greco FA, et al. Irinotecan (I), carboplatin (C), and radiotherapy (RT) followed by maintenance bevacizumab (B) in the treatment (tx) of limited-stage small cell lung cancer (LS-SCLC): Update of a phase II trial of the Minnie Pearl Cancer Research Network. *Proc Am Sc Clinic Oncol* 2006;24:385.
89. Grant SC, Kris MG, Houghton AN, Chapman PB. Long survival of patients with small cell lung cancer after adjuvant treatment with the anti-idiotypic antibody BEC2 plus Bacillus Calmette-Guerin. *Clin Cancer Res* 1999;5:1319–1323.
90. Giaccone G, Debruyne C, Felip E, et al. Phase III study of adjuvant vaccination with Bec2/bacille Calmette-Guerin in responding patients with limited-disease small-cell lung cancer (European Organisation for Research and Treatment of Cancer 08971-08971B; Silva Study). *J Clin Oncol* 2005;23:6854–6864.
91. McClay EF, Bogart J, Herndon JE 2nd, et al. A phase III trial evaluating the combination of cisplatin, etoposide, and radiation therapy with or without tamoxifen in patients with limited-stage small cell lung cancer: Cancer and Leukemia Group B Study (9235). *Am J Clin Oncol* 2005;28:81–90.
92. Le QT, McCoy J, Williamson S, et al. Phase I study of tirapazamine plus cisplatin/etoposide and concurrent thoracic radiotherapy in limited-stage small cell lung cancer (S0004): A Southwest Oncology Group study. *Clin Cancer Res* 2004;10:5418–5424.
93. Garkavij M, Samarzija M, Ewers SB, et al. Concurrent radiotherapy and tumor targeting with 111In-HMFG1-F(ab')2 in patients with MUC1-positive non-small cell lung cancer. *Anticancer Res* 2005;25:4663–4671.

94. Anscher MS, Garst J, Marks LB, et al. Assessing the ability of the antiangiogenic and anti-cytokine agent thalidomide to modulate radiation-induced lung injury. *Int J Radiat Oncol Biol Phys* 2006;66:477–482.
95. Adusumilli PS, Stiles BM, Chan MK, et al. Radiation therapy potentiates effective oncolytic viral therapy in the treatment of lung cancer. *Ann Thorac Surg* 2005;80:409–416.
96. Cerna D, Camphausen K, Tofilon PJ. Histone deacetylation as a target for radiosensitization. *Curr Top Dev Biol* 2006;73:173–204.

9 *Targeted Therapies in Pancreatic Cancer*

SUNIL KRISHNAN
VISHAL RANA
CHRISTOPHER H. CRANE

Pancreatic cancer is the third most common gastrointestinal malignancy and the fourth leading cause of cancer death in the United States. In 2006, an estimated 33,730 new cases of pancreatic cancer were diagnosed and a roughly equal number of deaths were attributable to pancreatic cancer (1). Pancreatic cancer has the poorest prognosis of any common gastrointestinal malignancy, with a 5-year overall survival of less than 5% (2). The absence of validated screening biomarkers and imaging tools to detect pancreatic cancer at an early stage and the inherent aggressiveness of pancreatic cancers contribute to the advanced stage of presentation of most patients by the time a diagnosis is established. At least half of all pancreatic cancer patients have radiographically detectable metastatic disease at the time of diagnosis. These patients are treated primarily with chemotherapy, with radiation therapy reserved for palliation of symptomatic disease. Surgery, the only potentially curative treatment for nonmetastatic patients, confers a 15–25% rate of 5-year overall survival (3). However, only approximately 10% of patients are candidates for surgery. The roughly 40% of patients without evidence of metastatic disease but ineligible for surgery comprise a heterogeneous group defined as locally advanced pancreatic cancer (LAPC) (4). Chemoradiation therapy, the conventional treatment approach for these patients, confers a 5-year overall survival rate of less than 5% (4). These sobering statistics clearly underscore the urgent need for better treatment strategies to effectively treat this devastating disease. This chapter focuses on the role of combining biologic therapies with chemoradiation therapy in the treatment of pancreatic cancer.

■ CURRENT ROLE OF CHEMORADIATION THERAPY

Adjuvant Therapy for Resected/Resectable Pancreatic Cancer

Although surgery is a critical component of curative treatment in resectable pancreatic cancers, the high incidence of locoregional and distant metastases contribute to the low cure rates seen even among resected patients. Both chemotherapy and radiation therapy have been widely used to maximize the probability of survival following surgery by addressing the high likelihood of distant and locoregional failures in these patients. The rates of locoregional failure of greater than 50% in published series (5–8) arise from the challenges posed by dissecting along the retroperitoneal margin (the proximal 3- to 4-cm of the superior mesenteric artery), the celiac trunk, the confluence of the superior mesenteric vein and portal vein, and the difficulty with pathologic assessment of margin status intraoperatively. Positive surgical margins, involved regional lymph nodes, and tumor size are key prognostic factors that contribute to poorer overall survival outcomes (3). In other tumor sites where combined modality therapy is routinely undertaken (rectal, breast, and head and neck cancers), the locoregional control rate consistently exceeds 90%. Therefore, it is not unreasonable to expect chemoradiation therapy to address the locoregional component of failure following surgery for pancreatic cancer. In parallel with the increased risk of locoregional failure, rapidly metastatic subclinical residual disease and the presence of occult metastatic disease at the time of surgery account for the competing risk and high rate of systemic metastatic disease. Distant metastatic disease frequently manifests as hepatic and peritoneal metastases in more than 75% of patients, often within 6 months of surgery (9). This argues for the consideration of systemic chemotherapy in these patients.

In the United States, adjuvant treatment with fluorouracil-based chemoradiation is frequently recommended postoperatively based on an early Gastrointestinal Tumor Study Group (GITSG) randomized study that demonstrated a significantly better overall survival among patients treated with adjuvant chemoradiation therapy than among those randomized to observation alone (20 versus 11 months, $p = 0.03$) (10). In the updated report, in which additional patients were treated with adjuvant chemoradiation therapy, this benefit was maintained. Unlike the GITSG trial, however, the European Organization for Research and Treatment of Cancer (EORTC) trial did not find a statistically significant overall survival benefit among patients treated with adjuvant chemoradiation compared with those randomized to observation alone (17.1 versus 12.6 months, $p = 0.099$) (11). More recently, the results of the European Study Group for Pancreatic Cancer-1 (ESPAC-1) trial employing a 2 × 2 factorial design questioned the role of chemoradiation as a component of adjuvant therapy (12,13). Patients treated with chemoradiation therapy had a worse overall survival than those who did not receive chemoradiation therapy (15.9 versus 17.9 months; $p = 0.05$), whereas patients treated with chemotherapy had a significantly better overall survival than those randomized to observation alone (20.1 versus 15.5 months; $p = 0.009$) (12,13). A similar benefit was documented for adjuvant gemcitabine chemotherapy when compared to observation alone in the Charité Onkologie (CONKO)-001 trial, in which a statistically significant improvement in disease-free survival (14.2 versus 7.5 months, $p < 0.001$) but not overall survival was noted regardless of nodal status or margin status (14). In Europe, these results establishing the role of chemotherapy in the adjuvant setting have led to the initiation of the ESPAC-3 trial, in which nearly 1000 patients are randomized to 5FU/leucovorin or gemcitabine with no radiation therapy in either arm. It is difficult to interpret and draw conclusions from these trials because of the less than optimal design and execution of these trials, which is most evident from the choice of radiation fractionation and equipment, chemotherapy schedule, delays in initiating treatment, compliance with radiation and chemotherapy delivery, surgical and pathologic quality assurance, and marginal statistical power. The likelihood of imbalances in persistent residual disease is best illustrated by the high rates of locoregional failure as a component of the first site of failure in these trials that did not require surgical, pathologic, and radiotherapeutic quality control or postoperative pretreatment reimaging of the tumor bed. For these reasons, it seems most reasonable to conclude that suboptimal chemoradiation therapy regimens administered adjuvantly to incompletely restaged patients is unlikely to translate to a substantial survival benefit. To some extent, the recently reported Radiation Therapy Oncology Group (RTOG) 9704 trial comparing two adjuvant therapy regimens addresses some of the shortcomings of earlier trials (15). The doses and schedules of chemoradiation therapy were more optimal and a post-hoc radiation quality assurance was performed (16). When adjuvant 5FU-based chemoradiation therapy was sandwiched between two chemotherapy regimens, patients with pancreatic head adenocarcinomas who received gemcitabine before and after chemoradiation had improved overall survival compared with patients who received 5FU before and after chemoradiation (18.8 versus 16.7 months; $p = 0.047$) (15). A promising alternative strategy is that of concurrent radiation therapy and multidrug chemotherapy using 5FU, cisplatin, and interferon. At a mean follow-up of 31.9 months, 67% of patients were still alive, and the 5-year overall survival rate was 55% in this phase II study (17). A confirmatory study is ongoing at the American College of Surgeons Oncology Group (ACOSOG).

Preoperative chemoradiation therapy has been evaluated at some centers because of the difficulty of administering postoperative adjuvant treatment in patients recovering after a major surgical procedure, the ability to preclude ineffective pancreaticoduodenectomies in patients with oligometastatic or subclinical metastatic disease who progress distantly during chemoradiation therapy, the greater efficacy with lower toxicity when chemoradiation therapy is administered preoperatively (as documented in rectal cancer), and the potential beneficial impact of tumor downstaging on resection margin status (18). This is particularly relevant since overall survival of patients with positive margins after tumor resection is no better than that of unresectable patients treated with chemoradiation therapy (19,20). An alternative approach has been to administer intraoperative radiation therapy (IORT) to the tumor bed at the time of resection. Intraoperative radiation therapy alone nearly halves the rate of local recurrence, but this does not translate into a survival benefit (21).

Unfortunately, these strategies have not substantially improved survival outcomes in resected/resectable pancreatic cancer patients. Further, a clear standard has not been established for adjuvant treatment of these patients. Based on the CONKO-001 and RTOG 9704 trials, it seems reasonable to use gemcitabine-based chemotherapy up-front to select out patients who develop an early systemic recurrence and to administer consolidative chemoradiation therapy to those who do not.

Treatment of Locally Advanced Pancreatic Cancer

For LAPC, treatment with radiation therapy, with or without chemotherapy, has not been prospectively compared to best supportive care in a randomized study. Early randomized trials by the GITSG combining split-course radiation therapy with bolus 5FU established that combined-modality therapy was more effective than radiation therapy alone. The chemoradiation therapy regimens nearly doubled the median survival over radiation therapy alone (10 versus 5.5 months, $p < 0.05$) and marginally improved median survival over chemotherapy alone (22). In a follow-up study comparing chemoradiation therapy to chemotherapy alone, the group receiving chemoradiation therapy had a superior 1-year overall survival rate of 41% compared with 19% for the group receiving chemotherapy alone (23). In contrast to these studies, an Eastern Cooperative Oncology Group study comparing 5FU chemotherapy to chemoradiation therapy showed no difference in median survival between the two groups, while toxicities were significantly higher in the chemoradiation therapy group (24). Streptozocin, mitomycin, methyl lomustine, and doxorubicin, the other chemotherapy regimens used during this period, were not superior to 5FU. Since then, the promising antitumor activity observed with gemcitabine in locally advanced and metastatic pancreatic cancer and its potential for radiosensitization have led to renewed interest in combining newer agents with radiation therapy (25–29). The increased toxicity of combining radiation therapy with gemcitabine has been addressed either by decreasing the dose of gemcitabine or by reducing the radiation dose and volume (30–32). Other cytotoxic agents, singly or in combination, have failed to demonstrate convincing and consistent improvements in clinical outcomes (33–38). An alternative approach that is increasingly employed is one of sequencing treatments such that patients receive chemoradiation therapy only after they receive induction chemotherapy. In light of the high propensity of patients with pancreatic cancer to develop metastatic disease, this strategy, by excluding patients with rapid, distant progression during induction chemotherapy, selects patients with truly locally advanced disease for optimal benefit from consolidative chemoradiation therapy. Using this approach of enriching the population of patients who receive a locoregional treatment modality, a retrospective analysis of 323 patients with LAPC treated at M.D. Anderson demonstrated significantly better median overall survival among patients treated with induction chemotherapy than among those treated with chemoradiation therapy alone (11.9 versus 8.5 months) (39). The efficacy of this strategy does not necessarily rely on the increased systemic potency of the induction chemotherapy regimen, but the induction regimen may serve merely as a therapeutic screening test for the inherent biology of LAPC that initially is deemed to have no radiographically identifiable metastatic disease. Patients who fail this screening test because of systemic progression are most likely to be patients who already had micrometastatic disease and were never optimal candidates for a locoregional treatment such as chemoradiation therapy. This strategy serves to preferentially select for chemoradiation therapy those patients who are most likely to benefit from a locoregional therapy.

It is evident that further advances in the treatment of pancreatic cancer will require screening of high-risk populations for early detection of pancreatic cancer; the use of molecular markers including genomic, proteomic, methylomic, and/or metabolomic profiling to predict response to chemoradiation therapy so as to facilitate treatment stratification and/or clinical decision-making and/or adaptive modification of treatment strategies; and improved treatment strategies based on a better understanding of the molecular underpinnings of signaling pathways that drive the development and progression of pancreatic cancer.

THE ARGUMENT FOR TARGETED THERAPIES

Over the last three decades, the results of trials evaluating cytotoxic chemotherapy combinations in the treatment of metastatic pancreatic cancer and cytotoxic chemotherapy combined with radiation therapy for LAPC have been singularly disappointing. The first and, until recently, the only drug approved specifically for metastatic pancreatic cancer was gemcitabine. Notably, even gemcitabine was approved largely based on its greater clinical benefit response (combining measurements of pain, Karnofsky performance status, and weight) than 5FU in symptomatic patients with metastatic pancreatic cancer. This improvement in clinical benefit was associated with a modest improvement in median survival (5.6 versus 4.4 months) and 1-year survival rates (18% versus 2%) when compared to 5FU (40). Since then, a number of studies have investigated combination therapies of gemcitabine and other cytotoxic chemotherapeutic agents, but none of these has demonstrated convincing improvements in survival over gemcitabine alone. Furthermore, combination cytotoxic therapies have a narrow therapeutic index; responses are usually partial, often disappointingly short-lived, and unpredictable.

In recent years, advances in our understanding of neoplastic transformation and progression at the genetic, biochemical, cellular, and molecular level have led to the development of specific molecules to target these aberrant processes that are unique to cancer cells. The resulting explosion in the supply of novel, rationally designed, molecularly targeted cancer therapies has prompted considerable excitement in the oncology community, particularly in light of the spectacular successes in treating certain cancers with such agents (41–43). In the case of pancreatic cancer, although its genetic signature has been extensively characterized, the molecular mechanisms linking these genetic changes to the aggressive malignant phenotype of pancreatic cancer and the inherent resistance to treatment with traditional cytotoxic therapies has not been fully elucidated (44). What is recognized is that mutations in oncogenes, inactivation of tumor suppressor genes, and overexpression of growth factors and their receptors with constitutive activation of downstream signal transduction pathways contribute to the creation and perpetuation of the malignant phenotype. Common genetic modifications in pancreatic carcinomas include activation of the K-*ras* oncogene (85%–95%); inactivation of the p16/RB1 (>90%), p53 (75%), DPC4 (55%), and *BRCA2* tumor suppressor genes; and overexpression of specific growth factors/cytokines and their associated receptors (45,46). The most commonly overexpressed of these growth factors/cytokines include epidermal growth factor, vascular endothelial growth factor (VEGF), fibroblast growth factor, transforming growth factor β, interleukin 1, interleukin 6, tumor necrosis factor α, and interleukin 8 (44). These aberrant processes confer a survival advantage to pancreatic cancer cells by achieving self-sufficiency in nutritional and proliferative signals, evasion of programmed cell death, promotion of invasion and angiogenesis, and development of metastases.

Despite the complexity and heterogeneity of these hallmarks of pancreatic cancer, the elucidation of these signaling aberrations, beginning at the level of the genome and involving cell surface receptors and intracellular switches, offers researchers and clinicians a veritable array of potentially "druggable" targets. Agents that target aberrant overexpression of growth-regulatory molecules such as growth factors and their receptors (for example, bevacizumab, cetuximab, erlotinib, and gefitinib) are now being used in clinical practice and evaluated in clinical trials in combination with chemotherapy in various tumor types. By focusing on molecular and cellular changes that are specific to the tumor and/or the tumor vasculature, targeted cancer therapies may possibly be more effective than current treatments, less harmful to normal cells, and less prone to the development of resistance.

INCORPORATION OF TARGETED THERAPY WITH RADIATION

The recent shift to the development of anticancer therapies that target specific alterations in cancer cells, fueled by the clinical success of monoclonal antibodies (mAb) targeting growth factors or their receptors and inhibitors of receptor tyrosine kinase (TK), has also sparked an interest in combining molecular targeted therapies with radiation therapy. Encouraging radiosensitization effects have been documented when targeted therapies have been combined with radiation therapy, both in the preclinical (47–51) and early clinical settings (52–55). This radiosensitization has the potential to not only selectively improve local disease control but may also improve disease-free and overall survival.

Cetuximab, a humanized mAb directed against the epidermal growth factor receptor (EGFR), is the only targeted agent approved by the U.S. Food and Drug Administration (FDA) for use specifically as a radiosensitizer, based on a phase III trial in patients with locally advanced head and neck cancer. Patients were randomized to receive definitive radiation alone versus the same treatment with concurrent cetuximab. The median duration of local tumor control was 24.4 months among patients treated with cetuximab plus radiotherapy and 14.9 months among those given radiotherapy alone (hazard ratio for locoregional progression or death, 0.68; $p = 0.005$). With a median follow-up of 54.0 months, the median duration of overall survival was 49.0 months among patients treated with combined therapy and 29.3 months among those treated with radiotherapy alone (hazard ratio for death, 0.74; $p = 0.03$) (53). Although similar efficacy improvements have been achieved with the use of concurrent cisplatin in head and neck cancer, the locoregional control and overall survival benefit in this study was achieved with increases in toxicity limited to rash and infusion reactions. These results have paved the way for renewed enthusiasm for the development of targeted therapeutics as radiosensitizers and have initiated a plethora of early clinical trials invoking this paradigm for improvement of locoregional control and possibly disease-free and overall survival.

Two areas of particular interest in advancing this paradigm in pancreatic cancer have been the combination of traditional chemoradiation therapy with inhibitors of VEGF and EGFR.

Vascular Endothelial Growth Factor Inhibition

Increased levels of VEGF expression in tumors has been correlated with invasiveness, vascular density, metastasis, and recurrence (56,57). Randomized trials have demonstrated the efficacy of bevacizumab, a humanized anti-VEGF mAb that effectively prevents VEGF from binding to its receptors, VEGFR-1 (Flt-1) and VEGFR-2 (Flk-1 and KDR). It is the first antiangiogenic agent to be approved by the FDA. In a pivotal trial, bevacizumab was found to increase survival in patients with metastatic colorectal cancer when added to irinotecan, 5FU, and leucovorin (58). Bevacizumab also increased survival in patients with metastatic colorectal cancer when added to 5FU and leucovorin (59). Most investigations of these and other drugs have focused on their benefits as components of systemic therapy in patients with advanced disease, although investigation of their benefits in the adjuvant setting are now underway in colon cancer. However, these molecular therapies may play important roles as radiosensitizers. The possible mechanisms of radiosensitization are not clear, but could include enhanced lethality of the endothelial cell (60) or tumor cell (61), or an improvement in vascular physiology leading to a reduction in tumor hypoxia (62). Expression of VEGF has been shown to be enhanced by radiation, and in vitro studies indicate that the enhanced cytotoxicity of the combination of radiotherapy and antibody-mediated VEGF neutralization may be due to the potentiation of endothelial cell death rather than to direct tumor cell cytotoxicity (60). These results seemed to suggest that VEGF is protective of endothelial cells exposed to the stress imposed by ionizing radiation and that VEGF blockade could overcome this protective effect. However, recent investigation has also demonstrated expression of VEGFR-1 protein, mRNA, and its ligands as well as protein kinase signaling in pancreatic cancer cell lines as well as endothelial cells. VEGFR-1–mediated migration and invasion that is blocked by a VEGFR-1–neutralizing antibody have been also been demonstrated (61,63). Thus, VEGFR-1 is not only present on tumor cells, but also apparently can mediate their biologic behavior. It is therefore possible that the preliminary clinical evidence of enhancement of radiotherapy by bevacizumab may be due to a direct effect on tumor cells. Last, although an antiangiogenic agent may, in principle, reduce blood supply to the tumor, depriving it of nutrients and oxygen, this has the potential to increase tumor hypoxia and make tumors suboptimally accessible to drug delivery. Despite these concerns, antiangiogenic agents have not only been shown to decrease hypoxia in preclinical models (64) but also to potentiate the effects of chemotherapy and radiation therapy in preclinical and clinical studies (47,58–60,64,65). One explanation for this apparent paradox is the concept that structurally and functionally aberrant tumor vasculature is transiently normalized by antiangiogenic agents, improving tumor blood flow via reduction of interstitial pressure (62,66).

The role of bevacizumab as a radiation response modifier was systematically evaluated by Willett and colleagues, who performed a phase I trial of bevacizumab and 5FU with concurrent preoperative radiotherapy in rectal cancer (52,67). Bevacizumab was well-tolerated with protracted venous infusional 5FU and radiotherapy at a dose of 5 mg/kg (n = 6), but there were two grade 3 gastrointestinal adverse events at the dose of 10 mg/kg, leading authors to recommend the 5-mg/kg dose level. A complement of correlative studies showed that bevacizumab decreased tumor perfusion, interstitial pressure, and microvascular density in rectal cancers (52). Five (83%) of six patients had only microscopic residual disease on thorough histologic evaluation. By comparison 192 (45%) of 431 of patients treated at our institution with a similar chemoradiotherapy regimen (without bevacizumab) had only microscopic residual disease (68). Correlative studies supported the hypothesis that antiangiogenic therapy normalizes tumor vascular physiology by reducing permeability and eliminating immature and inefficient blood vessels (62). The relationship of the results of the correlative studies to response is not clear; one possibility is that a more efficient tumor vasculature could improve oxygenation, which is well known to improve radiation response (64,65). The final results of the study included 11 patients. Interestingly, 10 out 11 patients had clinical complete responses. Eight patients had microscopic residual disease and two had complete histologic responses. Compared to historical controls, there appear to be fewer patients with gross residual disease and approximately the same number of complete histologic responses as with 5FU-based chemoradiation (68).

Bevacizumab has been evaluated in combination with radiation therapy in a large phase I dose escalation study in patients with locally advanced, unresectable pancreatic cancer conducted at M. D. Anderson. Forty-seven patients received capecitabine (650 mg/m^2 –825 mg/m^2 twice daily) and bevacizumab in combination with radiation (50.4 Gy) to the gross tumor alone (55). The study demonstrated that bevacizumab is generally safe when combined with chemoradiation in patients with locally advanced pancreatic cancer. The acute toxicity was minimal and easily managed with dose adjustments of capecitabine, without interruption or attenuation of either the bevacizumab or radiation dose. Bevacizumab did not appear to enhance acute toxicity; however, tumors with invasion of the duodenum appeared to be at higher risk for bleeding or perforation. Among the first 30 patients enrolled, three bleeding events were associated with tumor invasion of the duodenum. After this was recognized, these patients were excluded from protocol entry and there were no further bleeding events among the final 16 patients enrolled. Overall, the tumors in nine (20%) of 46 evaluable patients had an objective partial response to initial therapy. This included six of 12 tumors treated at a dose of 5 mg/kg of bevacizumab. Based on that trial, the recommended dose of bevacizumab for further study was 5 mg/kg every 2 weeks with radiotherapy (50.4 Gy in 28 fractions) and concurrent capecitabine (825 mg/m^2 twice daily Monday through Friday) (55). Notably, four of these patients who were initially deemed unresectable went on to undergo margin-negative pancreaticoduodenectomies without any complications. The RTOG has completed accrual to a phase II trial evaluating capecitabine-based chemoradiation with bevacizumab followed by systemic therapy with concurrent gemcitabine and bevacizumab (RTOG PA04-11). Ninety-four patients were treated, and preliminary analysis indicates that the treatment was generally well tolerated in comparison to previous RTOG phase II studies with similar inclusion criteria (69). Specific exclusion of patients with tumor invasion of the duodenum seemed to have avoided significant problems with bleeding thus far. Overall, 35.4% of patients had grade 3 or greater treatment-related gastrointestinal toxicity (16.0% during chemoradiation, 17.0% during maintenance chemotherapy, and 2.4% during both phases), and 52% patients had grade 3 or greater treatment-related hematologic toxicity, mostly during maintenance chemotherapy (43%). Median overall survival duration was 11.9 months (95% confidence interval, 10.1–14.2 months) and 1-year survival rate was 47% (95% confidence interval, 35%–57%). The authors concluded that the addition of bevacizumab to chemoradiation therapy followed by bevacizumab and gemcitabine resulted in median and 1-year overall survival and acute toxicity rates similar to studies conducted by the RTOG in the past (69). In an analysis of the potential benefit of the addition of bevacizumab to chemoradiation therapy, the outcomes of locally advanced pancreatic cancer patients treated with a combination of bevacizumab, capecitabine, and radiation therapy were compared to that of a large historical cohort of patients treated with chemoradiation with or without induction chemotherapy at M.D. Anderson (70). Among 371 patients treated with concurrent chemoradiation therapy, 47 patients received concurrent bevacizumab. On univariate analysis, the addition of bevacizumab to chemoradiation appeared to improve overall survival compared to historical regimens containing fluoropyrimidines or gemcitabine alone (15.0 months versus 9.0 months, $p = 0.005$). The magnitude of this difference was clinically significant, but did not hold up on multivariate analysis, possibly due to the relatively small numbers in this group (70).

Bevacizumab has also been combined with gemcitabine-based chemoradiation therapy in pancreatic cancer patients, and two recent reports describe early experiences with this approach. In the first report, presented at the 2008 GI Cancers Symposium, 29 of planned 30 nonmetastatic pancreatic cancer patients received gemcitabine (1000 mg/m^2), bevacizumab (10 mg/kg), and radiotherapy (gross tumor volume only, 36 Gy at 2.4 Gy/fraction) at Northwestern University between October 2005 and July 2007 (71). This was preceded and followed by a cycle of gemcitabine and bevacizumab before response assessment on week 10 with cross-sectional imaging and CA 19-9 tumor marker. Of 26 evaluable patients, 22 (76%) experienced grade 3 toxicities that included cytopenias, nausea, diarrhea, deep vein thrombosis, dehydration, and increased liver function tests, and one patient experienced grade 4 leukopenias. Among 26 patients evaluable for response at week 10, one patient had a radiographic complete response, three had partial responses, fourteen were stable, and three had progressive disease. Five patients underwent resection, with two complete pathologic responses. The authors concluded that the combination of full-dose gemcitabine, bevacizumab, and radiotherapy was generally well tolerated, with all but one patient completing all three cycles. The pathologic complete responses noted among resected patients were promising, and additional outcomes and survival data should be forthcoming in the near future. In a similar experience reported from M. D. Anderson, bevacizumab was combined with gemcitabine-based radiation in the preoperative setting in an attempt to maximize the number of patients who receive multimodality therapy and undergo a complete R0 pancreaticoduodenectomy (72). Eleven patients received six weekly cycles of gemcitabine (400 mg/m^2) and three infusions of bevacizumab (10 mg/kg, every 2 wks) with concomitant radiotherapy, 50.4 Gy at 1.8 Gy/fraction. Four to six weeks later, patients without disease progression and with good performance status underwent surgery. All completed chemoradiation therapy; ten underwent restaging and one patient died from cardiac arrest before restaging. At restaging, one patient had distant metastases, and the remaining nine underwent successful R0 pancreaticoduodenectomies. The pathologic partial response rate (>50% tumor kill) was 56%. Preoperative grade 3–4 toxicities were infrequent and included neutropenia, stent-related cholangitis, gastrointestinal toxicity, hypertension, and pulmonary embolism. However, major postoperative complications occurred in five of the nine patients (56%), who underwent pancreaticoduodenectomy and included wound dehiscence requiring reoperation (three), large ventral hernia related to fascial dehiscence (one), and biliary anastomotic leak (one). On a planned interim analysis, the study was terminated due to the unforeseen and significant rate of major postoperative complications attributable to poor wound healing caused by the combined use of bevacizumab and radiation therapy. These studies confirm that the optimal use of anti-VEGF therapy in the treatment of pancreatic cancer requires further refinement.

Inhibition of Epidermal Growth Factor Receptor Signaling

The EGFR signaling pathway represents another attractive target for biologic therapies. Its downstream signaling pathways, including the RAS-RAF-MEK-ERK axis and the phosphatidylinositol 3' kinase (PI3K)/AKT axis control proliferation, resistance to apoptosis, invasiveness, angiogenesis, metastasis, and resistance to therapy of pancreatic cancer. Blockade of this signaling pathway is readily accomplished by inhibition of the receptor using mAbs and/or small-molecule inhibitors of the intracellular TK domain. As noted earlier, radiosensitization via blockade of the EGFR pathway has already proven to be a viable strategy for improving clinical outcomes in head and neck cancer. Similar strategies for radiosensitization are being employed in pancreatic cancer. Notably, however, none of the currently available EGFR inhibitors (erlotinib, gefitinib, and cetuximab) have been evaluated in completed multi-institutional trials in combination with radiation therapy in LAPC. Outlined below are some of the early experiences with the combination of EGFR inhibitors with radiation therapy in LAPC.

Monoclonal Antibodies

A randomized trial of patients with irinotecan-refractory colorectal cancer was the first study to document the significant clinical activity of the anti-EGFR antibody, cetuximab (73). Since then, cetuximab has become an integral part of the treatment of metastatic colorectal cancer and has changed the standard of care for patients with advanced disease. A couple of studies incorporate cetuximab with chemoradiation regimens in LAPC patients (74). In the first such study (PARC) that is currently accruing patients, 66 patients are being randomized to treatment with intensity-modulated radiation therapy, gemcitabine, and cetuximab followed by four weekly cycles of gemcitabine versus intensity-modulated radiation therapy, gemcitabine, and cetuximab, followed by four weekly cycles of gemcitabine with 12 weeks of cetuximab. In our own experience with treatment of LAPCs with cetuximab and capecitabine-based chemoradiation therapy, patients underwent initial chemotherapy with gemcitabine, oxaliplatin, and cetuximab before receiving chemoradiation therapy. The preliminary analysis of outcomes in these patients should be available shortly.

Receptor Tyrosine Kinase Inhibitors

The recent FDA approval of erlotinib in the treatment of metastatic pancreatic cancer has renewed interest in receptor TK inhibitors. In a large trial that randomized more than 500 patients to receive a standard gemcitabine regimen plus placebo or gemcitabine plus oral erlotinib 100 mg/day, an improvement in both overall survival and progression-free survival was observed among patients who received the combination of gemcitabine plus erlotinib, compared with those who received only chemotherapy. The absolute benefit, however, was about a 2-week improvement in median overall survival. Although this may be a sobering statistic, this is the first and only positive trial in this disease since the approval of gemcitabine. Other studies have evaluated receptor TK inhibition in combination with radiation therapy in patients with LAPC. A phase I dose escalation study has recently been published from Brown University combining gemcitabine (75 mg/m^2), and paclitaxel (40 mg/m^2) weekly and daily erlotinib with 50.4 Gy to the primary tumor and regional lymphatics. The maximum tolerated dose of erlotinib was 50 mg/day. The median survival was 14.0 months, and six of 13 (46%) of locally advanced patients had a partial response, indicating that erlotinib-based chemoradiation regimens are possibly worthy of further study in pancreatic cancer (75). A significant amount of high-grade diarrhea occurred, which limited the inability to give full dose erlotinib. Toxicity could have been due to the concurrent gemcitabine and paclitaxel, the use of regional nodal irradiation, or the combination of radiotherapy and erlotinib. Another phase I study has recently been reported from Memorial Sloan Kettering evaluating gemcitabine-based chemoradiation therapy in combination with erlotinib (76). Escalating doses of erlotinib (100 mg, 125 mg) were combined with gemcitabine (40 mg/m^2, twice weekly) and radiation therapy (50.4 Gy in 28 fractions to the primary and regional nodes) followed by maintenance chemotherapy with gemcitabine 1000 mg/m^2 (days 1 and 8 every 21 days) and erlotinib 100 mg/day for four cycles. Among nine patients treated on this study, seven of eight evaluable patients had stable disease while one patient had disease progression. The maximum tolerated dose of erlotinib was 100 mg/day. Significant hematologic toxicity occurred with erlotinib at 125 mg/day. A phase I study at Duke University has been conducted evaluating concurrent gefitinib (250 mg/day), capecitabine (650–825 mg/m^2 b.i.d., 7 days/week), and radiotherapy in locally advanced pancreatic and rectal cancers. Patients were treated to a dose of 50.4 Gy (45 Gy in 25 fractions to the regional lymphatics followed by an additional 5.4 Gy in three fractions to the primary tumor). Dose limiting toxicity (DLT) was seen in two of six patients with rectal cancer and six of ten patients with pancreatic cancer. Diarrhea as well as nausea and vomiting with dehydration were common (77). A recommended dose was not established due to these toxicities. These data suggest that this combination of capecitabine-based radiation therapy with gefitinib should not be further studied in gastrointestinal malignancies.

■ LIMITATIONS OF TARGETED THERAPY

The early success of targeted therapy was derived from therapies that targeted molecules and/or signaling pathways that were preferentially overexpressed on specific tumors, such as trastuzumab for HER-2+ breast cancer, rituximab for CD20+ B-cell lymphomas, and imatinib for BCR-ABL+ chronic myeloid leukemia. In these instances, it seems likely that the target is a pivotal aberrant signaling moiety, the tumors are "addicted" to the given signaling pathway, and the targeted therapies directly affected signaling down the respective pathway. However, in the case of pancreatic cancer and most other solid tumors, multiple prosurvival, angiogenic, and antiapoptotic pathways are upregulated by tumor cells that confer them with a competitive advantage compared to surrounding normal cells. Highly targeted blockade of a single pathway may not sufficiently deter tumor growth or improve tumor control/cure rates because of the redundancy of signaling pathways that overcome single-pathway blockade. Therefore, the biologic relevance and antitumor efficacy of targeting one specific pathway may be intricately associated with the degree of addiction of the tumor to that particular pathway for progressive growth, in contrast to other pathways that are simultaneously overexpressed. In a particularly illustrative example of this phenomenon, it has recently been reported that metastatic colorectal cancer patients with tumors that express high levels of the EGFR ligands epiregulin and amphiregulin on gene expression profile analysis of biopsy specimens are more likely to have disease control with cetuximab (78). Among 110 patients treated with cetuximab monotherapy, median progression-free survival was 103.5 versus 57 days among epiregulin high- and low-expressers, respectively ($p = 0.0002$) and 115.5 versus 57 days among amphiregulin high- and low-expressers, respectively ($p < 0.0001$). These results suggest that elevated expression of EGFR ligands may stimulate an autocrine loop that is akin to EGFR pathway addiction. While this autocrine stimulatory loop confers a tumor growth advantage, the dependence on the EGFR signaling pathway also mediates sensitivity to cetuximab. Furthermore, patients whose tumors do not have *K-RAS* mutations were found to have a significantly higher disease control rate than patients with *K-RAS* mutations (78). In this case, activating mutations of *K-RAS* lead to downstream constitutive activation of the mitogen-activated protein kinase axis of the EGFR pathway. Since cetuximab blocks EGFR upstream of this constitutive activation of the downstream cascade of prosurvival signaling, it is not surprising that patients with tumors bearing *K-RAS* mutations are less responsive to cetuximab. In a similar study of 30 patients with metastatic colorectal cancer, a *K-RAS* mutation was found in 13 tumors (43%) and was significantly associated with the absence of response to cetuximab (*K-RAS* mutation in 0% of the 11 responders versus 68.4% of the 19 nonresponders; $p = 0.0003$) (79). The median overall survival of patients without *K-RAS* mutation in their tumor was significantly higher than that of patients with *K-RAS* mutations in their tumor (16.3 versus 6.9 months, $p = 0.016$). An increased EGFR copy number found in three patients (10%) was also significantly associated with an objective tumor response to cetuximab ($p = 0.04$). Similar results have also been reported with panitumumab, another mAb that targets EGFR (80). While all of these findings must be validated prospectively by the use of validated assays, these preliminary findings suggest that only a subgroup of patients benefits from targeted therapy, and identification of this subgroup may improve treatment outcomes, spare patients unnecessary toxicity, and reduce expenses associated with ineffective therapy.

■ RATIONAL DESIGN OF TRIALS TESTING TARGETED THERAPIES

Clearly, the identification of a response predictor would permit the rational design of trials in which only a subgroup of patients is treated with the targeted therapy agent. This would increase the probability of detecting a benefit to therapy, since trials in unselected patients may dilute the potential benefit seen in that subset of patients who have tumors expressing the target and/or are responsive to targeted therapy based on biologic relevance of the targeted signaling pathway. However, until specific selection criteria are identified, well-designed, focused, and robust empiric trials with rigorous assessment of the correlation between biologic attributes and clinical outcome are required. In the design of these trials, it would be instructive to know that the drug achieves and maintains adequate target tissue concentrations, that the drug inhibits (in target tissues) the process it is purported to inhibit, and that even a negative trial yields information about the mechanism of the drug's interaction with the tumor. This information would permit rational design of future trials that address these inadequacies using combination strategies and/or alternative sequencing/dosing strategies.

Specifically in the case of radiosensitizer studies using targeted agents, an opportunity exists for trials to specifically investigate one or more means of drug–radiation interaction, namely spatial cooperation, cytotoxic enhancement, biologic cooperation, temporal modulation, and normal tissue protection (81). Depending on the interaction being investigated, appropriate preclinical models, optimal sequencing/dosing strategies, clinical and correlative end-points, and surrogate translational components should be integrated into the design of rational trials. Where a pathway is known to mediate radiation resistance, targeting this specific pathway using optimal dosing and sequencing strategies with targeted agents based on preclinical models would be informative. Alternatively, where clear dependence on a specific pathway is not discernible, a multipathway-targeted approach may be undertaken to simultaneously block multiple redundant signaling pathways. This may be achieved by using single agents that target multiple pathways (multikinase inhibitors) or by combining single-target agents. Where target validation is not readily achievable in tissue because of the inability to obtain serial biopsies during treatment, newer molecular imaging modalities will need to be incorporated into these early clinical trials. Last, in contrast to constitutively activated prosurvival pathways that are the focus of current targeting strategies, the targeting of inducible prosurvival (radioresistance) pathways is an emerging concept that is worthy of consideration. To learn more about these mechanisms, it would be very beneficial to not only have preclinical models of inducible radioresistance but clinical information about tumor and microenvironmental changes that occur at the epigenetic, genetic, proteomic, methylomic, and metabolomic levels in response to radiation therapy. This could then guide future targeted therapies that address a specific inducible prosurvival signal or a spectrum of such signals.

■ CONCLUSIONS

The incorporation of targeted therapies with radiation has the potential to lead to improved responses, local control, and disease-free and overall survival without significantly increasing toxicity. The preliminary efficacy results for combining bevacizumab, cetuximab, gefitinib, or erlotinib with radiation therapy do not indicate a quantum increase in response rates, resectability rates, or overall outcomes. Although this does not argue against their use in future combination studies, there is a greater need for rational design of proof-of-concept studies based on sound preclinical rationales and rigorous and systematic characterization of clinical responses. Further study of the receptor TK inhibitors gefitinib and erlotinib with radiotherapy should be done with caution due to the possibility of a higher risk of severe diarrhea in gastrointestinal patients. In the future, multitarget therapies synergistically tackling several oncogenic pathways with either a combination of agents or multitarget agents will have to be evaluated in large studies. In addition, before initiation of a specific therapy directed against a specific pathway, rigorous and systematic characterization of the mechanism through which that pathway contributes to radioresistance should be undertaken; each tumor should be analyzed for the activation status of, and where possible, the addiction to multiple tumor-promoting pathways in order to apply an individually tailored therapeutic regimen that maximizes therapeutic efficacy and avoids side effects of drugs that may be ineffective in a particular patient.

■ REFERENCES

1. Jemal A, Siegel R, Ward E, et al. Cancer statistics 2006. CA *Cancer J Clin* 2006;56:106–130.
2. Sener SF, Fremgen A, Menck HR, et al. Pancreatic cancer: A report of treatment and survival trends for 100,313 patients diagnosed from 1985–1995, using the National Cancer Database. *J Am Coll Surg* 1999;189:1–7.
3. Yeo CJ, Cameron JL, Sohn TA, et al. Six hundred fifty consecutive pancreaticoduodenectomies in the 1990s: Pathology, complications, and outcomes. *Ann Surg* 1997;226:248–257; discussion 57–60.
4. Maheshwari V, Moser AJ. Current management of locally advanced pancreatic cancer. *Nat Clin Pract Gastroenterol Hepatol* 2005;2:356–364.
5. Tepper J, Nardi G, Sutt H. Carcinoma of the pancreas: Review of MGH experience from 1963 to 1973. Analysis of surgical failure and implications for radiation therapy. *Cancer* 1976;37:1519–1524.
6. Griffin JF, Smalley SR, Jewell W, et al. Patterns of failure after curative resection of pancreatic carcinoma. *Cancer* 1990;66:56–61.
7. Sperti C, Pasquali C, Piccoli A, et al. Recurrence after resection for ductal adenocarcinoma of the pancreas. *World J Surg* 1997;21:195–200.
8. Westerdahl J, Andren-Sandberg A, Ihse I. Recurrence of exocrine pancreatic cancer—local or hepatic? *Hepatogastroenterology* 1993;40:384–387.

9. Chua YJ, Cunningham D. Adjuvant treatment for resectable pancreatic cancer. *J Clin Oncol* 2005;23:04532–04537.
10. Kalser MH, Ellenberg SS. Pancreatic cancer. Adjuvant combined radiation and chemotherapy following curative resection. *Arch Surg* 1985;120:899–903.
11. Klinkenbijl JH, Jeekel J, Sahmoud T, et al. Adjuvant radiotherapy and 5-fluorouracil after curative resection of cancer of the pancreas and periampullary region: Phase III trial of the EORTC gastrointestinal tract cancer cooperative group. *Ann Surg* 1999;230:776–82; discussion 82-4.
12. Neoptolemos JP, Dunn JA, Stocken DD, et al. Adjuvant chemoradiotherapy and chemotherapy in resectable pancreatic cancer: A randomised controlled trial. *Lancet* 2001;358:1576–1585.
13. Neoptolemos JP, Stocken DD, Friess H, et al. A randomized trial of chemoradiotherapy and chemotherapy after resection of pancreatic cancer. *N Engl J Med* 2004;350:1200–1210.
14. Oettle H, Post S, Neuhaus P, et al. Adjuvant chemotherapy with gemcitabine vs observation in patients undergoing curative-intent resection of pancreatic cancer: A randomized controlled trial. *JAMA* 2007;297:267–277.
15. Regine WF, Winter KW, Abrams R, et al. RTOG 9704 a phase III study of adjuvant pre and post chemoradiation (CRT) 5-FU vs. gemcitabine (G) for resected pancreatic adenocarcinoma. *J Clin Oncol* 2006;24:4007.
16. Abrams RA, Winter KA, Regine WF, et al. RTOG 9704 - Radiotherapy Quality Assurance (QA) review and survival [Abstract]. *Int J Radiat Oncol Biol Phys* 2006;66:S22 (abstract).
17. Picozzi VJ, Kozarek RA, Traverso LW. Interferon-based adjuvant chemoradiation therapy after pancreaticoduodenectomy for pancreatic adenocarcinoma. *Am J Surg* 2003;185:476–480.
18. Spitz FR, Abbruzzese JL, Lee JE, et al. Preoperative and postoperative chemoradiation strategies in patients treated with pancreaticoduodenectomy for adenocarcinoma of the pancreas. *J Clin Oncol* 1997;15:928–937.
19. Nitecki SS, Sarr MG, Colby TV, et al. Long-term survival after resection for ductal adenocarcinoma of the pancreas. Is it really improving? *Ann Surg* 1995;221:59–66.
20. Willett CG, Lewandrowski K, Warshaw AL, et al. Resection margins in carcinoma of the head of the pancreas. Implications for radiation therapy. *Ann Surg* 1993;217:144–148.
21. Zerbi A, Fossati V, Parolini D, et al. Intraoperative radiation therapy adjuvant to resection in the treatment of pancreatic cancer. *Cancer* 1994;73:2930–2935.
22. Moertel CG, Frytak S, Hahn RG, et al. Therapy of locally unresectable pancreatic carcinoma: A randomized comparison of high dose (6000 rads) radiation alone, moderate dose radiation (4000 rads + 5-fluorouracil), and high dose radiation + 5-fluorouracil: The Gastrointestinal Tumor Study Group. *Cancer* 1981;48:1705–1710.
23. Treatment of locally unresectable carcinoma of the pancreas: Comparison of combined-modality therapy (chemotherapy plus radiotherapy) to chemotherapy alone. Gastrointestinal Tumor Study Group. *J Natl Cancer Inst* 1988;80:751–755.
24. Klaassen DJ, MacIntyre JM, Catton GE, et al. Treatment of locally unresectable cancer of the stomach and pancreas: A randomized comparison of 5-fluorouracil alone with radiation plus concurrent and maintenance 5-fluorouracil—an Eastern Cooperative Oncology Group study. *J Clin Oncol* 1985;3:373–378.
25. Oliani C, Padovani M, Manno P, et al. Gemcitabine and continuous infusion of 5-fluorouracil in locally advanced and metastatic pancreatic cancer: A phase I-II study. *Anticancer Res* 2004;24:2107–2112.
26. Ferrari V, Valcamonico F, Amoroso V, et al. Gemcitabine plus celecoxib (GECO) in advanced pancreatic cancer: a phase II trial. *Cancer Chemother Pharmacol* 2006;57:185–190.

27. Wang X, Ni Q, Jin M, et al. Gemcitabine or gemcitabine plus cisplatin for in 42 patients with locally advanced or metastatic pancreatic cancer. *Zhonghua Zhong Liu Za Zhi* 2002;24:404–407.
28. Okusaka T, Ito Y, Ueno H, et al. Phase II study of radiotherapy combined with gemcitabine for locally advanced pancreatic cancer. *Br J Cancer* 2004;91:673–677.
29. Wolff RA, Evans DB, Gravel DM, et al. Phase I trial of gemcitabine combined with radiation for the treatment of locally advanced pancreatic adenocarcinoma. *Clin Cancer Res* 2001;7:2246–2253.
30. Crane CH, Abbruzzese JL, Evans DB, et al. Is the therapeutic index better with gemcitabine-based chemoradiation than with 5-fluorouracil-based chemoradiation in locally advanced pancreatic cancer? *Int J Radiat Oncol Biol Phys* 2002;52:1293–1302.
31. Yavuz AA, Aydin F, Yavuz MN, et al. Radiation therapy and concurrent fixed dose amifostine with escalating doses of twice-weekly gemcitabine in advanced pancreatic cancer. *Int J Radiat Oncol Biol Phys* 2001;51:974–981.
32. Blackstock AW, Tepper JE, Niedwiecki D, et al. Cancer and leukemia group B (CALGB) 89805: Phase II chemoradiation trial using gemcitabine in patients with locoregional adenocarcinoma of the pancreas. *Int J Gastrointest Cancer* 2003;34:107-116.
33. Rich T, Harris J, Abrams R, et al. Phase II study of external irradiation and weekly paclitaxel for nonmetastatic, unresectable pancreatic cancer: RTOG-98-12. *Am J Clin Oncol* 2004;27:51–56.
34. Viret F, Ychou M, Goncalves A, et al. Docetaxel and radiotherapy and pancreatic cancer. *Pancreas* 2003;27:214–219.
35. Brunner TB, Grabenbauer GG, Klein P, et al. Phase I trial of strictly time-scheduled gemcitabine and cisplatin with concurrent radiotherapy in patients with locally advanced pancreatic cancer. *Int J Radiat Oncol Biol Phys* 2003;55:144–153.
36. Cohen SJ, Dobelbower R Jr., Lipsitz S, et al. A randomized phase III study of radiotherapy alone or with 5-fluorouracil and mitomycin-C in patients with locally advanced adenocarcinoma of the pancreas: Eastern Cooperative Oncology Group study E8282. *Int J Radiat Oncol Biol Phys* 2005;62:1345–1350.
37. Kornek GV, Potter R, Selzer E, et al. Combined radiochemotherapy of locally advanced unresectable pancreatic adenocarcinoma with mitomycin C plus 24-hour continuous infusional gemcitabine. *Int J Radiat Oncol Biol Phys* 2001;49:665–671.
38. Azria D, Ychou M, Jacot W, et al. Treatment of unresectable, locally advanced pancreatic adenocarcinoma with combined radiochemotherapy with 5-fluorouracil and cisplatin. *Pancreas* 2002;25:360–365.
39. Krishnan S, Rana V, Janjan NA, et al. Induction chemotherapy selects patients with locally advanced, unresectable pancreatic cancer for optimal benefit from consolidative chemoradiation therapy. *Cancer* 2007;110:47–55.
40. Burris HA 3rd, Moore MJ, Andersen J, et al. Improvements in survival and clinical benefit with gemcitabine as first-line therapy for patients with advanced pancreas cancer: A randomized trial. *J Clin Oncol* 1997;15:2403–2413.
41. Druker BJ, Talpaz M, Resta DJ, et al. Efficacy and safety of a specific inhibitor of the BCR-ABL tyrosine kinase in chronic myeloid leukemia. *N Engl J Med* 2001;344:1031–1037.
42. Vogel CL, Cobleigh MA, Tripathy D, et al. Efficacy and safety of trastuzumab as a single agent in first-line treatment of HER2-overexpressing metastatic breast cancer. *J Clin Oncol* 2002;20:719–726.
43. Slamon DJ, Leyland-Jones B, Shak S, et al. Use of chemotherapy plus a monoclonal antibody against HER2 for metastatic breast cancer that overexpresses HER2. *N Engl J Med* 2001;344:783–792.

44. Li D, Xie K, Wolff R, et al. Pancreatic cancer. *Lancet* 2004;363:1049–1057.
45. Bardeesy N, DePinho RA. Pancreatic cancer biology and genetics. *Nat Rev Cancer* 2002;2:897–909.
46. Jaffee EM, Hruban RH, Canto M, et al. Focus on pancreas cancer. *Cancer Cell* 2002;2:25–28.
47. Kozin SV, Boucher Y, Hicklin DJ, et al. Vascular endothelial growth factor receptor-2-blocking antibody potentiates radiation-induced long-term control of human tumor xenografts. *Cancer Res* 2001;61:39–44.
48. Bianco C, Tortora G, Bianco R, et al. Enhancement of antitumor activity of ionizing radiation by combined treatment with the selective epidermal growth factor receptor-tyrosine kinase inhibitor ZD1839 (Iressa). *Clin Cancer Res* 2002;8:3250–3258.
49. Milas L, Fan Z, Andratschke NH, et al. Epidermal growth factor receptor and tumor response to radiation: In vivo preclinical studies. *Int J Radiat Oncol Biol Phys* 2004;58:966–971.
50. Huang SM, Bock JM, Harari PM. Epidermal growth factor receptor blockade with C225 modulates proliferation, apoptosis, and radiosensitivity in squamous cell carcinomas of the head and neck. *Cancer Res* 1999;59:1935–1940.
51. Buchsbaum DJ, Bonner JA, Grizzle WE, et al. Treatment of pancreatic cancer xenografts with Erbitux (IMC-C225) anti-EGFR antibody, gemcitabine, and radiation. *Int J Radiat Oncol Biol Phys* 2002;54:1180–1193.
52. Willett CG, Boucher Y, di Tomaso E, et al. Direct evidence that the VEGF-specific antibody bevacizumab has antivascular effects in human rectal cancer. *Nat Med* 2004;10:145–147.
53. Bonner JA, Harari PM, Giralt J, et al. Radiotherapy plus cetuximab for squamous-cell carcinoma of the head and neck. *N Engl J Med* 2006;354:567–578.
54. Krishnan S, Brown PD, Ballman KV, et al. Phase I trial of erlotinib with radiation therapy in patients with glioblastoma multiforme: Results of North Central Cancer Treatment Group protocol N0177. *Int J Radiat Oncol Biol Phys* 2006;65:1192–1199.
55. Crane CH, Ellis LM, Abbruzzese JL, et al. Phase I trial evaluating the safety of bevacizumab with concurrent radiotherapy and capecitabine in locally advanced pancreatic cancer. *J Clin Oncol* 2006;24:1145–1151.
56. Ferrara N. Vascular endothelial growth factor: Basic science and clinical progress. *Endocr Rev* 2004;25:581–611.
57. Dvorak HF. Vascular permeability factor/vascular endothelial growth factor: A critical cytokine in tumor angiogenesis and a potential target for diagnosis and therapy. *J Clin Oncol* 2002;20:4368–4380.
58. Hurwitz H, Fehrenbacher L, Novotny W, et al. Bevacizumab plus irinotecan, fluorouracil, and leucovorin for metastatic colorectal cancer. *N Engl J Med* 2004;350:2335–2342.
59. Kabbinavar FF, Hambleton J, Mass RD, et al. Combined analysis of efficacy: the addition of bevacizumab to fluorouracil/leucovorin improves survival for patients with metastatic colorectal cancer. *J Clin Oncol* 2005;23:3706–3712.
60. Gorski DH, Beckett MA, Jaskowiak NT, et al. Blockage of the vascular endothelial growth factor stress response increases the antitumor effects of ionizing radiation. *Cancer Res* 1999;59:3374–3378.
61. Wey JS, Fan F, Gray MJ, et al. Vascular endothelial growth factor receptor-1 promotes migration and invasion in pancreatic carcinoma cell lines. *Cancer* 2005;104:427–438.
62. Jain RK. Normalization of tumor vasculature: An emerging concept in antiangiogenic therapy. *Science* 2005;307:58–62.
63. Fan F, Wey JS, McCarty MF, et al. Expression and function of vascular endothelial growth factor receptor-1 on human colorectal cancer cells. *Oncogene* 2005;24:2647–2653.

64. Winkler F, Kozin SV, Tong RT, et al. Kinetics of vascular normalization by VEGFR2 blockade governs brain tumor response to radiation: role of oxygenation, angiopoietin-1, and matrix metalloproteinases. *Cancer Cell* 2004;6:553–563.
65. Lee CG, Heijn M, di Tomaso E, et al. Anti-Vascular endothelial growth factor treatment augments tumor radiation response under normoxic or hypoxic conditions. *Cancer Res* 2000;60:5565–5570.
66. Jain RK. Normalizing tumor vasculature with anti-angiogenic therapy: A new paradigm for combination therapy. *Nat Med* 2001;7:987–989.
67. Willett CG, Boucher Y, Duda DG, et al. Surrogate markers for antiangiogenic therapy and dose-limiting toxicities for bevacizumab with radiation and chemotherapy: Continued experience of a phase I trial in rectal cancer patients. *J Clin Oncol* 2005;23:8136–8139.
68. Bonnen M, Crane C, Vauthey JN, et al. Long-term results using local excision after preoperative chemoradiation among selected T3 rectal cancer patients. *Int J Radiat Oncol Biol Phys* 2004;60:1098–1105.
69. Crane CH, Winter K, Regine W, et al. A Phase II study of bevacizumab with concurrent capecitabine and radiation followed by maintenance gemcitabine and bevacizumab for locally advanced pancreatic cancer: RTOG PA0411. *Int J Radiat Oncol Biol Phys* 2007;69: S77–S78.
70. Crane CH, Krishnan S, Rana V, et al. Does the addition of bevacizumab to chemoradiation prolong median survival in locally advanced pancreatic cancer patients? *Int J Radiat Oncol Biol Phys* 2006;66:S173.
71. Small W, Mulcahy M, Benson A, et al. A phase II trial of weekly gemcitabine and bevacizumab in combination with abdominal radiation therapy in patients with localized pancreatic cancer. *Proc GI Cancers Symposium* 2008: Abstract ID: 10764.
72. Varadhachary GR, Wolff RA, Crane CH, et al. Preoperative gemcitabine (gem) plus bevacizumab (bev) based chemoradiation for resectable pancreatic adenocarcinoma. *Proc GI Cancers Symposium* 2008: Abstract ID: 10570.
73. Cunningham D, Humblet Y, Siena S, et al. Cetuximab monotherapy and cetuximab plus irinotecan in irinotecan-refractory metastatic colorectal cancer. *N Engl J Med* 2004;351:337–345.
74. Krempien R, Muenter MW, Huber PE, et al. Randomized phase II study evaluating EGFR targeting therapy with cetuximab in combination with radiotherapy and chemotherapy for patients with locally advanced pancreatic cancer--PARC: Study protocol [ISRCTN56652283]. *BMC Cancer* 2005;5:131.
75. Iannitti D, Dipetrillo T, Akerman P, et al. Erlotinib and chemoradiation followed by maintenance erlotinib for locally advanced pancreatic cancer: A phase I study. *Am J Clin Oncol* 2005;28:570–575.
76. Kortmansky JS, O'Reilly EM, Minsky BD, et al. A phase I trial of erlotinib, gemcitabine and radiation for patients with locally-advanced, unresectable pancreatic cancer. *J Clin Oncol* 2005;23:4107.
77. Czito BG, Willett CG, Bendell JC, et al. Increased toxicity with gefitinib, capecitabine, and radiation therapy in pancreatic and rectal cancer: phase I trial results. *J Clin Oncol* 2006;24:656–662.
78. Khambata-Ford S, Garrett CR, Meropol NJ, et al. Expression of epiregulin and amphiregulin and K-ras mutation status predict disease control in metastatic colorectal cancer patients treated with cetuximab. *J Clin Oncol* 2007;25:3230–3237.
79. Lievre A, Bachet JB, Le Corre D, et al. KRAS mutation status is predictive of response to cetuximab therapy in colorectal cancer. *Cancer Res* 2006;66:3992–3995.

80. Amado RG, Freeman DP, M., Van Cutsem E, et al. Wild-type KRAS is required for panitumumab efficacy in patients with metastatic colorectal cancer: Results from a randomized, controlled trial. *Proc 4th Biannual European Cancer Conference (ECCO)* 2007: Abstract 0007.
81. Bentzen SM, Harari PM, Bernier J. Exploitable mechanisms for combining drugs with radiation: Concepts, achievements and future directions. *Nat Clin Pract Oncol* 2007;4:172–180.

10 *Targeted Therapies in Cervical Cancer*

CHRISTOPHER J. ANKER
DAVID K. GAFFNEY

There has been rapid growth and understanding of the biology of cancers of the cervix. Genomic, proteomic, and metabolomic techniques are increasing our understanding of tumor behavior significantly. The promise of personalized therapy may soon be on our doorstep. Remarkable breakthroughs have been achieved with targeted therapy in a variety of neoplasms. It certainly is plausible that this new biology will soon lead to improved therapy for cervical cancer treatment.

A variety of potential targeted agents may be available for the treatment of cancer of the cervix, including monoclonal antibodies (mAbs), small interfering RNA compounds, and small-molecule inhibitors. These various modes of protein inhibition affect cells at different components of the cellular machinery and, hence, advantages and disadvantages exist for each. A number of clinical trials have been performed with novel biologic agents, and a vast body of literature is available on molecular markers and their prognostic significance in cancer of the cervix.

The standard treatment for early-stage carcinoma of the cervix includes surgery or radiotherapy. Most patients are treated with a radical hysterectomy, including a lymph node dissection for patients with small-volume disease stage I–IIA. An advantage of surgery in early cervical cancer is that the late effects of radiation therapy are obviated. In a landmark trial by Landoni and colleagues, no difference in overall survival was noted in patients who received radiotherapy or surgery (1). However, for patients with tumors over 4 cm in size treated with surgery, 84% required postoperative radiotherapy. Additionally, morbidity was greatest for those patients who received both modalities. Hence, optimal treatment should include either surgery or radiation (including chemotherapy and possibly targeted therapy) for women with early carcinoma of the cervix.

For patients with more advanced disease [International Federation of Gynecologists and Oncologists (FIGO) stages IB2 through IVA], the traditional therapy is combination chemoradiotherapy (2–8). The National Cancer Institute (NCI) published a clinical alert in 1999 after the simultaneous release of five randomized trials, all of which documented a large overall survival benefit was documented for cisplatin-based chemotherapy. The most commonly used regimen is weekly cisplatin at 40 mg/m^2. Cisplatin in its own right serves as a radiation-sensitizing agent. The majority of clinical trials in the NCI clinical alert demonstrated a decrease in locoregional control, whereas a minority of trials demonstrated an improvement in distant metastatic disease with the addition of chemotherapy (2,4). Additionally, there have been several reports of less traditional chemotherapy along with radiotherapy for women with advanced disease (9,10).

CLASSES OF TARGETED AGENTS

Epidermal Growth Factor Receptor

The epidermal growth factor receptor (EGFR) has been widely studied in human carcinomas. This member of the HER-2/*neu* receptor family is a 170,000 kilodalton transmembrane glycoprotein. Both small-molecule inhibitors and mAbs target the EGFR. Upon binding to a ligand, the receptor undergoes either homo- or heterodimerization and subsequent phosphorylation of the intracellular tyrosine kinase (TK) domain. This leads to a downstream signaling cascade that affects cellular proliferation, angiogenesis, apoptosis, invasion, metastasis, and migration (11). Large-molecule inhibitors, such as mAbs, block the receptor function on the cell surface, whereas small-molecule TK inhibitors inhibit phosphorylation of the intracellular component of the EGFR receptor. The EGFR has also been found to interact with the human papilloma virus (HPV). HPV-E5 interacts with receptor processing by inhibiting an endosomal ATPase, thus blocking degradation of the EGFR molecule (12). When HPV+ cervical lesions were evaluated, EGFR was found in 98%, indicating significant expression of the receptor (13). In this study (13), no association was found between EGFR expression and HPV subtype, grade of cervical intraepithelial neoplasia, or clinical course. Overall, there appears to be significant data indicating a positive correlation between EGFR and HPV overexpression.

The incidence of EGFR overexpression varies widely in the literature. Overexpression has been identified in both squamous cell histologies and adenocarcinomas. The incidence of positive staining for EGFR ranged from 25.8% to 74.2% in different series, and in four of the six series listed in Table 10.1, EGFR expression had a negative impact on survival (14–19).

Inhibition of EGFR by antibodies or small molecules has shown antitumor activity in xenograft models (20,21). Inhibition of EGFR with the monoclonal

TABLE 10.1 Endothelial growth factor receptor (EGFR) expression versus survival

Marker	Evaluated Variable for Survival Analysis	Author/Year	Incidence of Positivity	Sample Size	Impact on Survival
EGFR	Immunohisochemistry: Any nuclear staining present	Cho, 2003	26.6%	84	Worsened extrapelvic failure ($p = 0.03$), OS ($p = 0.012$) and DFS ($p = 0.0165$)
	Immunohistochemistry: Intensity and area of staining	Gaffney, 2003	NS	55	Worsened OS ($p = 0.011$, MV)
	Immunohistochemistry: Intensity and number cells stained	Kersemaekers, 1999	54%	136	Worsened DFS ($p = 0.002$, UV) and OS ($p = 0.04$, MV)
	Immunohisochemistry: Membrane staining >10% cells	Kristensen, 1996	25.8%	132	Worsened DFS ($p = 0.014$, MV)
	Immunohistochemistry: >25% cells with moderate to intense staining	Ngan, 2001	74.2%	101	None
	ELISA	Kim JW, 1996	72.5%	40	None
c-ErbB-2/HER-2/neu	Positive immunohistochemical staining	Kersemaekers, 1999	8.8%	136	None
	Positive immunohistochemical staining	Kristensen, 1996	12.1%	132	None
	Marked cell membrane or cytoplasmic staining	Nakano, 1997	42.4%	64	Worsened DFS (p <0.01)
	Definitive membranous staining and >10% cells stained	Nishioka, 1999	33.6%	107	Worsened OS ($p = 0.019$) Worsened DMFS (p <0.001)
VEGF	Immunohistochemistry: Staining area and intensity	Gaffney, 2003	NS	55	Worsened DFS ($p = 0.014$, MV) and OS ($p = 0.005$, MV)
	Immunohistochemistry: Staining intensity	Loncaster, 2000	67%	100	Worsened OS ($p = 0.001$, MV) and DMFS (RR 2.3, MV)
	Immunohistochemistry: High intensity staining	Lee IJ, 2002	29.9%	117	Worsened OS ($p = 0.009$, MV) and DFS ($p = 0.001$, MV)

(continued on next page)

TABLE 10.1 Endothelial growth factor receptor (EGFR) expression versus survival

Marker	Evaluated Variable for Survival Analysis	Author/Year	Incidence of Positivity	Sample Size	Impact on Survival
	Immunohistochemistry: Strong VEGF-C staining	Ueda, 2002	73%	52	Worsened OS ($p = 0.0132$)
	ELISA: Serum VEGF >244 pg/mL (median)	Bachtiary, 2002	50%	23	Worsened PFS ($p = 0.003$)
	ELISA: VEGF >800 pg/mg protein	Cheng, 2000	24%	135	Worsened DFS ($p < 0.001$, MV) and OS ($p = 0.021$, MV)
	ELISA: VEGF and VEGF-C concentration vs. healthy control	Mitsuhashi, 2005	N/A	78	Increased disease recurrence and persistence ($p = 0.0112$)
	ELISA: Serum VEGF >581 pg/mL	Lebrecht, 2002	25%	84	None
	Immunohistochemistry: VEGF staining intensity	Lee JS, 2003	52% strong staining	86	None
	Immunohistochemistry: Staining > 50% slide	Tjalma, 2000	20%	130	None
HPV	ELISA, Any type (>1000 RLU/cutoff)	Datta, 2006	NS	21	Improved LC ($p = 0.0004$), DFS ($p = 0.0002$), OS ($p = 0.0001$)
	PCR, Any type	Harima, 2002	76.2%	84	Improved OS ($p = 0.007$, MV) and DFS ($p = 0.005$, MV)
	PCR, Any type	Lindel, 2005	70%	40	Improved OS ($p = 0.01$), DFS ($p = 0.02$), LC ($p = 0.047$)
	PCR, Any type	Pilch, 2001	73.4% Any; 45.3% HPV 16	93	OS worse only for HPV 16 on MVA ($p < 0.002$)
	PCR, 16/18	Schwartz, 2001	74%	399	Worsened CSS ($p = 0.001$) and OS ($p = 0.025$)for HPV 18, St. IB and IIA tumors
	PCR, Any type	Kersemaekers, 1999	87%	136	Worsened OS ($p < 0.001$)

TABLE 10.1 Endothelial growth factor receptor (EGFR) expression versus survival

Marker	Evaluated Variable for Survival Analysis	Author/Year	Incidence of Positivity	Sample Size	Impact on Survival
	PCR, 16/18/33	Fule, 2006	71%	150	None
	PCR, Any type	Graflund, 2004	78%	110	None
	PCR, Any type	Ikuta, 2005	76%	49	None
	PCR, 16/18/33	Ishikawa, 2001	76.9%	52	None
	PCR, Any type	Kristensen, 1996	93.3%	223	None
	PCR, 16/18	Ngan, 2001	79.2%	101	None
	PCR, 16/18	Tjalma, 2001	77%	111	None
		Microenvironmental Factors			
IFP	Divided by median (>19 mm Hg)	Fyles, 2006	51%	102	Worsened DFS ($p = 0.0005$, MV), Worsened pelvic failure ($p = 0.0346$, MV), Worsened extrapelvic failure ($p = 0.0014$, MV)
Hypoxic fraction (HP)	Hypoxic if >50% tumor cells have HP(5)	Fyles, 2006	49%	106	Worsened DFS ($p = 0.05$)
	Percentage cells with HP(5) divided by median	Knocke, 1999	NS	59	Worsened DFS ($p < 0.02$)
	Percentage cells with HP(2.5), HP(5), HP(10) divided by median and as continuous variable	Nordsmark, 2006	NS	105	None
Pimonidazole	Immunohistochemistry: Divided by median % staining score and as continuous variable	Nordsmark, 2006	49%	114	None
PO2	Divided by median (< 10 mm Hg)	Hockel, 1996	54%	89	Worsened DFS ($p = 0.0084$, MV) and OS ($p = 0.0039$, MV)
	Divided by median (≤ 10 mm Hg)	Knocke, 1999	51%	51	Worsened DFS ($p < 0.02$)
	Divided by median (≤ 4 mm Hg and as continuous variable)	Nordsmark, 2006	NS	105	None

(continued on next page)

TABLE 10.1 Endothelial growth factor receptor (EGFR) expression versus survival

Marker	Evaluated Variable for Survival Analysis	Author/Year	Incidence of Positivity	Sample Size	Impact on Survival
HIF-1α	Immunohistochemistry: moderate/strong staining	Bachtiary, 2003	47.7%	67	Worsened PFS (p = 0.049, MV) and CSS (p = 0.02, MV)
	Immunohistochemistry: % cells stained and intensity of staining	Birner, 2000	81.3%	91	Worsened OS (p = 0.0129, MV) and DFS (p = 0.0002, MV)
	Immunohistochemistry: % cells stained and intensity of staining	Burri, 2003	94%	78	Worsened local PFS (p = 0.04, UV), OS (p = 0.02, MV)
	Immunohistochemistry: staining above mean	Ishikawa, 2004	45%	38	Worsened recurrence free survival (p = 0.04) and DMFS (p = 0.03)
	Immunohistochemistry: staining positive for ≥2% tumor area	Haugland, 2002	50%	42	None
	Percent area with immunohistochemistry staining	Hutchinson, 2004	N/A	99	None
CA-IX	Immunohistochemistry: >1% cell area stained positive	Hedley, 2003	70%	102	None
	Immunohistochemistry: >1% cell area positive	Loncaster, 2001	71%	130	Worsened OS (p = 0.05, MV) and DMFS (p = 0.021, MV)
Lactate	Imaging bioluminescence lactate concentration, groups divided by median	Walenta, 2000	NS	34	Worsened OS (p = 0.015) and DFS (p = 0.014)
COX2	Immunohistochemistry: % cells stained	Ryu, 2000	100%	36	Increased lymph node or parametrial involvement (p = 0.013)
	Immunohistochemistry: ≥10% cell staining	Gaffney, 2001	50%	24	Worsened OS (p = 0.0126)
	Immunohistochemistry: Integrated density value above mean	Ferrandina, 2002	42.9%	84	Worsened OS (p = 0.0014, MV)
	Immunohistochemistry: Intensity and % cells stained	Chen, 2005	64.1%	167	Worsened DFS (p = 0.01, MV) and CSS (p <0.01, UV)

TABLE 10.1 Endothelial growth factor receptor (EGFR) expression versus survival

Marker	Evaluated Variable for Survival Analysis	Author/Year	Incidence of Positivity	Sample Size	Impact on Survival
	Immunohistochemistry: Area and intensity of staining	Kim JY, 2005	44%	318	None
		Apoptotic Markers			
Bax	>10% positive cells	Wootipoom, 2004	68.4%	174	Improved DFS (HR, 0.47; 95% CI 0.26–0.87)
	>70% positive cells	Crawford, 2001	20%	44	None
	>30% positive cells	Harima,1998	13%	37	None
	>10% positive cells	Ishikawa, 2004	45%	38	None
	>10% positive cells	Tjalma, 2001	83%	111	None
Bcl-2	>10% positive cells	Crawford, 2001	34%	44	Improved OS ($p = 0.03$)
	Staining intensity and number cells staining positive	Munakata, 2005	75.2%	125	Improved OS ($p = 0.0003$, MV) and DFS ($p = 0.01$, MV)
	>5% positive cells	Tjalma, 2001	68%	111	Improved OS ($p < 0.001$)
	>10% positive cells	Wootipoom, 2004	25.9%	174	Worsened DFS (HR, 2.51; 95% CI 1.03–6.12)
	>30% positive cells	Harima,1998	61.4%	37	None
	>10% positive cells	Ishikawa, 2004	45%	38	None
	Any positive cells	Jain, 2003	38.1%	76	None
Erythro-poetin	Immunohistochemistry for Epo	Leo, 2006	88%	48	Worsened OS ($p = 0.0084$)

LC, local control; DFS, disease-free survival; LDFS, local disease-free survival; PFS, progression-free survival; CSS, cause-specific survival; DMFS, distant metastases-free survival; OS, overall survival; MV, multivariate analysis; UV, univariate analysis; NS, not specified in manuscript; N/A, not applicable

Note: p-value refers to UV analysis unless otherwise specified.

antibody cetuximab (C225) has been found to improve survival in head and neck cancer patients (22). Cetuximab has been tested in the phase I setting by the Gynecologic Oncology Group (GOG) in combination with radiation for patients with advanced cervix cancer. No results have been published to date. In a preclinical experiment by Milas and colleagues evaluating tumor control with C225 in a xenotropic model, the authors demonstrated improved tumor cure with concurrent C225 and with maintenance therapy (23). The dose modification factor was 1.8 when given with radiation and 2.7 when given both during and after radiation. These data suggest a possible benefit of maintenance therapy for blockade of EGFR in future clinical trials. Recently, multiple agents have been developed that inhibit more than one target. This combinatorial therapy has significant promise in the curative treatment of cervical cancer.

C-ERBB-2/HER-2/neu

HER-2/*neu* staining has been identified in 8.8–42.4% of patients with carcinoma of the cervix (16,18,24,25). HER-2/*neu* overexpression has been found to correlate with diminished survival. Additional data is needed in both squamous cell carcinomas and adenocarcinomas correlating HER-2/*neu* with outcome. Multivariate statistics should be employed to determine the independent role of this marker.

Vascular Endothelial Growth Factor

Vascular endothelial growth factor (VEGF) is found to be overexpressed in many cancers, including cancer of the cervix. Hypoxia has long been studied in carcinoma of the cervix. Hypoxia is mediated by the hypoxia-inducible factor (HIF)-1 transcription factor. Increasing hypoxia is correlated with enhanced VEGF expression. Studies investigating VEGF overexpression in cervical cancer have found incidences ranging from 24% to 73% (15, 26–35). In a study of 100 patients by Loncaster and colleagues, the incidence of positive staining for VEGF was 67%, and this overexpression correlated with worsened overall survival in multivariate analysis (26). Similarly, worse overall survival with overexpression of VEGF on immunohistochemical staining was found in multiple other studies (28,34). A study by Cheng and coworkers demonstrated positive expression of VEGF using enzyme-linked immunosorbent assay (ELISA) in 24% of 135 patients, and this group had diminished disease-free survival in multivariate analysis (29). Elevated VEGF determined via ELISA has been seen to provide a significant risk of decreased progression-free survival (30,31). However, in addition to these positive reports, others show no effect of VEGF on survival (27,32,33). A mAb of VEGF [bevacizumab (Avastin)] has been shown to improve survival in concert with chemotherapy in breast and colon cancer. A phase II trial in women with stage IB2 through IVA is currently ongoing in the Radiation Therapy Oncology Group (RTOG). Fifty-eight patients are planned for this phase II trial, with the primary end-point being toxicity.

Human Papilloma Virus

Human papilloma virus serotypes 16 and 18 are frequently associated with cervical tumors, and these oncogenic subtypes clearly play a role in the pathogenesis of malignant transformation. The prognostic value of detecting HPV DNA in cervical cancer specimens is less clear. The incidence of HPV DNA positivity in studies evaluating the role of HPV DNA presence on outcome has ranged from 70% to 93.3% (16,19,35–45). The majority of studies that evaluated the presence of HPV DNA for subtypes 16 and 18 or even other subtypes, have found no impact on prognosis (19,36,39–41,45).

Although Graflund and colleagues (37) noticed a trend toward worse cause-specific survival with both HPV-16+ or HPV-18+ tumors, this was not significant ($p = 0.167$). Schwartz and coworkers (44) found that HPV-18 but not HPV-16 was a statistically significant predictor for worse cause-specific survival for early-stage tumors. However, Pilch and colleagues found overall survival to be worse for HPV-16 DNA positivity but not for the HPV-18 subtype (43). Kersemaekers and coworkers found HPV+ patients to have significantly worse overall survival (16). Contrary to these results portending worse prognosis, other studies have found improved overall survival with the presence of HPV DNA (35,38,42). Direct comparison of the varying results regarding prognostic significance is difficult, and differences between trials may be, in part, due to patient and treatment heterogeneity.

Microenvironmental Factors

Substantial literature exists regarding the impact of microenvironmental factors in cervical cancers, including interstitial fluid pressure, oxygenation status, and expression of hypoxia markers such as carbonic anhydrase IX (CA-IX), HIF-1α, and lactate. The significance of these various measurements is of interest, in part because hypoxia is considered to decrease radiosensitivity, which may lead to a worse patient outcome. In a recent trial by Fyles and colleagues, 107 eligible patients with cervical cancer were evaluated prospectively with tumor oxygenation measurements and interstitial fluid pressure measurements prior to radiotherapy (46). The authors identified interstitial fluid pressure as a strong independent prognostic factor for disease-free survival on multivariate analysis. However, the hypoxic portion defined as the percentage of Po_2 readings less than 5 mm Hg [HP(5)] was noted to be of borderline significance (p

= 0.05). In a separate, recently analyzed trial of 127 patients by Nordsmark and colleagues, there was no significance for any analyzed hypoxic portion including HP(2.5), HP(5), and HP(10) (47). In this study, evaluation with pimonidazole, a "hypoxia marker" that is reduced in cells with low oxygen tension forming stainable adducts, did not reveal tumors with worse prognosis. However, the authors report that these results do not preclude the potential prognostic utility of Eppendorf electrodes and pimonidazole, and that they should be evaluated under a more rigorous protocol with improved power. Other studies have demonstrated the negative prognostic impact of an elevated hypoxic fraction (48). Additionally, in studies evaluating the prognostic impact of Po_2 measurements, most studies identified low Po_2 as a negative prognostic factor (48–49).

The use of intrinsic markers may provide a relatively noninvasive method of evaluating tumor hypoxia compared with polarographic electrodes, as they only require pretreatment biopsy tissue. One such marker is HIF-1α, a subunit of the heterodimer HIF-1, which directly activates several hypoxia-inducible gene transcriptions. Multiple studies have shown worse outcome in terms of overall survival and progression-free survival with increased presence of HIF-1α (51–53). Another study showed significantly worse distant metastases-free survival (54). However, other studies show no correlation between HIF-1α and prognosis (55,56).

CA-IX is an HIF-1–responsive transmembrane glycoprotein that is also an intrinsic hypoxic marker. On multivariate analysis, Loncaster and colleagues found significantly worse overall survival and distant metastases-free survival in the 71% of patients whose cervical tumors were positive for CA-IX (50). Hedley and coworkers performed a similar analysis and observed 70% of the patients were positive for CA-IX. In contrast to the study by Loncaster, Hedley's revealed no correlation of CA-IX with prognosis (57).

The heterogeneous environment where tumors reside is due in part to abnormal vasculature. The altered permeability and distribution of blood vessels may lead to differences in the concentration of nutrients, such as glucose and oxygen, and by-products, such as lactic acid. In a study published by Walenta and colleagues in 2000, high lactate levels were found to be associated with the presence of metastases and worsened survival ($p = 0.015$) (58).

Cyclo-oxygenase 2

Cyclo-oxygenase (COX)-2 is an inducible enzyme required in the conversion of prostaglandins from arachidonic acid. COX2 has been correlated with angiogenesis, resistance to apoptosis, and cellular proliferation (59–61). In a landmark paper by Steinbach and colleagues, the authors observed a dose-dependent reduction of colon polyps in patients with familial polyposis adenosis treated with celecoxib (62). Inhibition of COX2 has been shown to sensitize tumors to radiotherapy (63). Preclinical studies by Ryu and coworkers (64) demonstrated that COX2 overexpression correlated with lymph node involvement in patients with cancer of the cervix. Multiple studies have demonstrated that overexpression of COX2 portended a worse prognosis (65–67), whereas other studies have shown no impact of COX2 expression on survival (68). A phase II protocol of celecoxib at 400 mg b.i.d. with standard chemoradiotherapy in women with advanced cervical cancer performed by the RTOG showed no apparent benefit compared to historical trials of chemoradiotherapy alone (69,70). A single-institution trial performed at Princess Margaret Hospital by Herrera and colleagues demonstrated similar findings (71). Despite the promising preclinical data indicating potential benefit of COX2 inhibition, the early clinical experience has not been positive. There may be multiple reasons for the lack of effect on COX2 inhibition in promoting improved disease-free survival, including poor understanding of the appropriate dose and length of treatment for COX2 inhibitors, and lack of enrichment in clinical trials for overexpressors of COX2. COX2 may be a nonspecific marker of inflammation and, hence, not rate limiting in the tumorigenic pathway. Similarly, tumors may display multiple routes of escape from COX2 inhibition.

Apoptotic Markers

Apoptosis, or the controlled cell death, has been studied extensively in gynecologic cancers. Bcl-2 and Bax are cytoplasmic proteins which have oppositional effects in regulating apoptosis. Bcl-2 overexpression could prevent initiation of this programmed cell death, whereas Bax overexpression could induce apoptosis. Although overexpression of Bax has been found to occur in 13–83% of tumors (45,54,72–74), the majority of studies have shown no impact on survival (45,54,72,73). Only one study, by Wootipoom and coworkers, revealed an improved disease-free survival (74). Enhanced expression of bcl-2 appears more useful as a prognostic factor, with several studies demonstrating an associated improved survival (45,72,75). However, several other studies have demonstrated no significant impact on outcome as well (54,73,76). Bcl-2 overexpression is variable as well, occurring in 25.9–75.2% of tumors (45,54,72–76).

Erythropoietin

Erythropoietin (Epo) has been studied to increase the oxygenation status of cervical cancers during radiotherapy. A phase III trial by GOG was discontinued due to concerns regarding toxicity. A recent trial by Temkin and coworkers found that Epo administration during radiotherapy for the treatment of locally advanced cervical carcinoma was associated with a poor treatment outcome

(77). This may be related to the expression of erythropoietin receptor (EpoR) on tumor cells. Hypoxia causes the expression of Epo in adult kidney cells, which then interacts with EpoRs in developing red blood cells to stimulate growth and prevent apoptosis. In a study by Leo and colleagues, cervical cancer patients with higher Epo expression showed a significantly reduced overall survival (78).

CONCLUSIONS

In summary, a number of promising targeted agents may have significant promise in the treatment of carcinoma of the cervix. Inhibition of EGFR has been studied by the GOG and in single-institution experiences. Additionally, the RTOG has an ongoing phase II trial with the addition of Avastin for women with advanced cervical cancer being treated with standard chemoradiotherapy. The treatment of squamous cell carcinomas in other sites has demonstrated significant improvements in survival with the addition of targeted agents, and it is quite likely this can be achieved as well for the treatment of carcinoma of the cervix.

REFERENCES

1. Landoni F, et al. Randomised study of radical surgery versus radiotherapy for stage Ib-IIa cervical cancer. *Lancet* 1997;350(9077):535–540.
2. Eifel PJ, et al. Pelvic irradiation with concurrent chemotherapy versus pelvic and para-aortic irradiation for high-risk cervical cancer: An update of radiation therapy oncology group trial (RTOG) 90-01. *J Clin Oncol* 2004;22(5):872–880.
3. Keys HM, et al. Cisplatin, radiation, and adjuvant hysterectomy compared with radiation and adjuvant hysterectomy for bulky stage IB cervical carcinoma. *N Engl J Med* 1999;340(15):1154–1161.
4. Morris M, et al. Pelvic radiation with concurrent chemotherapy compared with pelvic and para-aortic radiation for high-risk cervical cancer. *N Engl J Med* 1999;340(15):1137–1143.
5. Pearcey R, et al. Phase III trial comparing radical radiotherapy with and without cisplatin chemotherapy in patients with advanced squamous cell cancer of the cervix. *J Clin Oncol* 2002;20(4):966–972.
6. Peters WA 3rd, et al. Concurrent chemotherapy and pelvic radiation therapy compared with pelvic radiation therapy alone as adjuvant therapy after radical surgery in high-risk early-stage cancer of the cervix. *J Clin Oncol* 2000;18(8):1606–1613.
7. Rose PG, et al. Concurrent cisplatin-based radiotherapy and chemotherapy for locally advanced cervical cancer. *N Engl J Med* 1999;340(15):1144–1153.
8. Whitney CW, et al. Randomized comparison of fluorouracil plus cisplatin versus hydroxyurea as an adjunct to radiation therapy in stage IIB-IVA carcinoma of the cervix with negative para-aortic lymph nodes: A Gynecologic Oncology Group and Southwest Oncology Group study. *J Clin Oncol* 1999;17(5):1339–1348.
9. DiSilvestro PA, et al. Radiation therapy with concomitant paclitaxel and cisplatin chemotherapy in cervical carcinoma limited to the pelvis: A phase I/II study of the Gynecologic Oncology Group. *Gynecol Oncol* 2006;103(3):1038–1042.

10. Vrdoljak E, et al. Concomitant chemo brachyradiotherapy with ifosfamide and cisplatin followed by consolidation chemotherapy for women with locally advanced carcinoma of the uterine cervix--final results of a prospective phase II-study. *Gynecol Oncol* 2006;103(2):494–499.
11. Mendelsohn J. Blockade of receptors for growth factors: An anticancer therapy--the fourth annual Joseph H Burchenal American Association of Cancer Research Clinical Research Award Lecture. *Clin Cancer Res* 2000;6(3):747–753.
12. Yarden Y. The EGFR family and its ligands in human cancer. Signalling mechanisms and therapeutic opportunities. *Eur J Cancer* 2001;37(Suppl 4):S3–S8.
13. Tervahauta A, Syrjanen S, Syrjanen K. Epidermal growth factor receptor, c-erbB-2 proto-oncogene and estrogen receptor expression in human papillomavirus lesions of the uterine cervix. *Int J Gynecol Pathol* 1994;13(3):234–240.
14. Cho NH, et al. P63 and EGFR as prognostic predictors in stage IIB radiation-treated cervical squamous cell carcinoma. *Gynecol Oncol* 2003;91(2):346–353.
15. Gaffney DK, et al. Epidermal growth factor receptor (EGFR) and vascular endothelial growth factor (VEGF) negatively affect overall survival in carcinoma of the cervix treated with radiotherapy. *Int J Radiat Oncol Biol Phys* 2003;56(4):922–928.
16. Kersemaekers AM, et al. Oncogene alterations in carcinomas of the uterine cervix: overexpression of the epidermal growth factor receptor is associated with poor prognosis. *Clin Cancer Res* 1999;5(3):577–586.
17. Kim JW, et al. Expression of epidermal growth factor receptor in carcinoma of the cervix. *Gynecol Oncol* 1996;60(2):283–287.
18. Kristensen GB, et al. Evaluation of the prognostic significance of cathepsin D, epidermal growth factor receptor, and c-erbB-2 in early cervical squamous cell carcinoma. An immunohistochemical study. *Cancer* 1996;78(3):433–440.
19. Ngan HY, et al. Abnormal expression of epidermal growth factor receptor and c-erbB2 in squamous cell carcinoma of the cervix: correlation with human papillomavirus and prognosis. *Tumour Biol* 2001;22(3):176–183.
20. Birle DC, Hedley DW. Signaling interactions of rapamycin combined with erlotinib in cervical carcinoma xenografts. *Mol Cancer Ther* 2006;5(10):2494–2502.
21. Solbach C, et al. Cancer of the uterine cervix is susceptible to anti-EGF-R antibody EMD 55,900 therapy. *Anticancer Res* 2005;25(6B):4261–4267.
22. Bonner JA, et al. Radiotherapy plus cetuximab for squamous-cell carcinoma of the head and neck. *N Engl J Med* 2006;354(6):567–578.
23. Milas L, et al. Importance of maintenance therapy in C225-induced enhancement of tumor control by fractionated radiation. *Int J Radiat Oncol Biol Phys* 2007;67(2):568–572.
24. Nakano T, et al. Correlation of cervical carcinoma c-erb B-2 oncogene with cell proliferation parameters in patients treated with radiation therapy for cervical carcinoma. *Cancer* 1997;79(3):513–520.
25. Nishioka T, et al. Prognostic significance of c-erbB-2 protein expression in carcinoma of the cervix treated with radiotherapy. *J Cancer Res Clin Oncol* 1999;125(2):96–100.
26. Loncaster JA, et al. Vascular endothelial growth factor (VEGF) expression is a prognostic factor for radiotherapy outcome in advanced carcinoma of the cervix. *Br J Cancer* 2000;83(5):620–625.
27. Lee JS, et al. Expression of vascular endothelial growth factor in the progression of cervical neoplasia and its relation to angiogenesis and p53 status. *Anal Quant Cytol Histol* 2003;25(6):303–311.
28. Ueda M, et al. Correlation between vascular endothelial growth factor-C expression and invasion phenotype in cervical carcinomas. *Int J Cancer* 2002;98(3):335–343.

29. Cheng WF, et al. Vascular endothelial growth factor and prognosis of cervical carcinoma. *Obstet Gynecol* 2000;96(5 Pt 1):721–726.
30. Mitsuhashi A, et al. Serum vascular endothelial growth factor (VEGF) and VEGF-C levels as tumor markers in patients with cervical carcinoma. *Cancer* 2005;103(4):724–730.
31. Bachtiary B, et al. Serum VEGF levels in patients undergoing primary radiotherapy for cervical cancer: impact on progression-free survival. *Cancer Lett* 2002;179(2):197–203.
32. Lebrecht A, et al. Serum vascular endothelial growth factor and serum leptin in patients with cervical cancer. *Gynecol Oncol* 2002;85(1):32–35.
33. Tjalma W, et al. The association between vascular endothelial growth factor, microvessel density and clinicopathological features in invasive cervical cancer. *Eur J Obstet Gynecol Reprod Biol* 2000;92(2):251–257.
34. Lee IJ, et al. Prognostic value of vascular endothelial growth factor in Stage IB carcinoma of the uterine cervix. *Int J Radiat Oncol Biol Phys* 2002;54(3):768-779.
35. Datta NR, et al. Does pretreatment human papillomavirus (HPV) titers predict radiation response and survival outcomes in cancer cervix? A pilot study. *Gynecol Oncol* 2006;103(1): 100–105.
36. Fule T, et al. Prognostic significance of high-risk HPV status in advanced cervical cancers and pelvic lymph nodes. *Gynecol Oncol* 2006;100(3):570–578.
37. Graflund M, et al. HPV-DNA, vascular space invasion, and their impact on the clinical outcome in early-stage cervical carcinomas. *Int J Gynecol Cancer* 2004;14(5):896–902.
38. Harima Y, et al. Human papilloma virus (HPV) DNA associated with prognosis of cervical cancer after radiotherapy. *Int J Radiat Oncol Biol Phys* 2002;52(5):1345–1351.
39. Ikuta A, et al. Correlation p53 expression and human papilloma virus deoxyribonucleic acid with clinical outcome in early uterine cervical carcinoma. *Cancer Detect Prev* 2005;29(6):528–536.
40. Ishikawa H, et al. The effects of p53 status and human papillomavirus infection on the clinical outcome of patients with stage IIIB cervical carcinoma treated with radiation therapy alone. *Cancer* 2001;91(1):80–89.
41. Kristensen GB, et al. Human papilloma virus has no prognostic significance in cervical carcinoma. *Eur J Cancer* 1996;32A(8):1349–1353.
42. Lindel K, et al. Human papillomavirus status in advanced cervical cancer: Predictive and prognostic significance for curative radiation treatment. *Int J Gynecol Cancer* 2005;15(2):278–284.
43. Pilch H, et al. The presence of HPV DNA in cervical cancer: Correlation with clinico-pathologic parameters and prognostic significance: 10 years experience at the Department of Obstetrics and Gynecology of the Mainz University. *Int J Gynecol Cancer* 2001;11(1):39–48.
44. Schwartz SM, et al. Human papillomavirus and prognosis of invasive cervical cancer: a population-based study. *J Clin Oncol* 2001;19(7):1906–1915.
45. Tjalma WA, et al. The importance of biological factors (bcl-2, bax, p53, PCNA, MI, HPV and angiogenesis) in invasive cervical cancer. *Eur J Obstet Gynecol Reprod Biol* 2001;97(2):223–230.
46. Fyles A, et al. Long-term performance of interstitial fluid pressure and hypoxia as prognostic factors in cervix cancer. *Radiother Oncol* 2006;80(2):132–137.
47. Nordsmark M, et al. The prognostic value of pimonidazole and tumour pO2 in human cervix carcinomas after radiation therapy: A prospective international multi-center study. *Radiother Oncol* 2006;80(2):123–131.
48. Knocke TH, et al. Intratumoral pO2-measurements as predictive assay in the treatment of carcinoma of the uterine cervix. *Radiother Oncol* 1999;53(2):99–104.

49. Hockel M, et al. Association between tumor hypoxia and malignant progression in advanced cancer of the uterine cervix. *Cancer Res* 1996;56(19):4509–4515.
50. Loncaster JA, et al. Carbonic anhydrase (CA IX) expression, a potential new intrinsic marker of hypoxia: Correlations with tumor oxygen measurements and prognosis in locally advanced carcinoma of the cervix. *Cancer Res* 2001;61(17):6394–6399.
51. Bachtiary B, et al. Overexpression of hypoxia-inducible factor 1alpha indicates diminished response to radiotherapy and unfavorable prognosis in patients receiving radical radiotherapy for cervical cancer. *Clin Cancer Res* 2003;9(6):2234–2240.
52. Birner P, et al. Overexpression of hypoxia-inducible factor 1alpha is a marker for an unfavorable prognosis in early-stage invasive cervical cancer. *Cancer Res* 2000;60(17):4693–4696.
53. Burri P, et al. Significant correlation of hypoxia-inducible factor-1alpha with treatment outcome in cervical cancer treated with radical radiotherapy. *Int J Radiat Oncol Biol Phys* 2003;56(2):494–501.
54. Ishikawa H, et al. Expression of hypoxic-inducible factor 1alpha predicts metastasis-free survival after radiation therapy alone in stage IIIB cervical squamous cell carcinoma. *Int J Radiat Oncol Biol Phys* 2004;60(2):513–521.
55. Haugland HK, et al. Expression of hypoxia-inducible factor-1alpha in cervical carcinomas: Correlation with tumor oxygenation. *Int J Radiat Oncol Biol Phys* 2002;53(4):854–861.
56. Hutchison GJ, et al. Hypoxia-inducible factor 1alpha expression as an intrinsic marker of hypoxia: Correlation with tumor oxygen, pimonidazole measurements, and outcome in locally advanced carcinoma of the cervix. *Clin Cancer Res* 2004;10(24):8405–8412.
57. Hedley D, et al. Carbonic anhydrase IX expression, hypoxia, and prognosis in patients with uterine cervical carcinomas. *Clin Cancer Res* 2003;9(15):5666–5674.
58. Walenta S, et al. High lactate levels predict likelihood of metastases, tumor recurrence, and restricted patient survival in human cervical cancers. *Cancer Res* 2000;60(4):916–921.
59. Masferrer JL, et al. Antiangiogenic and antitumor activities of cyclooxygenase-2 inhibitors. *Cancer Res* 2000;60(5):1306–1311.
60. Tsujii M, DuBois RN. Alterations in cellular adhesion and apoptosis in epithelial cells overexpressing prostaglandin endoperoxide synthase 2. *Cell* 1995;83(3):493–501.
61. Tsujii M, Kawano S, DuBois RN. Cyclooxygenase-2 expression in human colon cancer cells increases metastatic potential. *Proc Natl Acad Sci USA* 1997;94(7):3336–3340.
62. Steinbach G, et al. The effect of celecoxib, a cyclooxygenase-2 inhibitor, in familial adenomatous polyposis. *N Engl J Med* 2000;342(26):1946–1952.
63. Milas L, et al. Enhancement of tumor response to gamma-radiation by an inhibitor of cyclooxygenase-2 enzyme. *J Natl Cancer Inst* 1999;91(17):1501–1504.
64. Ryu HS, et al. High cyclooxygenase-2 expression in stage IB cervical cancer with lymph node metastasis or parametrial invasion. *Gynecol Oncol* 2000;76(3):320–325.
65. Chen HH, et al. Increased expression of nitric oxide synthase and cyclooxygenase-2 is associated with poor survival in cervical cancer treated with radiotherapy. *Int J Radiat Oncol Biol Phys* 2005;63(4):1093–1100.
66. Ferrandina G, et al. Increased cyclooxygenase-2 expression is associated with chemotherapy resistance and poor survival in cervical cancer patients. *J Clin Oncol* 2002;20(4):973–981.
67. Gaffney DK, et al. Elevated cyclooxygenase-2 expression correlates with diminished survival in carcinoma of the cervix treated with radiotherapy. *Int J Radiat Oncol Biol Phys* 2001;49(5):1213–1217.
68. Kim JY, et al. Cyclooxygenase-2 and c-erbB-2 expression in uterine cervical neoplasm assessed using tissue microarrays. *Gynecol Oncol* 2005;97(2):337–341.

69. Gaffney DK, Winter K, Dicker AP. Celebrex (Celecoxib) and Chemoradiation in patients with locally advanced cervical cancer. An efficacy report of RTOG 0128. *Int J Radiat Oncol Biol Phys* 2006;66(3):S41.
70. Gaffney DK, et al. A Phase II study of acute toxicity for Celebrex (celecoxib) and chemoradiation in patients with locally advanced cervical cancer: Primary endpoint analysis of RTOG 0128. *Int J Radiat Oncol Biol Phys* 2007;67(1):104–109.
71. Herrera FG, et al. A prospective phase I-II trial of the cyclooxygenase-2 inhibitor celecoxib in patients with carcinoma of the cervix with biomarker assessment of the tumor microenvironment. *Int J Radiat Oncol Biol Phys* 2007;67(1):97-103.
72. Crawford RA, et al. Prognostic significance of the bcl-2 apoptotic family of proteins in primary and recurrent cervical cancer. *Br J Cancer* 1998;78(2):210–214.
73. Harima Y, et al. Bax and Bcl-2 expressions predict response to radiotherapy in human cervical cancer. *J Cancer Res Clin Oncol* 1998;124(9):503–510.
74. Wootipoom V, et al. Prognostic significance of Bax, Bcl-2, and p53 expressions in cervical squamous cell carcinoma treated by radiotherapy. *Gynecol Oncol* 2004;94(3):636–642.
75. Munakata S, et al. Expression of Fas ligand and bcl-2 in cervical carcinoma and their prognostic significance. *Am J Clin Pathol* 2005;123(6):879–885.
76. Jain D, et al. Evaluation of p53 and Bcl-2 expression as prognostic markers in invasive cervical carcinoma stage IIb/III patients treated by radiotherapy. *Gynecol Oncol* 2003;88(1):22–28.
77. Temkin SM, et al. Erythropoietin administration during primary treatment for locally advanced cervical carcinoma is associated with poor response to radiation. *Int J Gynecol Cancer* 2006;16(5):1855–1861.
78. Leo C, et al. Expression of erythropoietin and erythropoietin receptor in cervical cancer and relationship to survival, hypoxia, and apoptosis. *Clin Cancer Res* 2006;12(23):6894–6900.

11 Targeted Therapies in Endometrial Cancer

JERGIN CHEN
DAVID K. GAFFNEY

Endometrial cancer is the most common gynecologic malignancy in the United States. The primary management of this disease is surgical resection with hysterectomy and bilateral salpingo-oophorectomy, which provides both therapeutic benefit and prognostic information. Radiation therapy is typically used in an adjuvant setting to eliminate occult disease and reduce the risk of recurrence. In early stage disease, the majority of women are cured with surgery alone; however, subsets of patients are at high risk for recurrence. The established pathologic risk factors include high-grade histology, lymphovascular invasion, deep myometrial invasion, and cervical extension (1). Advanced-stage disease is associated with a high risk of recurrence. Despite adjuvant pelvic irradiation, the high risk of recurrence in the abdomen is 25–30% (2–5). Therefore, whole abdominal irradiation and systemic multiagent chemotherapy have been used to decrease the rate of recurrence and improve survival (6–8). Over the last two decades, there has been increasing enthusiasm for the use of therapies designed for specific biologic targets. These may be effective agents in improving the cure rates of endometrial cancers with minimal or no additional side effects.

■ HORMONAL THERAPY

Modulation of endogenous hormone activity has been successful in improving outcomes of patients with hormone-sensitive malignancies. The blockade of hormone production and receptors has been successful in improving the survival of patients with breast and prostate cancers without significant long-term morbidities (9–13).

The use of progestin has been studied in the management of endometrial cancers without much success. Long-term, unopposed exposure of the endometrium to estrogen has been associated with the development of endometrial cancer. Intermittent exposures to progestins are believed to have protective effects. Multiple trials utilizing progestins to treat advanced and recurrent endometrial cancers have been conducted. Initial studies resulted in promising response rates; however, Gynecologic Oncology Group (GOG) trials produced response rates of only 15–24% (14,15). GOG 081 compared different doses of medroxyprogesterone acetate (100 mg versus 1000 mg) in patients with advanced and recurrent endometrial cancers and found no difference in response rates between the low and high doses (14).

Despite some initial response to progestin, the benefits were short-lived without significant improvement in survival. The loss of survival benefit is thought to be partly due to the downregulation of progestin receptors with continuous use of progestins (16). Early studies have shown better responses in tumors with higher progestin receptor concentration. Tamoxifen has been shown to increase the concentration of progestin receptors (16,17). Therefore, GOG conducted a pair of phase II studies examining the effects of tamoxifen alternated with progestins. The results of both trials were similar to historic GOG trials with progestins alone, showing response rates, progression-free intervals, and median survivals of 27–33%, 2.7–3 months, and 13–14 months, respectively. In patients with stage I disease, adjuvant progestin therapy prevented relapses, increased the disease-free interval, and improved the endometrial cancer death rate, but did not improve overall survival because of increased rate of death from other causes (18).

■ VASCULAR ENDOTHELIAL GROWTH FACTOR

Angiogenesis is essential to the progression and growth of solid tumors (19). Vascular endothelial growth factor (VEGF) is one of the most well studied angiogenic factors in the growth of solid tumors. In endometrial cancer, stimulation of estrogen receptors has been linked to VEGF expression (20). Yokoyama and colleagues demonstrated increased frequency of VEGF receptor expression in endometrial cancer compared to normal endometrium and atypical endometrial hyperplasia (AEH) (21). In tumors with VEGF receptor expression, VEGF and its receptors stained with similar intensity in the endothelial cells of microvessels in adjacent stromal tissue. Tumor dissemination in endometrial cancer is primarily through lymphatic spread (22). VEGF-C has been identified to induce lymphatic endothelial proliferation and is highly restricted to lymphatic endothelial cells (23).

In 228 cases of endometrial cancers, Hirai and colleagues examined the relationship between cytosolic VEGF-A and VEGF-C concentrations with high-risk pathologic features (24). Both cytosolic VEGF-A and VEGF-C concentrations correlated with vascular invasion, parametrial-serosal invasion, lymphatic invasion, and lymph node metastasis. On multivariate analysis, VEGF-C expression, lymph node metastasis, and parametrial-serosal invasion were associated with worse progression-free survival. VEGF-C receptor expression has also been identified as an independent prognostic factor for overall survival in endometrial cancer (21). Chen and colleagues had similar results in their series of 53 cases of endometrial cancers (25). Higher concentrations of cytosolic VEGF correlated with advanced stage, lymph vascular invasion, and lymph node involvement. Six of the 53 cases developed recurrences during follow-up. The recurrent cases were associated with increased microvessel density and cytosolic VEGF concentrations. On multivariate analysis, only high histologic grade and VEGF overexpression was identified as an independent predictor for recurrence, with no correlation between histologic grade and cytosolic VEGF concentration.

In animal models, the inhibition of VEGF via monoclonal antibodies (mAbs) (26), suppression of VEGF expression (27), or binding of VEGF and VEGF receptors (28) causes decreased microvasculature, regression of tumors, and improved survival in animal models. Expression of VEGF antisense (29,30) and anti-VEGF antibodies (31) has also been shown to decrease tumor implantation and growth. In animal studies, irradiation of tumors induces production of VEGF within the tumor, while the inhibition of VEGF sensitizes the vascular endothelial cells to radiation (32). Gorski and colleagues demonstrated a threefold increase in VEGF levels after radiation treatments compared with nonirradiated cells. The elevations in VEGF were persistent even 2 weeks after irradiation. Anti-VEGF antibodies given prior to irradiation resulted in tumor volume reduction greater than the additive effects of irradiation or anti-VEGF antibodies alone.

■ ENDOSTATIN

Angiogenesis is a balance between proangiogenic factors and angiogenic inhibitors. Endostatin and angiostatin are protein fragments secreted by tumors; they inhibit angiogenesis at the primary site and downstream. Shaarawy and colleagues examined the preoperative serum levels of VEGF and endostatin in 72 women with endometrial cancer treated with surgery (33). Preoperative serum VEGF and endostatin were elevated in women with endometrial cancers compared with women with normal endometrium and atypical endometrial hyperplasia (AEH). The levels were significantly higher with increasing stage of disease. Both VEGF and endostatin levels were significantly decreased after hysterectomy. In addition, the ratio of serum VEGF to endostatin was slightly less than 1 in women without endometrial cancer and in stage I and II endometrial cancer, suggesting a balance between angiogenic and antiangiogenic factors. However, in women with stage III and IV, the ratio was greater than 1, favoring angiogenesis in advanced disease.

In animal studies, systemic introduction of endostatin resulted in decreased growth of tumor and metastases (34). Intramuscular injection of a formulated gene encoding endostatin resulted in sustained systemic expression of endostatin. The presence of endostatin was associated with reduction in tumor growth and in the development of lung metastases compared to controls. In another animal study, a short course of angiostatin injection during irradiation resulted in a synergistic reduction of tumor growth greater than angiostatin or irradiation alone (35). Additional angiostatin injection after irradiation resulted in no improvement and possibly less tumor reduction. This suggests that the maximal benefit of angiostatin occurs in the presence of irradiation.

■ CYCLO-OXYGENASE

Multiple studies have identified an association between cyclo-oxygenase (COX) activity with tumor growth and advancement of various tumors. Metabolites of COX, prostaglandins, have angiogenic activity and can induce VEGF production. In the endometrium, they may also promote tumorigenesis through a phospholipase C–mediated phosphorylation of the epidermal growth factor receptor (EGFR) and mitogen-activated protein kinase (MAPK) signaling pathway (36). Toyoki and coworkers identified a correlation between COX-2 and microvessel count in endometrial cancers, which has been identified as a negative prognostic factor (37). An elevation of COX-2 was found only in early-stage endometrial cancer and decreased in cancers with myometrial invasion. The authors theorized that COX-2 interacts with VEGF on angiogenesis only during early stages of the disease and diminishes with invasive disease. After a curative resection, residual disease is of low volume or microscopic. Hence, the initiation of angiogenesis may be similar to that in early primary tumors. Therefore, a COX-2 inhibitor may be useful as adjuvant therapy.

COX-2 inhibition has also been shown to improve tumor response to radiotherapy (38,39). The injection of a COX-2 inhibitor, SC-236, resulted in greater tumor growth delay in animal studies. When given prior and during irradiation, the growth delay was greater than the additive effects of radiation or SC-236 alone. In addition, treatment with SC-236 resulted in increased radiosensitivity of tumor with a decreased TD_{50}. Examination of tumors treated with SC-236, showed decreased neovascularization and no increase in apoptosis. The reduction in neovascularization preceded the delay in growth. Therefore, the mechanism of action is thought to be due to an inhibition on angiogenesis.

EPIDERMAL GROWTH FACTOR

Epidermal growth factor receptors have also been implicated in cancer development (40). The EGFRs are a family of tyrosine kinase (TK) cell surface receptors that are normally expressed in normal endometrium and may be overexpressed in endometrial cancers (41–43). EGFR overexpression is associated with higher-grade histology, metastasis, tumor stage, and invasion (44,45); however, there are conflicting results for it as an independent prognostic indicator (45–48). In vitro studies have shown that stimulation of EGFR induces downstream TK activity (49). In addition, the downstream effects can be inhibited by treatment with gefitinib (Iressa).

CLINICAL STUDIES

To date, no major clinical studies have used targeted therapies in conjunction with radiation treatment in the management of endometrial cancers. Based on preclinical studies, there are some potential uses with adjuvant radiotherapy. Preclinical studies have shown synergistic effects between radiation therapy and angiostatin and inhibition of COX-2, VEGF, and EGFR. Therefore, the concurrent use of these agents with radiation therapy may result in improved locoregional control and survival.

The use of adjuvant pelvic irradiation in patients with early-stage endometrial cancer is still being defined. Adjuvant radiotherapy decreases the risk of pelvic recurrence; however, whether it provides a survival benefit remains unclear. The randomized trial by Aalders and coworkers suggested a survival benefit only in women with both stage IC and high-grade histology (50). The Postoperative Radiation Therapy in Endometrial Carcinoma (PORTEC) trial showed no survival benefit of adjuvant pelvic radiotherapy in disease with low-grade histology or without invasion into the outer half of the myometrium (51). Analysis of the Surveillance Epidemiology and End Results (SEER) database (52) supported the use of adjuvant pelvic radiotherapy for women with stage IC disease. GOG 99 included women with intermediate-risk early-stage disease treated with hysterectomy and pelvic lymph node dissection (53). The results showed a reduction in the recurrence rate with radiation treatment, without a survival benefit. Subset analysis identified a group of women with higher risk for recurrence with a combination of poor risk factors, including older age, lymphovascular invasion, invasion of outer one-third of myometrium, and grade 2–3 histology. This group of women demonstrated a greater reduction in recurrence with radiation treatment. The authors indicated that the trial was not powered to detect a survival benefit.

In these discussed trials, the rate of pelvic recurrence with and without pelvic irradiation were 1–4% and 7–18%, respectively (50,51,53). Although the risk of pelvic recurrence is improved with pelvic radiation, a significant proportion of women would not benefit from additional treatment. Multiple molecular markers have been identified as independent predictive factor for recurrence, disease spread, and worse prognosis. These markers may act as a guide to who should be treated with adjuvant pelvic radiotherapy and who should receive concurrent targeted therapy, such as VEGF, COX-2, and the like. In the PORTEC trial (51) and the study by Aalders and coworkers (50), women who received pelvic irradiation had a higher rate of distant metastasis than did those who did not (10% versus 4–5%), although this was not statistically significant. Clinical trials evaluating systemic agents may be warranted in this population, either alone or in combination with radiation therapy.

Women with advanced-stage disease have high rates of recurrence. One of the most common sites of recurrence is within the abdomen, outside of the pelvic radiation field. Whole abdominopelvic irradiation (WAI) has been utilized in an attempt to decrease these failures (6,7). Despite some potential improvements, these treatments are still associated with significant failures within the abdomen and pelvis, particularly in patients with gross residual disease at the time of radiation therapy (6,7). The GOG recently published the results of a phase III randomized trial studying the use of WAI versus doxorubicin and cisplatin in patients with stage III and IV endometrial cancer (8). The results revealed an improvement in progression-free and overall survival with chemotherapy. However, chemotherapy was associated with greater rates of grade 3–4 toxicity. In addition, chemotherapy was associated with 4% treatment-related deaths versus 2% treatment related deaths in WAI arm. First site of recurrence in the abdomen and pelvis occurred in 16% and 13%, respectively, in the WAI arm and in 14% and 18%, respectively, in the chemotherapy arm. The high rates of recurrence within the radiation field may in part be due to the inadequate dose needed to sterilize tumors. The prescribed radiation dose is limited by the normal tissue tolerance of surrounding vital organs, such as kidneys and small bowel. In WAI protocols, the dose of radiation to the pelvis is commonly 45 Gy, and dose to the paraortic lymph nodes and abdomen are 45 Gy and 30 Gy, respectively (54). In addition, the doses to paraortics and abdomen are given at lower doses per fraction, resulting in a decreased radiobiologic effect. Radiosensitization with concurrent chemotherapy may be too toxic; therefore, the use of target therapies may be useful as a radiosensitizer with acceptable size effects.

■ REFERENCES

1. Kadar N, Malfetano JH, Homesley HD. Determinants of survival of surgically staged patients with endometrial carcinoma histologically confined to the uterus: Implications for therapy. *Obstet Gynecol* 1992;80:655–659.

2. Bedwinek J, Galakatos A, Camel M, et al. Stage I, grade III adenocarcinoma of the endometrium treated with surgery and irradiation. Sites of failure and correlation of failure rate with irradiation technique. *Cancer* 1984;54:40–47.
3. Eifel PJ, Ross J, Hendrickson M, et al. Adenocarcinoma of the endometrium. Analysis of 256 cases with disease limited to the uterine corpus: Treatment comparisons. *Cancer* 1983;52:1026–1031.
4. Genest P, Drouin P, Girard A, et al. Stage III carcinoma of the endometrium: A review of 41 cases. *Gynecol Oncol* 1987;26:77–86.
5. Hendrickson M, Ross J, Eifel P, et al. Uterine papillary serous carcinoma: A highly malignant form of endometrial adenocarcinoma. *Am J Surg Pathol* 1982;6:93–108.
6. Stewart KD, Martinez AA, Weiner S, et al. Ten-year outcome including patterns of failure and toxicity for adjuvant whole abdominopelvic irradiation in high-risk and poor histologic feature patients with endometrial carcinoma. *Int J Radiat Oncol Biol Phys* 2002;54:527–535.
7. Sutton G, Axelrod JH, Bundy BN, et al. Whole abdominal radiotherapy in the adjuvant treatment of patients with stage III and IV endometrial cancer: A gynecologic oncology group study. *Gynecol Oncol* 2005;97:755–763.
8. Randall ME, Filiaci VL, Muss H, et al. Randomized phase III trial of whole-abdominal irradiation versus doxorubicin and cisplatin chemotherapy in advanced endometrial carcinoma: A Gynecologic Oncology Group Study. *J Clin Oncol* 2006;24:36–44.
9. Fisher B, Dignam J, Bryant J, et al. Five versus more than five years of tamoxifen for lymph node-negative breast cancer: updated findings from the National Surgical Adjuvant Breast and Bowel Project B-14 randomized trial. *J Natl Cancer Inst* 2001;93:684–690.
10. Bolla M, Collette L, Blank L, et al. Long-term results with immediate androgen suppression and external irradiation in patients with locally advanced prostate cancer (an EORTC study): a phase III randomised trial. *Lancet* 2002;360:103–106.
11. D'Amico AV, Manola J, Loffredo M, et al. 6-month androgen suppression plus radiation therapy vs radiation therapy alone for patients with clinically localized prostate cancer: A randomized controlled trial. *JAMA* 2004;292:821–827.
12. Hanks GE, Pajak TF, Porter A, et al. Phase III trial of long-term adjuvant androgen deprivation after neoadjuvant hormonal cytoreduction and radiotherapy in locally advanced carcinoma of the prostate: The Radiation Therapy Oncology Group Protocol 92-02. *J Clin Oncol* 2003;21:3972–3978.
13. Roach M 3rd, DeSilvio M, Lawton C, et al. Phase III trial comparing whole-pelvic versus prostate-only radiotherapy and neoadjuvant versus adjuvant combined androgen suppression: Radiation Therapy Oncology Group 9413. *J Clin Oncol* 2003;21:1904–1911.
14. Thigpen JT, Brady MF, Alvarez RD, et al. Oral medroxyprogesterone acetate in the treatment of advanced or recurrent endometrial carcinoma: A dose-response study by the Gynecologic Oncology Group. *J Clin Oncol* 1999;17:1736–1744.
15. Lentz SS, Brady MF, Major FJ, et al. High-dose megestrol acetate in advanced or recurrent endometrial carcinoma: A Gynecologic Oncology Group Study. *J Clin Oncol* 1996;14:357–361.
16. Mortel R, Levy C, Wolff JP, et al. Female sex steroid receptors in postmenopausal endometrial carcinoma and biochemical response to an antiestrogen. *Cancer Res* 1981;41:1140–1147.
17. Carlson JA Jr., Allegra JC, Day TG Jr., et al. Tamoxifen and endometrial carcinoma: Alterations in estrogen and progesterone receptors in untreated patients and combination hormonal therapy in advanced neoplasia. *Am J Obstet Gynecol* 1984;149:149–153.
18. Martin-Hirsch PL, Jarvis G, Kitchener H, et al. Progestagens for endometrial cancer. *Cochrane Database Sys Rev* 1999;(4)CD001040.

19. Folkman J. What is the evidence that tumors are angiogenesis dependent? *J Natl Cancer Inst* 1990;82:4–6.
20. Cullinan-Bove K, Koos RD. Vascular endothelial growth factor/vascular permeability factor expression in the rat uterus: Rapid stimulation by estrogen correlates with estrogen-induced increases in uterine capillary permeability and growth. *Endocrinology* 1993;133:829–837.
21. Yokoyama Y, Sato S, Futagami M, et al. Prognostic significance of vascular endothelial growth factor and its receptors in endometrial carcinoma. *Gynecol Oncol* 2000;77:413–418.
22. Yokoyama Y, Maruyama H, Sato S, et al. Indispensability of pelvic and paraaortic lymphadenectomy in endometrial cancers. *Gynecol Oncol* 1997;64:411–417.
23. Joukov V, Pajusola K, Kaipainen A, et al. A novel vascular endothelial growth factor, VEGF-C, is a ligand for the Flt4 (VEGFR-3) and KDR (VEGFR-2) receptor tyrosine kinases. *EMBO J* 1996;15:290–298.
24. Hirai M, Nakagawara A, Oosaki T, et al. Expression of vascular endothelial growth factors (VEGF-A/VEGF-1 and VEGF-C/VEGF-2) in postmenopausal uterine endometrial carcinoma. *Gynecol Oncol* 2001;80:181–188.
25. Chen CA, Cheng WF, Lee CN, et al. Cytosol vascular endothelial growth factor in endometrial carcinoma: correlation with disease-free survival. *Gynecol Oncol* 2001;80:207–212.
26. Yuan F, Chen Y, Dellian M, et al. Time-dependent vascular regression and permeability changes in established human tumor xenografts induced by an anti-vascular endothelial growth factor/vascular permeability factor antibody. *Proc Natl Acad Sci USA* 1996;93:14765–14770.
27. Benjamin LE, Keshet E. Conditional switching of vascular endothelial growth factor (VEGF) expression in tumors: Induction of endothelial cell shedding and regression of hemangioblastoma-like vessels by VEGF withdrawal. *Proc Natl Acad Sci USA* 1997;94:8761–8766.
28. Goldman CK, Kendall RL, Cabrera G, et al. Paracrine expression of a native soluble vascular endothelial growth factor receptor inhibits tumor growth, metastasis, and mortality rate. *Proc Natl Acad Sci USA* 1998;95:8795–8800.
29. Cheng SY, Huang HJ, Nagane M, et al. Suppression of glioblastoma angiogenicity and tumorigenicity by inhibition of endogenous expression of vascular endothelial growth factor. *Proc Natl Acad Sci USA* 1996;93:8502–8507.
30. Claffey KP, Brown LF, del Aguila LF, et al. Expression of vascular permeability factor/vascular endothelial growth factor by melanoma cells increases tumor growth, angiogenesis, and experimental metastasis. *Cancer Res* 1996;56:172–181.
31. Melnyk O, Shuman MA, Kim KJ. Vascular endothelial growth factor promotes tumor dissemination by a mechanism distinct from its effect on primary tumor growth. *Cancer Res* 1996;56:921–924.
32. Gorski DH, Beckett MA, Jaskowiak NT, et al. Blockage of the vascular endothelial growth factor stress response increases the antitumor effects of ionizing radiation. *Cancer Res* 1999;59:3374–3378.
33. Shaarawy M, El-Sharkawy SA. Biomarkers of intrinsic angiogenic and anti-angiogenic activity in patients with endometrial hyperplasia and endometrial cancer. *Acta Oncol* 2001;40:513–518.
34. Blezinger P, Wang J, Gondo M, et al. Systemic inhibition of tumor growth and tumor metastases by intramuscular administration of the endostatin gene. *Nat Biotechnol* 1999;17:343–348.
35. Gorski DH, Mauceri HJ, Salloum RM, et al. Potentiation of the antitumor effect of ionizing radiation by brief concomitant exposures to angiostatin. *Cancer Res* 1998;58:5686–5689.
36. Sales KJ, Milne SA, Williams AR, et al. Expression, localization, and signaling of prostaglandin F2 alpha receptor in human endometrial adenocarcinoma: Regulation of prolifera-

tion by activation of the epidermal growth factor receptor and mitogen-activated protein kinase signaling pathways. *J Clin Endocrinol Metab* 2004;89:986–993.

37. Toyoki H, Fujimoto J, Sato E, et al. Clinical implications of expression of cyclooxygenase-2 related to angiogenesis in uterine endometrial cancers. *Ann Oncol* 2005;16:51–55.
38. Kishi K, Petersen S, Petersen C, et al. Preferential enhancement of tumor radioresponse by a cyclooxygenase-2 inhibitor. *Cancer Res* 2000;60:1326–1331.
39. Milas L, Kishi K, Hunter N, et al. Enhancement of tumor response to gamma-radiation by an inhibitor of cyclooxygenase-2 enzyme. *J Natl Cancer Inst* 1999;91:1501–1504.
40. Herbst RS. Review of epidermal growth factor receptor biology. *Int J Radiat Oncol Biol Phys* 2004;59:21–26.
41. Kraus MH, Issing W, Miki T, et al. Isolation and characterization of ERBB3, a third member of the ERBB/epidermal growth factor receptor family: Evidence for overexpression in a subset of human mammary tumors. *Proc Natl Acad Sci USA* 1989;86:9193–9197.
42. Libermann TA, Nusbaum HR, Razon N, et al. Amplification, enhanced expression and possible rearrangement of EGF receptor gene in primary human brain tumours of glial origin. *Nature* 1985;313:144–147.
43. Coussens L, Yang-Feng TL, Liao YC, et al. Tyrosine kinase receptor with extensive homology to EGF receptor shares chromosomal location with neu oncogene. *Science* 1985;230:1132–1139.
44. Niikura H, Sasano H, Kaga K, et al. Expression of epidermal growth factor family proteins and epidermal growth factor receptor in human endometrium. *Hum Pathol* 1996;27:282–289.
45. Khalifa MA, Abdoh AA, Mannel RS, et al. Prognostic utility of epidermal growth factor receptor overexpression in endometrial adenocarcinoma. *Cancer* 1994;73:370–376.
46. Nagai N, Oshita T, Fujii T, et al. Prospective analysis of DNA ploidy, proliferative index and epidermal growth factor receptor as prognostic factors for pretreated uterine cancer. *Oncol Rep* 2000;7:551–559.
47. Athanassiadou P, Petrakakou E, Liossi A, et al. Prognostic significance of p53, bcl-2 and EGFR in carcinoma of the endometrium. *Acta Cytol* 1999;43:1039–1044.
48. Niikura H, Sasano H, Matsunaga G, et al. Prognostic value of epidermal growth factor receptor expression in endometrioid endometrial carcinoma. *Hum Pathol* 1995;26:892–896.
49. Albitar L, Laidler LL, Abdallah R, et al. Regulation of signaling phosphoproteins by epidermal growth factor and Iressa (ZD1839) in human endometrial cancer cells that model type I and II tumors. *Mol Cancer Ther* 2005;4:1891–1899.
50. Aalders J, Abeler V, Kolstad P, et al. Postoperative external irradiation and prognostic parameters in stage I endometrial carcinoma: Clinical and histopathologic study of 540 patients. *Obstet Gynecol* 1980;56:419–427.
51. Creutzberg CL, van Putten WL, Koper PC, et al. Surgery and postoperative radiotherapy versus surgery alone for patients with stage-1 endometrial carcinoma: Multicentre randomised trial. PORTEC Study Group. Post Operative Radiation Therapy in Endometrial Carcinoma. *Lancet* 2000;355:1404–1411.
52. Lee CM, Szabo A, Shrieve DC, et al. Frequency and effect of adjuvant radiation therapy among women with stage I endometrial adenocarcinoma. *JAMA* 2006;295:389–397.
53. Keys HM, Roberts JA, Brunetto VL, et al. A phase III trial of surgery with or without adjunctive external pelvic radiation therapy in intermediate risk endometrial adenocarcinoma: A Gynecologic Oncology Group study. *Gynecol Oncol* 2004;92:744–751.
54. Fletcher G. *Textbook of Radiotherapy*. 3rd ed. Philadelphia, PA: Lea & Febiger; 1980.

Index

Note: Boldface numbers indicate illustrations; *t* indicates a table.